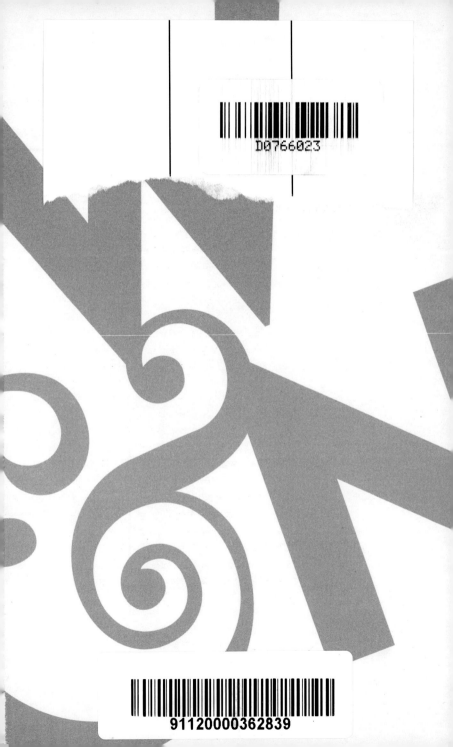

D0766023

9112000362839

Wendy Moore is a freelance journalist and author. Her first book, *The Knife Man*, won the Medical Journalists' Association Consumer Book Award in 2005 and was shortlisted for both Saltire and the Marsh Biography Awards. Her second book, *Wedlock*, has been highly acclaimed in reviews and was chosen as one of the ten titles in the Channel 4 TV Book Club. *How to Create the Perfect Wife* was published to rapturous reviews on both sides of the Atlantic.

ALSO BY WENDY MOORE

The Knife Man
Wedlock
How to Create the Perfect Wife

Praise for *The Mesmerist*

'**Engrossing** . . . [Moore's] social history of Victorian medicine, which struggled with innovation and provision for the poor, also feels **rivetingly topical** . . . [A] **witty and instructive** tale' *Daily Telegraph*

'**Lively** . . . Moore tells her story with gusto' *Observer*

'**Fascinating** . . . she brings the London medical world to vivid life. Elliotson's experiments were covered in lavish detail by contemporary journals, but **Moore has made this an altogether richer story** by judicious use of details gleaned from diaries, case reports and hospital archives' *TLS*

'Charles Dickens, as it happens, has a cameo role in Moore's book. Sceptical at first about the powers of mesmerism, the novelist became a convert after witnessing one of the many sessions run by John Elliotson, the doctor who helped to start a craze for putting Londoners, sick and healthy alike, into trances' *The Times*

'Wendy **Moore is an expert guide** to the world of early 19th-century medicine, and this **fascinating** book is packed with buccaneering, larger-than-life doctors and gruesome operations, as well as the minutely documented antics of the Okey sisters. UCH in those times was evidently a much livelier place than it is today under our dear old NHS' *Spectator*

'Wendy Moore has written **a thrilling account** of this odd byway of medical history . . . she has successfully taken a historical episode and used it to colour in the world of 19th-century scientific endeavour and its attempts to uncover the still-unexplained mysteries of the human unconscious' *Literary Review*

'As in all her works, **Moore provides evidence of meticulous research** with copious notes to be appreciated by the medical historian and her acknowledgements demonstrate the breadth of her consultation . . . **an invaluable addition to the literature on the struggle between science and superstition**' British Society For The History Of Medicine

'Elliotson, as Moore's **engrossing** study describes, became passionate about hypnosis, under which (he tried to prove) a patient could have surgery without pain. His demonstrations became as fashionable as any theatre – but was it fraud?' *Sunday Telegraph*

'The author's dry asides combined with the unsentimental light she sheds on medical experimentation make this **an informative and riveting page turner**' *Country Life*

'The idea of a higher, healing state took 19th-century society by storm but, as this **lively** book shows, it was to prove controversial'
History Revealed

THE MESMERIST

WENDY MOORE

The Society Doctor
Who Held Victorian London
Spellbound

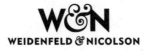

WEIDENFELD & NICOLSON

For Peter, Sam and Susie

First published in Great Britain in 2017
by Weidenfeld & Nicolson.
This paperback edition published in 2018
by Weidenfeld & Nicolson
an imprint of the Orion Publishing Group Ltd
Carmelite House, 50 Victoria Embankment
London EC4Y 0DZ

An Hachette UK Company

ISBN (Mas Market Paperback) 978 1 4746 0231 0
ISBN (eBook) 978 1 4746 0232 7

Internal artwork: eye drawing by Hemesh Alles

Typeset by Input Data Services Ltd, Somerset

Printed and bound in Great Britain by Clays Ltd, St Ives plc

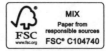

www.orionbooks.co.uk

CONTENTS

You're a fool, Dr Ellisson. Ha! Ha!

University College Hospital, Gower Street, London, 10 May 1838

The girl sat impassively at the centre of the stage while the lecture theatre filled with people.[1] As the spectators poured through the doorway and squeezed along the narrow wooden benches, she seemed oblivious to their presence, lost in a world of her own. Some of the men – for the audience was composed predominantly, if not entirely, of men – brought out spectacles or opera glasses so they could scrutinise the girl more closely as they took their seats. Through their lenses they could see her ghostly pale face with its dainty features and dark eyes fringed by long black lashes. She wore her hair piled on top of her head in 'a profusion of flaxen ringlets', which set off her handsome 'Grecian features', according to one observer. She had the head and face of a child but the mature body of a young woman, said another. In fact she was seventeen, though small for her age; she seemed poised on the point of puberty, an innocent child on the brink of womanhood. Silent and still, she appeared neither to notice the men's arrival nor to mind their attention.

The tiered benches that rose on three sides of the room were now filled to capacity yet still people arrived. Chairs were set out on the floor of the lecture theatre to accommodate more guests and once these were taken the latecomers had to stand at the back and in the aisles. As the excited chatter grew, so the temperature in the room rose. Although the morning had started out unseasonably frosty, it had turned into a bright, warm, dry afternoon. At last, the theatre was filled to bursting and the door was closed. The spectators shifted in their seats and craned their necks for a better view. The journalists lifted their pens in readiness. All were impatient for the performance to begin. In the summer of 1838 there was no more thrilling place to be. For the 300 or so invited guests who crowded the lecture theatre in Gower Street this was the hottest ticket in town.[2]

At theatres and entertainment halls across London, audiences could laugh at pantomime or cower at melodrama, gasp at daring acrobatics or blush at risqué cabaret. Yet none of these could match the novelty of the spectacle set to unfold in the lecture theatre of the capital's newest hospital. Those lucky guests who had begged, beseeched or bartered an invitation had been promised theatre and pantomime, farce and cabaret, all rolled into one. The display they had come to watch was the chief talking point in every gentlemen's club and scientific society, every plush dining room and plain servants' hall throughout the nation. As one journal remarked, it was 'scarcely possible to join a dozen persons in any society' where the topic was 'not a subject of serious discussion'.[3] But this was not titillation for the masses; this was not entertainment for entertainment's sake. The spectacle the distinguished audience had come to see was being staged in the name of Science. For they had all gathered to bear witness to an extraordinary force of nature, which held out the prospect of a significant advance in medicine.

Heaven knows it was needed. Many in the audience knew from bitter experience the dismal failings of orthodox medicine to prevent or relieve the raft of diseases and ailments which unleashed suffering daily and despatched thousands to an early grave. Some had even endured the brutality of surgery without pain relief or basic hygiene. It was no wonder that the public resorted to buying quack medicines in high street chemists or turned to more outlandish alternatives in the desperate hope of finding relief. It was little wonder either that many regarded the medical profession with cynicism and muttered darkly about loved ones who might have lived longer or suffered less without medical interference. So the unveiling of a powerful new treatment, which some of the profession's most respected leaders believed could conquer both pain and disease, was welcome news indeed.

Not surprisingly, with so much at stake, the audience included some of the best-known names in scientific and intellectual society. Michael

Faraday, the brilliant director of the laboratory at the Royal Institution, had taken time out from his research on electricity to watch the demonstration. Sir James South, the renowned astronomer who had recently described Mars, had interrupted his stargazing to attend. Sir Joseph de Courcy Laffan, physician to the late Duke of York, the young queen's father, was taking a keen professional interest. And squeezed among these illustrious personalities were assorted peers and MPs, scientists and journalists, medical practitioners and medical students, all eagerly awaiting the exhibition.

Some had already witnessed strange scenes during the past few months on the hospital's wards. Faraday, for one, had devoted many hours to studying the patients involved, in an attempt to find a logical explanation. Teachers and students from almost every medical school in London had flocked to see the extraordinary sights for themselves along with innumerable members of the prominent scientific institutions and medical societies. What they had seen divided them equally into zealous evangelists convinced a new scientific wonder had been discovered and outright sceptics adamant that it was all a grand delusion. One visitor, the radical MP Sir William Molesworth, had been so impressed he had donated 30 guineas (worth more than £3,000 today) to the hospital's coffers. Another, Lord Henry Brougham, the political reformer and co-founder of University College London, which ran the hospital, had stormed out in disgust.[4]

Even Charles Dickens, the young journalist and author who was fast gaining celebrity following the serialisation of his first novel, *The Pickwick Papers*, had joined one of these private parties huddled around the hospital beds with his collaborator, the artist George Cruikshank, in tow.[5] Dickens had been so enthralled that he had come back a few weeks later with his actor friend William Macready. Many drawn to the demonstration on 10 May would have heard of even more bizarre experiments – involving cats, mirrors and electricity – which had taken place over recent months within the walls of the hospital. All would have read the incredulous reports in their newspapers and scientific journals. Now they were ready to judge for themselves.

At last the chatter fell away and attention turned to the man who stood beside the girl's chair waiting for silence. Professor John Elliotson was a familiar figure to all. At forty-six, Elliotson was in his prime; he was at the pinnacle of his medical career and the peak of his popularity.[6]

Although the doctor was below average height and walked with a limp following a carriage accident some years earlier, he was still strikingly handsome with his curling jet-black hair, dark brown eyes, prominent eyebrows and abundant side whiskers. His high forehead, long straight nose and strong chin were all suggestive of authority. Having held the post of Professor of Medicine at the university for seven years, Elliotson was regarded as one of the most successful and respected teachers and physicians in London, as popular with his patients as he was with his students. The influential weekly medical journal *The Lancet* would admit no equal. Elliotson was quite simply 'not surpassed by any physician in the metropolis'.[7]

Every day well-dressed members of the aristocracy and gentry flocked to consult the doctor at his elegant house in Conduit Street in London's West End. According to *The Times*, Conduit Street was choked with the carriages of Elliotson's patients as thickly as St James's Street on the day of a royal reception. A fervent patron of the arts, the doctor drew just as many people to his house for the 'splendid musical parties' he hosted for his friends in high society. On the other side of London and at the opposite end of the social scale, desperately poor labourers and their families, who scratched a living in the capital's northern slums, packed the waiting room at University College Hospital where the doctor treated them for free. Indeed it was only through Elliotson's persistence that the hospital had been built at all. It was Elliotson who had mobilised support for the loan that had financed the bricks and mortar; it was Elliotson who had insisted on the name to reflect its academic origins. Just as devoted were the professor's students who crowded his lectures and followed him around the wards, hanging on his every word. The doctor's lectures and case studies were avidly reported in the medical press, and his book, *Human Physiology*, was the standard medical textbook of the day.

Yet for all his wealth and success, Elliotson was not uncritical of the establishment. Shocked by the poverty and injustice he witnessed daily, the professor had backed campaigns to reduce factory working hours, ban army flogging and end capital punishment. Just as he supported free healthcare for all, so he advocated education for the masses. And he was equally determined to reform the medical world. One of a new breed of uncompromising medical mavericks, he was impatient to shake up the antiquated and corrupt institutions which stifled progress and suffocated genuine talent. Well aware, from his own experience, of the difficulties in scaling the slippery career ladder, he was determined to help create a forward-looking profession based on open and meritocratic principles. Central to this vision was medical practice founded on sound scientific evidence. Elliotson was at the forefront of testing new techniques and therapies that might one day provide effective treatments and replace the centuries of reliance on blistering and bleeding, cupping and purging, and the hotchpotch of toxic potions that comprised the official pharmacopoeia. As a frequent traveller on the Continent, the professor was always on the lookout for promising innovations, and was even ready to try out some of the more outlandish ideas. In short, if anything novel was happening in the world of science and medicine, the audience in the lecture hall of UCH could be sure that Elliotson would be first to investigate it. Today, they were not going to be disappointed.

Elliotson began defensively. He had been attacked in the press by sceptics who scorned his latest discoveries as a deception or an absurdity, he said. He had been ostracised by some sections of the medical profession who refused to accept his work. He had even been warned by some of his university colleagues to stop his demonstrations, despite the fact that those same colleagues had not even deigned to witness his experiments. Indeed, at this very moment, some of his fellow professors were raising a petition demanding an end to his work.

But Elliotson refused to be cowed. He believed it was his duty to research the startling new phenomenon he had stumbled upon and to present the results of his experiments in the full glare of the public eye. The hospital in which they were sitting had been opened four years earlier as a 'liberal institution' to 'throw light on truth and nature'; he therefore believed it was wrong to perform experiments on its patients 'with closed doors'.[8] In his own mind there was no doubt about the veracity of his discoveries. For he was convinced he had found a 'powerful remedial agent' with the potential to treat numerous ailments and even to conquer pain. Indeed, he had already used the therapy to cure several of his patients.

A child who had been paraplegic and incontinent for nine months had recently walked out of the hospital fit and well, the doctor revealed. A patient who had suffered epileptic seizures had been cured after just one application. A patient with St Vitus's dance (Sydenham's chorea), the so-called 'dancing mania', had been perfectly cured. And now the professor was ready to demonstrate the effects of this remarkable therapy before his largest audience to date.

Throughout the professor's speech the girl sitting beside him had remained motionless and silent, seemingly immune to the crowd's curiosity. Yet immediately he ceased speaking she rose abruptly from her seat. The guests were transfixed; a change had come over her. Nobody was quite sure what had occasioned this change, noted a journalist from *The Lancet*, but there was no doubt that the placid composure of her face was suddenly transformed. She began to stroll and skip around the stage, stopping every so often to examine individuals and objects, exclaiming at them in childish language or meaningless babble, yet all the while she remained apparently unaware of the presence of the massed audience. She was now, the professor explained, in a state of 'delirium' or 'sleep-waking' as he sometimes termed it. In fact, one of his fellow enthusiasts, a professor from a rival medical school, had recently suggested the term 'trance'.[9]

The girl, Elliotson explained, was a patient who had been admitted into the hospital some twelve months earlier, suffering epileptic fits. Her name was Elizabeth Okey.[10] Yet she scarcely needed any introduction, for Elizabeth had become something of a celebrity over the past year. Her surname was routinely misspelled 'O'Key' by journalists so that her origins were widely assumed to be Irish. Inevitably this gave rise to the lazy assumption that she came from one of the numerous poor, illeducated, unskilled Irish families that had gravitated to London over the past few decades – and triggered popular prejudice as a result. In fact her family boasted a long English pedigree – although they had certainly seen better times. Over the past year her starring role in Professor Elliotson's experiments at UCH had been excitedly reported in newspapers and journals as far afield as Dublin and Belfast.[11] Elizabeth Okey had become a household name in dining clubs and gin palaces, mansions and garrets up and down the land. The demonstration at UCH on 10 May was set to become one of her most virtuoso performances.[12]

First Elizabeth headed towards the Marquess of Anglesey, Henry Paget, who was seated in the front row. The marquess, who was nearly seventy, had famously had his right leg amputated on a cottage dining table after his knee was shattered by grapeshot during a reckless charge at the Battle of Waterloo.[13] Known affectionately as 'One-Leg', the old campaigner sported a fine pair of buff-coloured trousers, which concealed an artificial limb that had been designed expressly for him and was patented as 'the Anglesey Leg'. Having stoically endured his battlefield amputation without so much as flinching, the marquess still suffered dreadful pain from the stump. More recently he had become victim to excruciating facial pain due to the nerve disorder tic douloureux (trigeminal neuralgia) for which he had tried numerous therapies, including homoeopathy and hydrotherapy. Few people in the audience had more experience of the inadequacies of conventional medical care, or such a personal interest in its improvement.

Elizabeth greeted the veteran soldier like an old friend with: 'Oh! how do ye?' To the audience's amusement, she continued: 'White trowsers! Dear! you do look so tidy, you do. What nice things. You *are* a nice man.' Since contemporary prudishness dictated that 'trousers' were frequently referred to with a euphemism such as 'unutterables', it was clear the girl had a sense of humour.[14] She then turned to the marquess's brother, Sir Charles Paget, who sat nearby, and tartly asked: 'Why do you wear your hat?' At that point she grasped Sir Charles's hand and enfolded it in her own. But this move was evidently a step too far for a young single woman in front of an all-male audience and Elliotson swiftly intervened. Stepping behind the girl, the professor theatrically lifted his hand and brought it slowly down. As if by magic, her eyes closed, she teetered on her heels, and then fell straight backwards like an axed tree. She was only saved from crashing to the floor by Elliotson's assistant, a young medical student called William Wood, who caught her in his arms. She awoke in less than a minute and was safely returned to her chair. Elliotson waved his hand again and Elizabeth's eyelids dropped like shutters. She was roused by the doctor blowing on her face and then she was up and off again, chatting, joking, flirting and cavorting with the enraptured men.

For the next two and a half hours, Elizabeth Okey amazed and entertained the audience with a heady mixture of childlike naivety and flagrant sexuality as Elliotson presided over the event like a master of ceremonies. The girl's extraordinary behaviour, the fascinated spectators were informed, represented a complete change of personality. For, as the *Monthly Chronicle* reported, in her natural state Elizabeth was timid and modest in the 'manner proper to her age and sex'.[15] Ordinarily, the journal added, 'she is silent and reserved, never speaking except in answer to questions directly put to her' and then giving her answers 'in a low and gentle tone with rather a downcast expression of countenance, apparently resulting from great modesty of disposition'. Yet, acting under the professor's strange power, the girl lost all her inhibitions and was transformed into a saucy minx of the type more familiarly seen prancing about in a pantomime chorus or, worse still, beckoning from a street corner.

In this half-childlike, half-coquettish condition, Elizabeth seized a walking stick from one guest, snatched a pair of gloves from another and plucked a set of opera glasses from a third. Throughout these frolics she kept up a lively commentary. Holding the opera glasses aloft, she exclaimed: 'Oh, Dr Elliotson, see what I've got.' Instructed to return them to their owner, she turned to one ruddy-faced gentleman and announced: 'Tisn't yours, beauty cheeks.' To another spectator, who sported a breastpin in his handkerchief, she declared: 'Oh, what a beautiful oyster!' The doctor explained that he had once told her, while she was in this trance-like state, that a brooch was an oyster – although he did not see fit to explain why he should have done that. Greeting the doctor's assistant, Elizabeth exclaimed: 'Oh, Mr Wood, dear, how do ye?' Then she pointed at the feet of the men in the front row and added: 'Look here, what lots of feet!' Casting around for the marquess again, she asked: 'Where's that beauty white gentleman?' By turns charming and impudent, skittish and provocative, she held her audience rapt as surely as any actress on the London stage.

Yet each time Elizabeth's behaviour transgressed too far, she was smartly sent back to sleep with a deft wave of Elliotson's hand before being restored again by the doctor blowing on her face. At one point, when she collapsed lifelessly into the lap of one surprised visitor, she was rapidly roused. Likewise, when she made a sudden lunge for some gloves inside a guest's hat which rested on his lap, she was quickly returned to her chair and sleep.

At this point Elliotson crouched behind the chair, out of Elizabeth's sight, and snapped his jaws three or four times. The girl mimicked him exactly. While she was still apparently asleep, a wooden board was placed under her chin so she could see nothing below it. As the doctor raised and lowered his arms out of her sight, her own arms mirrored his actions perfectly. Now the doctor pointed his hand towards her and drew his right arm upwards and outwards. In a few seconds the girl's right arm moved in the same direction. When the doctor wriggled his fingers, hers followed suit. When he raised his left arm, hers went up too. When he pointed to her right foot, her leg magically rose.

She was now in a state of 'catalepsy', the doctor informed his audience. But it was not just the doctor who could produce these strange reactions. A volunteer from the audience moved his hand upwards and the girl's left leg obediently rose. She was now sitting on the chair with both legs stuck stiffly out, both arms raised, and her eyes closed, to all appearances like a china doll. Elliotson then invited members of the audience to come forward and examine her limbs. They did not need asking twice. Several volunteers, including the eager reporter from *The Lancet*, stepped forward to prod and poke the girl's arms and legs. They were all 'rigidly fixed', the journalist confirmed, and Elizabeth continued to sit for several minutes balanced only on the seat of her chair. At last the doctor blew in her face. Instantly her limbs dropped and she awoke.

As the exhibition progressed, Elizabeth's reactions became wilder and more exotic. When Elliotson or Wood waved their hands, her hands became fixed so she could not separate them. When Wood backed away behind her, she twitched and jerked then suddenly shot backwards in her chair as if being yanked towards him by an invisible rope. And when *The Lancet* journalist pulled her hair and pinched her neck, she sat un-flinching and unresponsive. As he later remarked, 'she did not notice it, or evince the slightest symptom of pain'. This was scarcely surprising since it was widely reported that she had previously withstood electric shocks without betraying the least sign of pain.

While Elliotson earnestly explained each response to his actions as a manifestation of the mysterious power he was manipulating, Elizabeth enlivened proceedings with impromptu turns supplemented by a repertoire of rude comments and ribald jokes that kept the audience enthralled. It was a formidable double act. At one point she whistled a popular air, 'The Green Hills of Tyrol', from Rossini's 1829 opera *William Tell*, 'perfectly as regards both time and tune'. Then she abruptly switched style and hummed two psalms 'in an exceedingly delicate tone' while absent-mindedly picking at the flowers sewn on her dress. At an-other point she chattered away in French – muttering *'méchant diable'* – in apparent mimicry of a French woman who was being treated on the same ward. Then she began spouting a stream of gobbledegook which sounded, *The Lancet* suggested, like 'misce crutis, crece croo'.

Most amusing, however, was the 'innocent familiarity' with which Elizabeth treated her audience. As the journalist from the *Morning Post* noted, 'she speaks truth with all the *naivete*, and non-reservation of a person half seas over' – or, in plain words, drunk. She addressed one generously proportioned spectator as 'a nice large gentleman, with white legs'. Then she turned to his neighbour and remarked: 'You are not so big, are you? No, for that gentleman has the advantage of being stuffed. Stuffed? Pray with what? Is it with a good dinner? For that's the best of all good stuffing.' To another well-fed guest she proclaimed: 'Oh! How do ye? You're a very fat gentleman. Stand up on your understandings, and let me see how you look then. If I'd got such a pair, I'd not sit down I can tell you.' Plainly preoccupied with food or rather the lack of it – doubtless a reflection of the austere hospital diet – she spoke to her own hands and mused: 'S'pose I give you no dinner. You'd be very glad to talk then.' She addressed Professor Elliotson, or 'Ellisson' as she pronounced his name, as 'You beauty white man'. She even spoke to the wooden board in front of her as if it were alive saying: 'Such a dirty beast you are. I don't like you. Does your mother know you're out?'

As Elizabeth's behaviour progressed from the comic to the absurd, at one point she woke from her artificially induced sleep and asked where the doctor had gone. 'I'm in that boot,' answered Elliotson. 'Are you?' she replied. 'Yes, and I ate Mr Wood for breakfast today, and have got in there.' Obligingly Elizabeth trotted over to one of the guests and began running her hand up the man's trousers while protesting: 'Oh! come out. Don't live in that nasty hole.' She was hastily returned to sleep. It was hard, admittedly, at times to determine who was behaving the more bizarrely, the revered doctor or his patient. Absurd or not, the audience loved it.

At length two more patients were brought into the theatre. The first was a girl, aged between two and three, who had recently been admitted to the hospital with a 'nervous complaint' – though quite what nervous complaint a child of three could be subject to was not elucidated. The professor's attempts to induce sleep in her merely produced a yawn, though when the child sat facing Elizabeth and mimicked the professor's hand movements, she managed to send Elizabeth to sleep. The third patient was Okey's younger sister, Jane, who had also been admitted to the hospital the previous year with epilepsy. Jane, who was fifteen, was even more susceptible to the mysterious influence than her sister, explained the professor, since she could be sent to sleep simply by being pointed or looked at – as he immediately proved when Jane fell motionless into the lap of the nearest spectator.

With the audience's appetite for novelty undimmed, Elliotson repeated his experiments on both Jane and the child and even demonstrated how the invisible influence could be multiplied by strength of numbers. Volunteers from the audience queued up to place their hands on the child's shoulders as they successively put Elizabeth to sleep more quickly. Before long the floor of the theatre was so crowded that *The Lancet* reporter had difficulty seeing what was happening.

Yet for all the variety on stage it was Elizabeth who was undeniably the star of the show. Even if her sister was more responsive, it was Elizabeth who produced the most amusing, the most daring, the most outrageous antics. Her talents were manifold, her repertoire was wide, suggesting a keen interest in the popular entertainment of the day. In particular, the audience was thrilled when she gave a rendition of 'Jim Crow', a well-known song recently imported across the Atlantic by the American vaudeville performer Thomas Dartmouth Rice.[16] Rice had made a name in his native country as a 'negro' impersonator. With his face blacked-up by burnt cork, he danced and sang in supposed imitation of a black slave from the American south, or a 'right down Yankee nigger' as the newspapers would have it.[17] Two years previously Rice had brought his act to London where it had enjoyed a successful run at the Surrey Theatre in Lambeth and his signature song had become an instant hit.

Whether Elizabeth had managed to see Rice at one of his shows or heard the song elsewhere, she was plainly familiar with the lyrics. In mid-verse she suddenly halted to ask Elliotson whether he had also 'come over from Kentucky' and then offered to 'wheel about, and turn about' in accordance with the song's chorus. This proposal was peremptorily rejected by the doctor, to the spectators' manifest disappointment.

As her performance drew to its close, everyone agreed: Elizabeth Okey was the indisputable prima donna of the day. Whatever the doctor wanted her to do she complied with. She was a puppet responding to every twitch and tweak of her puppet master; she was putty in the hands of a sculptor. She appeared to be completely responsive to his gestures, totally under his power. For most of the time at least.

During the course of the afternoon there were certain interludes when Elizabeth suddenly asserted her independence and defied the professor's commands, even to the point of casting ridicule on him. At one stage, Elliotson ordered: 'Pray don't sing.' But Elizabeth smartly retorted: 'I may sing "Buy a black sheep", for Mr Wood told me so.' And she duly belted out a verse. When the doctor tried to incite her to mimic his wriggling fingers, she declared: 'Oh, but you're a fool, Dr Ellisson. Ha! Ha! How do ye? Mine won't go like yours. They ain't so silly.' Another time she coyly remarked: 'Poor Dr Ellisson, would you like some sop, with some milk in it?' And Elliotson, pre-empting the joke, replied: 'No, for then I should be a milksop.'

It was plain, too, that when her sister and the child were introduced Elizabeth took umbrage at sharing the limelight. Laughing at the young girl's efforts to place her in a trance, Elizabeth scolded: 'Suppose, my little dear, I was to knock you off your perch.' Then she turned to the professor and said: 'I say, Dr Ellisson, 'spose I was to knock you off *your* perch; how funny you'd look.' Quickly she added: 'But I won't do that; I wouldn't hurt you.' Each rude outburst only excited the audience to more hilarity.

Finally, as the guests gathered their belongings to leave the lecture theatre late that afternoon, Elliotson attempted to restore Elizabeth Okey to her normal, lucid state in order to send her back to the ward. Ordinarily, this process was accomplished by simply rubbing her forehead with his thumbs. But this time all his efforts were in vain. Elizabeth, it seemed, did not want the show to end. Neither the professor nor his assistant, Wood, could wake her. Then Wood had a bright idea. He asked Elizabeth herself how and when she would awake. 'In five minutes,' she muttered in her sleep. 'Shall you awake of yourself?' 'No.' 'How then?' asked Wood. 'You must wake me.' 'In what way?' he asked. 'By rubbing my neck.' Fascinated by this new development, the assembled guests waited patiently until five minutes had elapsed. At that point Elliotson attempted to rouse the girl by rubbing her neck. There was no response. A few seconds later, Wood tried his luck and Elizabeth awoke to her natural state.

The transformation was entire. Elizabeth's countenance and manner underwent such a complete change it was 'as if she had risen from the dead', said the *Morning Post*. She was suddenly transfigured into the meek young girl they had all heard about who kept her head bowed in fitting modesty. She seemed to have no recollection of anything that had happened in the theatre, only complaining of a headache. As the guests filed out, many of them stopped to shake hands with her and she responded with a demure curtsey. She appeared, said *The Lancet*, 'greatly wearied, depressed, and much abashed at her situation'.

*

There was no doubt the demonstration had provided a perfect afternoon's entertainment. But were the bizarre capers authentic? Did this peculiar exhibition truly represent a major advance in medicine? Almost everybody present agreed: they were convinced the patients' responses were genuine. And although nobody could explain the scientific cause of the phenomena they had witnessed, all were satisfied that Elliotson's experiments provided ample proof of the reality of animal magnetism, or mesmerism as the doctor preferred to call it.

The *Morning Post* reporter – who had already witnessed similar scenes on the wards – had no hesitation. 'Our own opinion is already formed, by frequent and attentive observation, that the extraordinary effects produced in Dr Elliotson's lecture-room are real and unsophisticated, however inexplicable they may be on any known theory of disease.'[18] The journalist from *The Lancet* was equally convinced. Having similarly observed Elizabeth Okey on several previous occasions, he attested: 'The question of deception was at once met by a conviction, derived from appearances, that the most accomplished actor that ever trod the stage could not have presented the change with a truer show of reality.'[19]

The alternative explanation – that a seventeen-year-old girl with a rich line in comic repartee could fool not only a renowned university professor but some 300 distinguished gentlemen – was simply unthinkable. Less than a year earlier an eighteen-year-old girl had ascended the British throne. Preparations were currently well advanced for the coronation of Queen Victoria as head of the British Empire in June. But the young queen had, of course, been born with blue blood in her veins and been bred for her future role. The possibility that a young girl from a poor labouring family could deceive the whole country was utterly absurd.

The timing was crucial. Elizabeth Okey's theatrics had certainly mesmerised the audience but it was John Elliotson's status within the scientific world that gave mesmerism its credibility. Outside the lecture theatre, within the medical establishment and beyond, Elliotson knew that opposition to his work was growing. His enemies in the university were conspiring to stop his experiments, fearful that the regular extravaganzas and feverish press interest were bringing the medical school into disrepute. Other medical professionals remained deeply sceptical about the supposed effects of mesmerism. They argued that the patients' responses were either a trick or a fraud, and they believed that Elliotson truly was, in Okey's words, a 'fool'. Some even dared to suggest that the professor himself was in on the trick. At a time when scepticism towards orthodox medicine was rife, these critics were anxious that the medical profession should win public confidence for its conventional methods, and assert its superiority over the raft of charlatans peddling their alternatives – or else face extinction. With its mysterious origins and theatrical displays, mesmerism seemed to be precisely the kind of absurdity they wanted to distance themselves from. If allowed to continue, they feared mesmerism could prove the profession's death knell and the gullible professor its destroyer.

Yet Elliotson believed he was unassailable. Fiercely obstinate and famously single-minded, he was never one to shrink from controversy or buckle in the face of hostility. He had devoted his career to seeking out new medicines and techniques that might help conquer disease and suffering. Finally he was convinced he had identified a treatment that doctors could harness to treat a range of illnesses and banish pain. It was his duty, he believed, to research mesmerism's potential to the full in order to reduce this new 'science' to 'certain fixed principles'.

Facing his critics squarely, he was certain he could rely on the continuing support of his devoted students, his wealthy private patients, his well-connected political patrons, his friends in the arts and his allies in the scientific world. But above all, he was confident he could count on the unwavering loyalty of his good friend Thomas Wakley, the radical MP and founding editor of *The Lancet*. A fellow crusader in the campaign for medical reform, Wakley had nurtured Elliotson's career from its infancy, publicising his discoveries and lauding his progress with unstinting zeal. Wakley had approached the professor's latest enthusiasm with the same fervent attention. Since Elliotson's investigations into mesmerism had begun, *The Lancet* had published hundreds of pages detailing the sensations unfolding at UCH, and had stoutly defended the professor against accusations of credulity. In the trials that inevitably lay ahead, Elliotson was sure Wakley would not fail him. It was a battle, no less, for the future of medicine, and Elliotson was braced for the onslaught. All his life so far had been a rehearsal for this moment. It had been a long uphill struggle and he was determined not to go back from where he had come.

2

The Sign of the Golden Key

Southwark, Surrey, 30 September 1806

Most people who arrived in Southwark left again as quickly as they could. The medieval inns which lined Borough High Street were popular staging posts for travellers crossing London Bridge into the capital or heading in the opposite direction for Kent and the Continent. Few stayed beyond a single night in the squalid and lawless district which spread like a disease along the south bank of the filthy Thames. For anyone with an ambition to succeed in London, Southwark was very definitely the wrong side of the river.

Having spent most of his short life so far in Southwark, fourteen-year-old John Elliotson was determined to escape as soon as he could. On 30 September 1806, a few weeks short of his fifteenth birthday, he embarked on one of the most important journeys of his life. Leaving his home at 106 Borough High Street, where his father ran a prosperous chemist and druggist business, he walked a few hundred yards up the road, turned right into St Thomas Street and entered under the imposing stone archway of Guy's Hospital. Here he enrolled as a pupil under the pre-eminent surgeon of the day, Astley Cooper.[1] Yet the student was already set on surpassing his teacher. For despite his youth, the boy had already spent a year at Edinburgh University studying for a medical degree as the first step towards qualifying as a physician at the top of the medical tree. For the son of a chemist from Southwark, this was a grand ambition indeed.

John Elliotson was born in Southwark on 24 October 1791, the eldest surviving son of John and Elizabeth Elliotson.[2] John's father, Elliotson senior, had inherited his chemist shop from his own father, Thomas Elliotson, and had built up a lucrative business.[3] Sandwiched between cheesemongers, tea dealers, brandy merchants and tobacco sellers, the Elliotson shop was easily distinguished by the sign of the golden key that swung outside.

Although Southwark was not the best starting point for personal advancement, it was the ideal location for a druggist. Fronting Borough High Street, the Elliotson business was close to the docks where traders imported the raw ingredients for preparing medicines – opium from India, aloes from Africa, cinchona from South America – as well as being convenient for the riverside kilns which fired the beautiful English Delftware jars to contain them. The shop was ideally situated for customers too. The proximity of two of London's biggest hospitals, Guy's and St Thomas', assured a ready market for pills and potions while the surrounding slums guaranteed long queues of sickly patients.

Since precious few people could afford a physician's exorbitant fees, the majority of Londoners brought their aches and pains, their coughs and fevers to apothecaries or chemists such as Elliotson. Even those with ample funds often preferred to choose their own medication at a high street chemist over the foul purges and enemas prescribed by qualified doctors. One contemporary, who was also the son of a Southwark druggist, said his father's shop was filled every morning by people of all classes queuing with their sick children for 'a twopenny powder of compound senna' or a 'grain of calomel' or 'a little syrup of poppies'.[4] In addition to preparing popular remedies such as syrup of poppies, the Elliotson business sold ready-made patent medicines such as 'Grant's Lisbon Tonic Pills' for bowel complaints and 'Cundell's Improved Balsam of Honey' for 'violent coughs, colds, asthmas, and consumptions'.[5] And as a profitable sideline, chemists and druggists sold household staples such as soap powder, toothbrushes and rat poison.

Growing up above the shop, young John would have helped his father grind minerals and pound herbs, mix potions and roll out pills to dispense to the sick hordes who thronged at the door. Surrounded by giant flasks filled with colourful liquids and domed porcelain jars labelled 'Rhubarb' and 'Magnesia', he would have learned to weigh ingredients, handle poisons and refresh the water in the perforated urns that stored the leeches. The experience must have imprinted the notion of a pill for every ill on the young lad's mind. Yet the all-too-evident failure of his father's potions to cure or alleviate the innumerable diseases which scythed down the local population – not least his own siblings – must have made him determined to do better.

In practice, it made little difference whether a patient consulted the most expensive university-trained physician and took his scrawled Latin prescription to be dispensed by a licensed apothecary, or wandered into a high street chemist to buy a cheap concoction advertised in the newspaper or recommended by a friend. Almost none of these remedies worked. Aside from vaccination to prevent smallpox, digitalis to control heart disease, and cinchona – or Peruvian bark – to treat malaria, there were no effective medicines to combat the battery of infectious diseases that assailed rich and poor alike. There were similarly no useful therapies to treat chronic conditions ranging from cancer and diabetes to rheumatism and gout, although at least the syrup of poppies – effectively opium – helped dull the pain. The golden key was no guarantee of good health.

By the time he reached fourteen, four of John's siblings – an older boy and three girls – had already died, most likely from one of the many infectious diseases that killed nearly forty per cent of children under five at the beginning of the nineteenth century.[6] Another sister, born later in 1806, would live only six months. There was a long gap, therefore, between John and his only surviving siblings: Thomas, born in 1800, and Emma, born in 1802.[7] A second sister, Eliza, would arrive in 1808. Alone then for much of his childhood, John grew used to being the centre of his parents' attention and – as the little coffins of his siblings were carried one by one to St Saviour's churchyard – the focus of their anxieties too. Growing up in Southwark, he was perfectly placed to study the medical problems of the age.

Although medieval palaces once lined the south bank, Southwark had always had a reputation for low-life and bawdy behaviour.[8] Venereal diseases were rife in the dockside brothels while typhus fever stalked the Marshalsea and King's Bench prisons at the southern end of Borough High Street. Contagious diseases, such as measles, whooping cough and scarlet fever, ran rampant in the tenement blocks that lined murky alleyways with names such as Foul Lane and Dark Entry. The prevalence of rickets – caused by a deficiency of vitamin D, most commonly from lack of sunlight – was starkly spelled out in the alley named Crooked Bandyleg Walk.

In this fruitless battle against death and disease the profits of Elliotson's chemist shop mounted high. According to one contemporary, he had 'amassed a considerable fortune'.[9] Yet despite his prosperity, Elliotson senior did not want his eldest son to follow in his footsteps and take over the family business. Instead he determined to use his hard-earned wealth to buy – in the words of one contemporary – 'the best education that money could procure' to launch his son on a more elevated path.[10] So John was educated at a reputable local school and tutored privately in Latin and Greek to prepare him for admission to university. Only by attaining a degree in medicine would he be allowed to practise as a physician in London and scale the heights of the medical hierarchy.

And so it must have been a wrench when, at barely fourteen, in autumn 1805, John had set off on the long journey to Edinburgh, leaving his home and family – his mother preoccupied with five-year-old Thomas and three-year-old Emma, his father preparing to teach young Thomas the tricks of the trade.[11] Although students often started university early, fourteen was still unusually young and John was small for his age. Moreover, while most students came from middle-class professional backgrounds – the sons of physicians, lawyers and clergymen – John's origins bore the unwholesome taint of trade. His father, after all, was essentially a shopkeeper. But what he lacked in years, stature and pedigree, John Elliotson made up for in determination and hard work.

Widely regarded as the best medical school in Britain, if not the world, Edinburgh attracted students from across Europe and America. John duly enrolled for lectures in anatomy, chemistry, theory and practice of medicine, botany and *materia medica* – or pharmacy – and put his Latin and Greek to immediate use, poring over medical texts from Ancient Rome and Greece. Medical theory had remained fundamentally unchanged since Hippocrates outlined his belief, more than 2,000 years earlier, that the body contained four 'humours' which needed to be kept in balance. More practical were the twice-weekly visits to Edinburgh Royal Infirmary where the professors discussed the progress of selected patients.

As well as attending lectures and bedside lessons, the young scholar 'made a point of devoting three or four hours a day to studies not medical'.[12] He would always be proud of his rounded education and never missed a chance to proffer a pertinent literary quotation at an opportune moment.

John returned home to Southwark the following spring, putting the rest of his medical degree on hold for a few years – a not uncommon practice – with his interest in medicine increased, his fascination for chemistry heightened and his belief in his own talents considerably enlarged. Now he was ready to gain hands-on experience in a London hospital through the customary practice of 'walking the wards' – a vital step towards obtaining a permanent post.

Queuing up to sign the pupils' register at Guy's after that short walk from his home in Borough High Street, John handed over 44 guineas (roughly £3,500 today) for weekly lectures in surgical and medical subjects – much the same as at Edinburgh – as well as permission to follow ward rounds, observe operations and learn dissection. Since Guy's had amalgamated its medical school with neighbouring St Thomas', becoming the United Hospitals some years previously, he would gain experience at two hospitals for the price of one. Anatomy and surgery were taught at St Thomas' while medical and other subjects were the province of Guy's. It was a profitable, if somewhat uneasy, partnership.

Founded in 1215, St Thomas' was one of the oldest hospitals in London.[13] Behind its wrought-iron gates on Borough High Street, four elegant courtyards extended along the riverside, each surrounded by segregated male and female wards. Just as impressive, though comparatively modern, Guy's had been founded in 1721 by Thomas Guy, a governor of St Thomas', to treat the 'incurables' rejected by its neighbour. Facing St Thomas' across St Thomas Street, its stone façade was adorned with statues of Hygeia and Aesculapius, the Greek gods of health and medicine, in homage to the ancient wisdom its doctors still followed.

Yet for all their grandeur, both hospitals – like hospitals everywhere at the time – were charities that catered only to the poor. Anyone with sufficient means paid for treatment in the comparative safety of their own homes. Even operations were generally performed on a kitchen table in a patient's house, rather than running the risk of entering the overcrowded, infested and perilous public hospitals. Hospital treatment was free, though patients had to guarantee the cost of a funeral in the – relatively likely – event that they did not emerge alive. Mortality ran at more than ten per cent. In return for this charitable care, patients had to submit to the experimental efforts of the medical staff and excited attentions of the students. It was an arrangement that efficiently married philanthropy with utility. For, as George Eliot would wryly note in her novel *Middlemarch*, the gentry liked their doctors to try 'experiments on your hospital patients, and kill a few people for charity' since they preferred treatment 'that has been tested a little'.[14]

Twice a week John joined the ward rounds, when packs of students followed the physicians and surgeons from bed to bed. As each teacher scrutinised their patients, the pupils 'pushed and jostled, and ran and crowded round the bed', according to one student.[15] For all the commotion, there was little to see or hear of any value. Since physicians considered themselves above such menial tasks as prodding flesh – that was the work of surgeons – they never performed a physical examination.[16] Diagnosis consisted merely of questioning the patient and inspecting their urine, stools and blood. Of his time at Guy's and St Thomas', John would later say: 'I never saw a physician dirty his hands with the living.'[17] Aside from caustic drugs to purge the patient or induce vomiting, the standard therapies were bloodletting – by splicing a vein or applying leeches – cupping and blistering, all designed to rebalance the bodily humours. Under this brutal regime, recovery depended as much on surviving the treatment as beating the disease.

There was even less decorum when John joined his fellow pupils in the tiny St Thomas' operating theatre. Packed like 'herrings in a barrel', according to one student, the 'crowding and squeezing was oftentimes unbearable' and the atmosphere 'almost stifling'.[18] In the days before anaesthesia, patients were held down by muscular assistants or tied to the operating table. As the patient writhed and screamed, the surgeon's speed and precision were vital to success. These were harrowing scenes for a fourteen-year-old boy. One pupil wrote that 'so long as the patient did not make much noise I got on very well, but if the cries were great, and especially if they came from a child, I was quickly upset, had to leave the theatre, and not infrequently fainted'.[19] Another, professing more bravado, scoffed, 'the more the poor devils cry the more I laugh with the rest of them'. Whether John laughed or fainted went unrecorded but the sight and sound of patients suffering on the operating table with no form of pain relief left a deep impression on him.

The most fortunate patients in the operating theatre came under Astley Cooper's knife. Handsome and self-assured, thirty-eight-year-old Cooper was rising rapidly in prowess and fame; he would later be created a baronet after removing a cyst from George IV's head.[20] A keen anatomist, Cooper liked to fit in several hours of dissection before breakfast to hone his surgical skills. As a surgeon he was not only speedy, but kind and sympathetic. Those less fortunate braced themselves for the cold steel of Henry Cline's knife. Cline's operations were slow and cautious – and therefore all the more painful – though he was generally considered competent. The unluckiest patients found themselves staring up from the table at the quivering lancet of William Lucas.

A scruffy, ungainly man, William – or Billy – Lucas shuffled into the operating theatre with stooped shoulders. As a student he had complained that the foul atmosphere of the dissecting rooms made him ill, so consequently he never studied anatomy. This rather basic deficiency had not prevented him being appointed a surgeon, however, purely on account of his father having previously held the post. So began his long career in butchery. As one pupil recorded: 'His surgical acquirements were very small, his operations generally very badly performed, and accompanied with much bungling, if not worse.' On one occasion Lucas amputated a leg then painstakingly stitched the skin to cover the exposed bone on the part he had removed, leaving the patient with a raw, bleeding stump. It was lucky, for Lucas at least, that he was profoundly deaf and therefore immune to his patients' dying groans.

The hospitals' physicians were scarcely more prepossessing. William Babington and James Curry were both Irish and lived in the same house but shared no other characteristics. Babington was good-tempered and well-liked by the students though a 'very untidy dresser' who 'rejoiced in dirty hands'.[21] Curry was fierce and severe, a fluent lecturer but a harsh critic, who was feared and despised. He believed all illness stemmed from the same complaint – liver disease – and accordingly recommended the same medicine, calomel (a form of mercury), in every case. Convinced he too suffered from liver disease, he sprinkled calomel on his sandwiches – and hence acquired the nickname 'Calomel Curry'.

Scuttling back and forth between the two hospitals through the dimly lit tunnel which ran under St Thomas Street, John attended lectures, watched operations and walked the wards. And on 1 October, having just turned fifteen, he took his place in the St Thomas' dissecting room for the start of the dissection season. Bungling Billy Lucas was not the only one to object to the noisome atmosphere of the tiny room. In this airless space, between seventy and eighty pupils, dressed in blood-soaked gowns, crowded round a dozen corpses laid out on tables so there was 'literally scarce possibility of moving'.[22] Since there was no means of preserving the cadavers, long before the introduction of formaldehyde, the rotting flesh tainted the air with its foul odour. Almost as unsavoury as the stench was the presence of the grave-robbers who mingled among the students.

Prior to the 1832 Anatomy Act there was no legal source of bodies for dissection beyond the half a dozen or so hanged murderers whose corpses were granted annually to the medical profession.[23] Having emerged in the mid-eighteenth century to supply cadavers for the first private anatomy schools, by the early 1800s body-snatching had become big business. The grave-robbers – or 'Resurrection Men' – were roundly despised for their work, though they earned a grudging respect from Astley Cooper who acknowledged their vital contribution to medical education. He helped them with legal costs if they were caught and looked after their families if they were sent to jail.

Awed by the charismatic Cooper, Elliotson would always make a habit of performing autopsies on patients who died in his care and carry out dissection for his own research. It was plain, however, that for all Cooper's status and wealth, real recognition and riches lay with medicine not surgery. There seemed little hope of improving the field of surgery without some means of rendering operations painless as well as countering the virulent infections which frequently killed those patients who survived the surgeon's knife. Medicine, it seemed, held more promise.

On the Continent advances were being made in understanding and diagnosing disease, even if effective treatment lagged lamentably behind. Spurred by the shortcomings he had witnessed trailing after Babington and Calomel Curry, young John became convinced that better diagnosis and more effective medicine held the key to improving medical care. 'I conceived practical medicine was to be perfected by improvements in our knowledge of the nature of diseases,' he explained, 'and by improvements in our acquaintance with remedies and their application.'[24] Qualifying as a physician would allow him, moreover, to escape his humble origins and provide a passport out of Southwark.

Even at the age of fifteen, young Elliotson tendered high hopes. Asked by family friends about his ambitions over dinner one evening, he grandly replied: 'I'll be a physician, and ride in my carriage.'[25] And yet this youthful pomposity was tempered by a strong social conscience. According to one story, at sixteen he encountered a local family in desperate straits. He not only raised a sizeable sum of money from family and friends to help them but secretly donated his own pocket money to pay school fees for the eldest son.[26] In this heady combination, a fierce self-importance would always vie for priority with a compulsion to do good.

After a second year at Guy's and St Thomas', John returned to Edinburgh and two years later he emerged with a degree in medicine.[27] Already he had shown clear signs of intellectual rigour and leadership. He was elected a junior president – there were four each year – of the Royal Medical Society of Edinburgh, the students' own club, for 1809–10. Now, at just eighteen, he was qualified to practise medicine. Yet despite Edinburgh's enviable reputation, a degree from a Scottish university only entitled him to become a licentiate – a second-class member – of the Royal College of Physicians in London.[28] Only graduates from Oxford or Cambridge were entitled to become full fellows, enjoying the highest status and rights, despite the fact the English universities provided neither medical tuition nor medical lectures. So, still only eighteen, Elliotson enrolled at Cambridge to study a second degree in medicine for the next three years.[29]

In truth, escaping to Cambridge was probably a welcome release from the confines of the family home. Though he was a dutiful son who plainly adored his 'dear mother' – she was 'one of the finest characters in existence' and 'endowed with every thing that is excellent in the female half of human nature' – there seemed little love lost between John and his father.[30] And while he was always protective of his siblings, the differences in age meant they would never be close. The two girls, Emma and Eliza, now eight and two years old, would forge a tight bond with each other – they would be inseparable till death – and maintain a fond affection for Thomas, now ten. Thomas would follow in John's footsteps, to Edinburgh and Cambridge on the road to becoming a physician, but his achievements would always be a pale imitation of his clever brother's glowing career.

With no lectures to trouble him, Elliotson kept busy at Cambridge by reading eight hours a day.[31] It was not all dreary study, however. As a diversion, he often took himself to the West End to see the gaslights in Pall Mall. The only street in London to be lit by gas at the time – everywhere else used foul-smelling whale oil – Pall Mall was viewed as an aberration; it was thought impractical to install gaslight more widely. 'This was a bright spot in London,' he recalled, 'for comparative darkness prevailed in every other street.'[32] Drawn to novelty and innovation, Elliotson imbued this scepticism towards gaslight with symbolic importance. As London streets were belatedly lit by gas over the ensuing years, he would compare 'the progress of illumination' with the painfully slow advance of medicine.

In the meantime he travelled Europe, discovering an appetite for alpine hikes as well as a fascination for the new Continental approach to medicine. While medicine and medical education in Britain were still encased in a medieval cocoon, the revolution in France had swept away archaic institutions and practices. At the new medical school in Paris, students were being taught to compare the appearance of the dead body at post-mortem with the signs and symptoms of disease in living patients.[33] Contrary to the ancient principles of humoral medicine, it was becoming blindingly obvious that specific diseases originated in specific organs and tissues. Inexplicably, and in the absence of any effective alternative, this startling realisation only spurred French doctors to bleed their patients all the more enthusiastically. At the same time, French and German chemists were analysing common compounds to isolate their active ingredients and produce pure medicines for the first time.

Now that the long Napoleonic Wars were over, the young Elliotson was among the first in a tranche of British and American medical students who gravitated to France and Germany to embrace this new scientific approach. In his early twenties he visited hospitals and universities in France, Germany, Italy, Spain and Switzerland, becoming fluent in French, German and Italian in the process, as well as making friends abroad.[34] The experience was cathartic. He not only discovered a love of foreign travel – he would take off for long summer vacations in Europe every year throughout his life – but would always place a higher value on Continental ideas than home-grown ones, with profound consequences.

Inspired by his veneration of all things Continental and impatient to make his mark on the medical world, Elliotson was confident enough in 1815, at just twenty-four, to translate from Latin to English a major medical book by Johann Friedrich Blumenbach, distinguished Professor of Medicine at Göttingen University and a world authority on physiology.

First published in 1787, Blumenbach's book, *Institutiones Physiologicae*, was regarded as the principal textbook on the living human body.

Elliotson's translation, *The Institutions of Physiology*, published anonymously at first, added twenty pages of notes to update Blumenbach's research.[35] The book sold rapidly and a second edition, published under his own name two years later, not only added a further 150 pages of notes but was the first book ever printed on a revolutionary new press, driven by steam, which put out 900 sheets an hour. The book – another nod to Elliotson's love of novelty – was advertised as a 'typographical curiosity'. Though he was still a novice in medical practice, Elliotson drew on his extensive reading to correct the veteran professor's errors and confidently assert his own views, resulting in the most up-to-date and comprehensive summary of knowledge on human physiology at the time. It was a remarkable achievement – at any age – and a testament to his extraordinary scholarship and enormous self-confidence. The book also laid out his humanitarian outlook for the first time.

Elliotson bluntly rejected the prevailing view that Africans represented the lowest of Blumenbach's five human 'races', arguing that the slave trade might lead 'the poor Negro' to believe white people were not only inferior to himself but 'below apes in intellect'. He backed the controversial theory, which was then gathering pace, that different species produced offspring better adapted to their environment and that the human species probably originated in Africa. At the same time, he clearly marked himself out as a materialist, if not yet an atheist, by declaring that science and religion should be kept separate.

The book established the young Elliotson as an authority on current medical knowledge as well as an outspoken maverick. Medical journals acclaimed the work and even Blumenbach was generous with his praise. Elliotson crowed to a friend that 'the old gentleman himself has sent me a letter full of delight'.[36] And although he was fully aware his open avowal of materialism was 'dangerous ground', he promised the next edition would go even further: 'I have begun to throw off some of the prejudices which I imbibed with the milk of the breast & which grew up with me, mistaken for unbiased legitimate conclusions.'

Elliotson's translation would go through a total of five editions, his own contribution augmented in each one, until the final edition, published in 1840, was so transformed from the original Blumenbach text that he published it under a new title, *Human Physiology*, as his own work.

*

In rejecting his religious upbringing, young Elliotson was plainly distancing himself from familial obligations. He was distancing himself from his family too. By 1816, at the age of twenty-five, he had moved out of the family home and taken lodgings in Grafton Street, in London's fashionable West End.[37] Two letters – to a druggist in the City of London and a surgeon in Royston, Hertfordshire – survive from these early days when he was establishing himself in practice. He would always describe himself as a 'cockney' and boast that he had lived all his life within the sound of Bow bells, but in truth those bells were becoming exceedingly faint, especially during the summers when he fled the London stink for his father's country retreat in Clapham.[38]

Charming and urbane, with his dark good looks and suave self-assurance, John Elliotson was ready to establish himself as a respectable physician and a serious man of science. He had made connections at Edinburgh and Cambridge among the privileged sons of landed England, and he would use these connections to tout for private patients.[39] He was likewise forging alliances with the most forward-thinking figures in scientific circles. Already, when he was twenty, he had been elected to the Medical and Chirurgical Society, recently set up by reformers to debate new advances in medicine. At these exhilarating meetings he met rising stars such as Humphry Davy and Michael Faraday from the Royal Institution.[40] Yet despite his qualifications and connections, he was still struggling to gain a foothold in the brutally competitive medical marketplace. And he was still, humiliatingly, dependent on Papa for financial support. His chances of progressing further depended on one thing: obtaining a post within a large London hospital.

Securing a hospital post was a vital stepping stone to professional success in the nineteenth-century medical world. Firstly, such posts helped a physician establish his reputation; secondly, although the appointments were part-time and unpaid, a position in a medical school could provide a healthy income through pupils' fees as well as vital teaching and research material in the flow of poor patients who streamed through the hospital doors. But obtaining such a position was far from easy.

There were only three or four posts for physicians at each of the large London hospitals, a total of just over twenty positions throughout the capital.[41] Since these jobs were for life, vacancies arose only when a post-holder retired or, more usually, died. They were filled, more often than not, by the relatives of the presiding medical staff – regardless of merit. On the rare occasions when nepotism did not prevail, posts were generally awarded to a staff member's apprentice.

John Elliotson boasted neither blood ties nor apprenticeship bonds, and so, when the first vacancy for an assistant physician arose at St Thomas' in 1816, he was soundly beaten by a rival in the ballot.[42] The following year, when a new vacancy came up, he was ready. Though he lacked the family connections that guaranteed success in medicine, as in all walks of public life, he possessed something else: the clout new money was bringing to the middle classes. Elliotson used his father's influence as a local businessman and the support of wealthy friends to swing the vote and secure the job. Appointed assistant physician to George Gilbert Currey – no relation to Calomel Curry – his tasks included prescribing for patients and leading students on ward rounds. Now began the long wait for a senior post. It was going to prove a bumpy ride, for the young Elliotson was not only adept at making friends, he was careless in making enemies.

Frustrated with the nepotistic regime and its blinkered approach, Elliotson was impatient to carve out his own path. With his passion for chemistry undimmed, he collaborated with an old Edinburgh university friend, a chemist named William Prout.[43] In 1819 Prout suggested that Elliotson give iodine, isolated eight years earlier by a French chemist, to patients with goitre, an enlarged thyroid gland. The medication had the 'most striking effects'. Impressed by the results, Elliotson publicised the benefits of iodine for goitre and recommended its use to students. It was his first major advance, albeit at someone else's suggestion, and a significant breakthrough; although with the characteristic slowness of medical discoveries, it would be more than a century before iodine was routinely added to table salt.

It was a fruitful partnership. Elliotson and Prout founded a medical journal, *Annals of Medicine and Surgery*, which ran for several years, to publicise their research. Yet as long as he was denied a senior physician's post, Elliotson was subordinate to Currey, and could therefore not test his more controversial theories on patients, or lecture students on his radical ideas. Impatient as ever, he was determined to remedy the latter at least.

*

Ever since Guy's and St Thomas' had united, all lectures on medicine had been delivered at Guy's by the Guy's physicians; to stifle competition, the physicians at St Thomas' were forbidden from lecturing on medicine, even within their own hospital. The ruling had long caused friction. When Elliotson's superior, Currey, asked the governors in 1820 for permission to lecture at St Thomas' he was briskly rebuffed.[44] Slinking away, Currey launched a series of private classes in a nearby schoolroom. His junior colleague was not so easily subdued.

The following year Elliotson requested permission to give lectures at St Thomas' on 'state medicine'. The subject, essentially forensic medicine, had fast been gaining popularity on the Continent and Elliotson was adamant that it was a vital topic since medical men were increasingly being called to give evidence in court cases and inquests. Even though his proposal presented no conflict of interest – since the subject was not offered at either hospital – the governors bluntly refused. Elliotson, however, would not take no for an answer. He continued to bombard the governors with requests until finally he was warned that his letters to the treasurer, Abel Chapman, should be 'expressed in language more temperate and decorous'. It was a taste of battles to come; Elliotson's temper often got the better of him when he was opposed. As he confided to a friend, the 'pain of disguising my opinions of things or of persons is so intense that I despair of ever being prudent in this respect. Intense feeling causes great freedom of spirit & this is my besetting sin.'[45] Nonetheless he was incapable of giving way. A month later, he began lecturing on forensic medicine at a rival anatomy school right on St Thomas' doorstep.

The Webb Street anatomy school had been opened a few years earlier by Edward Grainger, a former St Thomas' pupil who had studied under Cooper.[46] Grainger had been furious when he was passed over for an anatomy post in favour of Cooper's nephew, and had set up his rival school in revenge, even paying the body-snatchers higher fees. When Elliotson joined forces with Grainger, opening his course in 'state medicine' on 1 November 1821, it was a blunt rejection of the age-old patronage system and a kick in the teeth for the St Thomas' establishment.

Defiantly, Elliotson began his introductory lecture by lambasting the governors for refusing to allow him to deliver his course at St Thomas'.[47] Then, in the characteristic manner he would adopt throughout his career, he set out his ideas in concise plain English, backed by solid scientific evidence. Tapping into the early nineteenth-century appetite for true crime, especially cases of bloody murder, he illustrated his points using real-life examples from contemporary court cases.

One such case was the trial of Elizabeth Fenning, a twenty-year-old servant found guilty in 1815 of attempting to murder three members of the household in which she worked by putting arsenic in some dumplings.[48] She was hanged chiefly on the evidence of one medical witness, who testified that his tests proved the dumplings contained arsenic. Fenning's plight became a *cause célèbre*, attracting support from leading public figures who were convinced the forensic evidence was flawed. Elliotson agreed, arguing that the prosecution had laid too much stress on the dumplings being dark and not having risen although arsenic produced neither of these effects (he had plainly conducted his own tests). Likewise he related the tale of a widower, recently found guilty of murdering his young housekeeper by helping her procure an abortion; there were evidently suspicions of an illicit liaison. Three doctors had testified that the woman had been poisoned despite a complete absence of chemical evidence and no sign of a foetus. Had they been properly trained in forensic medicine, the doctors would not have 'thus ruined the investigation of truth', said Elliotson.

Even more controversially, Elliotson cited the case of a man who had died following injuries at the notorious Peterloo Massacre in 1819. The young man, one of the 60,000-strong crowd at the peaceful meeting calling for electoral reform in St Peter's Field, Manchester, had suffered multiple wounds when sabre-wielding cavalry charged the gathering. He died three weeks later. The doctor who attended him had stated categorically that his death was caused by the sabre wounds, but as a Quaker he was not permitted to give evidence at the subsequent inquest because he refused to swear on the Bible. Three rather more compliant doctors testified that the man's death was not due to his injuries at all, but to a pre-existing lung condition.

Such miscarriages of justice were rife, Elliotson told his students. 'I could adduce hundreds of other instances. Indeed every assize furnishes them.' Not only were doctors' reputations at stake in such cases, but also people's lives. 'The life, of an accused individual may depend entirely upon the opinions you deliver,' he said. 'The part you act, is acted openly. You may blast your reputation, or you may acquire honour.'

It was clear that Elliotson was nailing his colours to the mast in exposing the unfair treatment of the labouring classes and supporting their demands for greater rights and representation. Growing up in Southwark had given him a deep compassion for the poor and vulnerable that would stay with him all his life. But he also used his lectures on forensic medicine to vent his anger at his own unfair treatment – in being blocked by the oligarchy that ruled the capital's hospitals and medical institutions. A man 'with inferior knowledge' could rise above another, he fumed, simply by being a member of a particular party along with 'a canting, hypocritical earnestness in religious matters; a disgusting system of fawning and crouching to persons from whom any thing is likely to be obtained, and always united, according to my observation, with gross negligence and barbarous asperity towards the poor'.

The long wait for a senior post clearly rankled. Elliotson was desperate for professional and financial independence; the reliance on parental aid was chafing. He was ill the following summer too – perhaps with the bladder stones that would plague him for many years – and repaired to the seaside to recover.[49] But Elliotson was not about to debase himself by 'fawning and crouching' to those in authority to achieve his aims. Finally his chance came.

At the end of 1822 Currey died – tragically on his honeymoon – and Elliotson put himself forward for the vacancy. Promotion was generally a formality for the assistant physician, but Elliotson's obstinacy and alliance with Grainger had spawned fierce enemies among the medical staff and hospital officials. These opponents 'raised a great hubbub' and warned him that 'I should have very little chance of being appointed physician, if I continued lecturing out of doors'.[50] Not only had he offended the St Thomas' treasurer, Chapman, with his indecorous language, he had riled an even more dangerous opponent: the despotic Guy's treasurer Benjamin Harrison. Having inherited the post from his father – of course – Harrison ran Guy's with an iron fist and held huge sway over St Thomas' too; his enemies called him the 'Boro' King'. Now King Harrison seized his opportunity for revenge.

Marshalled by Harrison, Elliotson's enemies put up an alternative candidate, an ex-pupil named John Spurgin. But Elliotson's independent spirit and intellectual vigour had won him friends among the governors too and – with Papa's help again – he recruited supporters to his flag. Realising he lacked sufficient votes, Spurgin stood down, and on

22 January 1823 Elliotson was duly appointed. At the instigation of King Harrison, however, the board insisted on a malicious caveat to Elliotson's appointment.

In front of the board, Elliotson was forced to sign a declaration promising he would not lecture outside the hospital, despite the fact that he was halfway through his second year of teaching at Webb Street. Reluctantly he agreed. Yet when other governors heard of this imposition they were 'indignant', and at the next full meeting they ordered the document to be 'torn to pieces'. Now Elliotson was at liberty to lecture outside the hospital walls when and where he liked – 'I was free as air' – though he was still forbidden from lecturing within his own hospital's premises.

It had been a tough battle and Elliotson meant to make full use of the spoils. He was now thirty-one, having served five years without remuneration as an assistant physician, and he was determined to make up for lost time. At last he possessed the platform through which to test his theories to the full, and to promote his views on medical treatment to his students – on ward rounds at least. He proved himself both a diligent and caring physician and a skilled and inspirational teacher. 'No man in London ever attended to his hospital duties with greater punctuality and assiduity,' wrote one contemporary.[51] 'The wards became to him storehouses of profitable knowledge, and he gathered abundantly from their wealth.' The father of one student, asked to account for Elliotson's popularity, explained that he 'devoted himself heart and soul to the common interests of the hospital and the pupils'. A colleague said his popularity among the Irish patients was so great that they 'considered him next to God in the cure of disease and felt disposed to invoke him as a saint!'

Emboldened by his success, Elliotson was more determined than ever to embrace novelty and flout convention. As a dedicated follower of fashion, he not only shocked fellow medics by striding around the hospital in trousers instead of the traditional silk stockings and black breeches but also grew luxuriant, under-the-chin whiskers in the latest style.[52] Shaving, he later wrote, was 'a custom most insulting to nature' while a beard 'completes the perfection of man's face'. And just as he was drawn to originality in his personal appearance, so he was quick to adopt new ideas in his professional work.

Beginning in the early 1820s, Elliotson became one of the first men in Britain to use the latest innovation from the Continent: the stethoscope. Listening for sounds in the chest (auscultation) and tapping the chest to produce sounds (percussion) had been advocated by Hippocrates, but with their usual aversion to touching the human body, physicians had long scorned the idea.[53] The new emphasis, in post-revolutionary France, on physical examination revived the practice so that students in Paris had to learn the art of distinguishing different sounds to detect different diseases. One Parisian physician, René Laennec, was having difficulty, in 1816, listening to the chest of a woman due to her excessive size, but then he had a bright idea. He rolled a sheet of paper into 'a sort of cylinder' and discovered he could hear the sounds much more distinctly. Laennec perfected his 'cylinder', renamed it the stethoscope, and published his discovery in 1819.

The invention of the stethoscope triggered a revolution in medicine just as surely as the guillotine had enabled a revolution in government. The instrument formalised the idea of examining patients for outward signs of disease and this in turn produced a climactic shift in the doctor–patient relationship which prevails to this day. Instead of illness being understood chiefly through the experience of its sufferer – by the symptoms patients described – now the doctor could discern the problem using his professional expertise. The humoral theory with its holistic approach, which conceived illness as affecting the whole person, gradually became replaced by a more localised view. Even if the idea of specific diseases affecting distinct parts of the body did not change treatment one iota – bloodletting continued unabated – the almost mystical gift of seeing inside the body conveyed a new power and status on medical men.

As with all innovations, the stethoscope was not immediately embraced by ecstatic practitioners leaping up and down with glee. Most doctors were sceptical, dismissing the stethoscope as another form of quackery, while others found it difficult to master or simply could not be bothered to learn a new technique when unctuous words had always sufficed. In a typical response, one Guy's physician placed a stethoscope on a table, stuck a flower in it, and exclaimed, 'What a capital bouquet holder!'[54] Patients were often equally wary of this intimidating instrument – early models were large and heavy – with its disturbing ability to see inside the body, not to mention their shock at their doctors' sudden intimacy. It would be two decades before the stethoscope was routinely used in British hospitals. When George Eliot wanted to mark her hero Dr Lydgate as a modern man in *Middlemarch* – set in 1829 – she armed him with a stethoscope. The stethoscope was symbolic of a new era in medicine, a new kind of doctor.

John Elliotson has been credited as the very first doctor to use the stethoscope in Britain.[55] This is almost certainly untrue. Various candidates for that accolade include John Forbes, a Scottish army physician, who published an English translation of Laennec's book in 1821, and Thomas Hodgkin, a Guy's student, who brought a stethoscope back from Paris and presented it to a student society in 1822. But Elliotson did something far more significant. He was not only one of the first physicians routinely to use the stethoscope, he did more than any other medical man to promote its benefits among his peers.

Using the stethoscope was not a simple matter of sticking one end to an ear and the other to a chest. It was a complicated skill, gleaned through careful study and long practice in order to distinguish the telltale sounds of one disease from another, discerning the subtle difference between a wheeze and a murmur, between a rattle and a hiss. Elliotson became adept at its use and, more importantly, in teaching its application to others, not only to his pupils at St Thomas' but in a series of lectures at the Royal College of Physicians, employing eloquent and often lyrical descriptions. A healthy heartbeat could be likened to 'the purring of a cat', while pericarditis sounded like 'the cooing of a dove'. Influenza produced a sound 'something like a faint snoring, or the base chord of a musical instrument', while fluid in the lungs produced a 'metallic tinkling'.[56] In a letter to a referring surgeon in 1829, Elliotson proudly asserted that he had examined the chest of his patient 'carefully by the ear & find the heart perfectly sound'.[57]

For his pains in promoting the stethoscope Elliotson met with opposition and ridicule. One colleague pronounced the instrument 'an absurdity', while another boasted he never used 'these French fooleries'.[58] At one point he even overheard the president of the RCP, Sir Henry Halford, remark: 'Oh, it is a thing which will do for Elliotson to rave about.' Never one to be put off by hostility, Elliotson was just as ready to 'rave about' an even less conventional idea that had emerged from the Continent.

*

Ever since his appointment as an assistant physician, Elliotson had been fascinated by the field of phrenology imported from France.[59] Over the ensuing years he would become the foremost advocate of the theory within British medical circles and its chief ambassador in London. Phrenology had first been outlined in the 1790s by Franz Gall, a German physician who had settled in Paris. Gall argued that different parts of the brain governed different mental characteristics and that these could be assessed by measuring the contours – or bumps – on a person's skull. So a pronounced bump in the cerebellum area above the nape of the neck indicated a large sexual appetite, while a protuberance on the forehead suggested a tendency towards benevolence. A phrenologist could therefore 'read' a person's head – or a plaster cast of their skull – to reveal aspects of their personality and their innermost emotions.

Gall's disciple, Johann Spurzheim, first introduced phrenology to Britain when he visited Edinburgh in 1816 and performed a series of brain dissections. Watching these demonstrations, a Scottish lawyer, George Combe, became an instant convert. Combe founded the Edinburgh Phrenological Society – the first of its kind in Britain – in 1820 and was largely responsible for the spread of the practice throughout the British Isles. Phrenology was to captivate British intellectual and fashionable society for decades to come. The Duke of Wellington had a cast made of his head and Queen Victoria would later invite Combe to read the young Prince of Wales's bumps. Some followers refused to hire servants without first measuring their heads, while one man tried to reduce his baby son's overlarge organ of 'firmness' by leaving him floundering on a sideboard.[60]

But phrenology was not just a popular cult. In British intellectual circles, phrenology was regarded as a genuine science. Eminent lawyers believed that measuring the heads of criminals could help identify villainous tendencies, while leading medical practitioners thought phrenology could help them diagnose a propensity towards certain diseases and mental conditions. Phrenology was widely hailed as a 'new science of the mind', and not completely without justification. Although the notion of determining character by reading bumps on the head would ultimately be discredited, scientists would later confirm that different functions are indeed located in specific parts of the brain, and that some parts which are used more frequently can even become enlarged.[61]

It was only natural that Elliotson should be drawn to phrenology, given his fascination for forensics as well as his growing interest in the relationship between the mind and body. In 1821 he sent a cast of his own head, and later those of his mother and two teenage sisters, to Combe in Edinburgh for a reading – known as a 'development' – and the following year he joined the Edinburgh Phrenological Society as a corresponding member.[62] In fact his younger brother, Thomas, had already met Combe in Edinburgh and had become a member a year earlier. From this point Elliotson began a voluminous and highly revealing correspondence with Combe that would continue for the next eight years.

As Elliotson's conviction in phrenology increased, so he drew friends, students and associates to the cause. In January 1823, the same month he became a senior physician, he founded the Phrenological Society of London with a handful of fellow devotees and they met once a fortnight to read papers and examine the heads of suitable volunteers. 'A few of us cocknies have long desired to act in concert for the good of the new science,' he told Combe.[63] Soon after, he reported: 'I believe you may say that there is a small band of devoted phrenologists in London & a very large number of persons favourable to the science.' His collaborators included a fellow physician, Dr Robert Willis, an engineer named Bryan Donkin and Donkin's friend James Deville, who owned a shop in the Strand that produced phrenological casts in plaster.

Over the next few years Elliotson bombarded Combe with reports of the society's swelling numbers, parcelled up with the assorted skulls and casts that fell his way. As well as sending the casts of three good friends – 'all highly educated & elegant fellows' – on whose characters he wanted Combe's opinion, and a cargo of Greek skulls donated by a friendly Greek aristocrat, Elliotson furnished the casts of several notorious murderers and other villains.[64] Among them were Philip Stoffel and Charles Keppel, famously known as the 'Clapham murderers', who were executed in July 1823 for suffocating Stoffel's seventy-five-year-old aunt with her own apron in order to steal a paltry sum of money. Elliotson told Combe he had actually been passing the house where the murder took place at the time of the crime as it was near his father's Clapham retreat.

Shortly afterwards, Elliotson sent a cast of the head of John Thurtell, found guilty in October 1823 of killing a gambling associate in Radlett, Hertfordshire, by cutting his throat with a penknife then bludgeoning his skull with a pistol.[65] The case had created a sensation in the press and Thurtell was executed the following January. 'We all consider Thurtell's development in complete unison with his deeds,' Elliotson assured Combe. Of course it was easy, with hindsight, to assign villainous traits to a criminal's bumps and bulges. Elliotson used his connections in clubs and societies to gain access to such criminals. He had obtained Thurtell's cast from a friend who was one of the magistrates hearing the case, while another friend, a magistrate in York, sent him the cast of a murderer executed there. At other times he procured the skulls of felons after they were executed and these too were packed up in hampers and sent to Combe. As his renown in phrenology rose, Elliotson would become a familiar figure in Newgate and other jails.

Elliotson believed phrenology could shed light not only on criminality but also on medical matters if investigated scientifically. He told Combe: 'I love truth, & believing phrenology to be founded in truth, study it as a science connected with my professional pursuits.'[66] He was convinced the mind held the key to treating various medical problems – including conditions such as hysteria, epilepsy and St Vitus's dance – which had no apparent physical cause, as well as ailments, such as dyspepsia, which he believed to be exacerbated by anxiety. 'It is right to look out for Disease in Various Organs,' he told his students, but added: 'You should also look to the state of the mind.'[67] He examined his patients' heads for clues to their conditions and reported his findings in medical journals. As he told Combe: 'I impress all my pupils at the hospital with the truth of Phrenology & invite them to our meetings.'[68] But he was not completely naive. When he hoped to be elected a fellow of the Royal Society in 1823 – prematurely, as it turned out – he urged Combe to keep quiet his role in the Phrenological Society of London, since he feared 'being blackballed, if stigmatised'.

The long correspondence between Elliotson and Combe reveals as much about Elliotson's complex character and contradictory temperament as it does about his dedication to phrenology.[69] While Combe maintains a friendly but polite formality throughout, Elliotson's responses swing erratically between a cool, professional tone and gushing, affectionate confidences detailing his deepest doubts and private furies. Combe repeatedly endeavours to calm him with flattery and rational advice backed up by his astute reading of Elliotson's character. At one point he writes encouragingly: 'Your brain is large enough to give you natural weight, and if you display knowledge, for you have talent, the others will act under your guidance without reluctance.'[70] But Elliotson's replies reveal him by turns as being oversensitive, insecure, overconfident, vain, defensive and argumentative. 'I was really hurt you made no comment on the two heads of my acquaintance,' he complains petulantly in one letter.[71] Another time he confides: 'I cannot think or read as formerly: my intellect is confused & I have an irresistible [longing] & restlessness.' Most of all the letters reveal a tragic pattern in the young Elliotson's management of personal relationships. One after another, he falls out with his closest friends as each relationship runs through the same cycle of admiration, even infatuation, quickly cooling to harsh criticism, then bitter rivalry, descending ultimately into total animosity.

At first, for example, Elliotson was 'much pleased' with Dr Willis, the society's first secretary, but before long he was describing him as 'a conceited, overbearing fellow' who is 'but half educated'. Similarly he became embroiled in a petty argument with Deville who simply wanted credit for helping Elliotson to found the new society. Refusing to allow this 'mental hallucination', Elliotson complains that Deville is 'really deranged' and had 'attacked' him in his shop. Giving full vent to his snobbery, he describes Deville as 'an illiterate vulgar being' whose 'arrogance is abominable, his whole conversation ridiculous & his knowledge of phrenology equally so'. Within a year of establishing the society, Elliotson argued with Willis at a public meeting, stormed out of the room and promptly resigned. He immediately founded a new London Phrenological Society and enticed twenty members of the former organisation to join him, leaving its predecessor to wither on the vine.

Elliotson even found himself at loggerheads with the two founding fathers of the discipline, Gall and Spurzheim. When he first met Gall, who was visiting London, he looked 'the finest philosopher that ever existed', but before long Elliotson was accusing him of a grasping greediness – though later he would venerate the old man once more. At first, he also admired Spurzheim, but once the young disciple had established himself as a popular lecturer in London, Elliotson denounced him as a 'vile pilferer' from his former teacher. Inevitably, in time, he would argue with Combe too.

It was a cycle that was set to be repeated many times throughout Elliotson's life. Just as he was dogged, forthright and single-minded in his scientific pursuits, so he was unforgiving, jealous and intolerant in his personal relationships. He could be a loyal friend and a strong ally to those who supported his endeavours, but once he felt himself to have been crossed or slighted he became a fierce and vindictive enemy. His sense of self-belief frequently bordered on arrogance, yet he was also highly sensitive and could be easily offended by a chance remark or trivial jibe. It was as if he needed to prove himself because of his inauspicious origins, yet he could be obnoxiously snobbish about other people's lack of education or breeding. At one point he describes Deville as 'the most unprincipled lying grasping quack & cockney tradesman in existence' even though Elliotson often called himself a 'cockney' and owed his own success to his father's work as a tradesman.[72] All his life he would demonstrate compassion for the sick and poor, yet he could also display contemptuous disdain for those he deemed beneath him, socially or intellectually.

Combe probably summed up Elliotson's personality best when he told him that his head suggested he could be 'a second Gall' except that certain qualities – numbered 9, 11, 12 and 13 – 'predominate too much over other organs to enable you to act fully up to your moral & intellectual endowments'.[73] The offending organs governed secretiveness, love of approbation, cautiousness and veneration. Later, an exasperated Combe rebuked him: 'Your late letters strongly impress me with the conviction that your organs of Love of approbation, and some others are in a state of morbid excitement. Matters of very little moment appear to affect you as if they involved your whole existence present & to come.' It was a warning Elliotson would have done well to heed.

Ultimately Elliotson would break off correspondence with Combe entirely, in 1829, when Combe had supposedly failed to defend him against a critic. At that point he would accuse Combe of 'injustice', 'cold selfish coarseness' and 'sophistry' and announce that he 'here terminates his conversation with that gentleman'.

Yet although Elliotson made enemies and alienated those who should have been his allies, he generally won more friends and supporters to his side. Secure in his new position at St Thomas', Elliotson's reputation as an upcoming medical practitioner and a serious man of science was rising. At last he possessed the prestige and position to forge a name for himself. And he was ready to make common cause with a brilliant young firebrand who had the power to raise his prospects to the highest summit.

3

The Talk of the Town

The Strand, London, 5 October 1823

Thomas Wakley watched with pride as the printing press turned out the first edition of his new magazine, *The Lancet*.[1] He had chosen the title with care. As a qualified surgeon he intended to use the weekly publication to lance the boil of corruption and malpractice he had witnessed in the capital's hospitals and medical schools. At the same time, like a lancet window in a church, he wanted his journal to shed light on the best contemporary medical advances and practice. He had staked everything on this gamble. For only three years earlier, his home, his career and his reputation had all been in ruins.

Just as Wakley was getting ready for bed in the early hours of 27 August 1820 he had heard a knock on the front door of his house, which also served as his practice, in Argyll Street in London's West End.[2] Newly married, the twenty-five-year-old surgeon had recently taken over the large house and consulting rooms from a retiring medical practitioner, thanks to the generosity of his father-in-law who had paid a substantial sum for the property and goodwill of the business. That night, Wakley's wife, Elizabeth, was staying with family in South Kensington and, suffering from a slight headache, he had applied leeches to his temples prior to retiring to bed. When he heard the knocker he wound a bandage around his head to keep the leeches in place; that bandage probably saved his life.

Opening the door, Wakley was greeted by a frantic man who begged him to come immediately to visit a sick patient. Yet the mission was apparently not quite so urgent since the caller first requested a drink. When Wakley returned from his cellar with a draught of cider he was hit on the head, knocked to the ground then viciously kicked and beaten. He awoke nearly one hour later – the bandage having prevented a fatal head injury – to the smell of smoke. As fire raged through his home Wakley escaped through a skylight and raised the alarm. Yet despite the best efforts of the fire brigade, the house was gutted and all its furnishings destroyed. Wakley's splendid marital home and fledgling medical business were both destroyed. But worse was to come.

The motive for this seemingly random attack was mysterious but rumours soon began to circulate. Six months earlier a band of around thirty men had gathered in an attic room in west London to hatch a plot to assassinate the Prime Minister, Lord Liverpool, and his entire Cabinet at a forthcoming dinner party. The so-called 'Cato Street Conspirators' were arrested and the plot was foiled – in fact they had been set up by a police informer all along. Five of the men were sentenced to be hanged and mutilated as the ancient penalty for treason. After hanging for half-an-hour before a large crowd, the bodies were taken down and a masked man appeared who deftly beheaded them to angry jeers from the onlookers. Such was the decapitator's skill that some had speculated he was surgically trained and one newspaper had even gone so far as to suggest that he was a 'young surgeon of Argyll Street'. In fact the masked man was probably an assistant, and erstwhile body-snatcher, at the Webb Street anatomy school where John Elliotson taught. Shortly afterwards, Wakley had received an anonymous letter, threatening to burn down his house and murder him. Shrewdly he had doubled the insurance value of his property to £1,200. But now that the threat had been enacted, the insurance company contested his claim as inflated. Even more seriously, gossipmongers suggested that Wakley had set fire to his own house – and presumably beaten himself up – in order to make a fraudulent claim.

Not the kind of man to back down meekly, Wakley had sued the insurance company and won his claim in full, but the victory could not repair the damage to his business or his reputation. Veiled accusations of arson and fraud would dog him all his life.[3] For the next two years he and his wife had shifted fretfully across London, from one rented property to another, as he struggled to rebuild a respectable practice. Eventually they settled in Norfolk Street, off the Strand, but the house was neither as spacious nor as elegant as their former residence and the patients neither as numerous or as affluent as his previous clients. Relations with his father-in-law had become strained, his wife disliked the down-at-heel district and Wakley despaired of ever succeeding in the competitive London medical world.

As the youngest son in a family of eleven children, Wakley – he always pronounced it 'Wackley' – knew he had no chance of inheriting property or capital.[4] Although his father was a successful Devon farmer, the family lacked sufficient funds to give the eighth son a helpful shove up the social or professional ladder. Tall, muscular and athletic, young Thomas had worked with his brothers on the farm. With a keen spirit of adventure, he had even persuaded his father to let him go to sea at the age of twelve or thirteen on an East Indiaman bound for Calcutta. Both experiences had imprinted a deep respect for labouring people on the young lad's mind. He would later say that he had 'felt a great interest in the welfare of the working class' since boyhood.[5] Although he had attended good grammar schools he did not progress to university – he never studied Latin or Greek – and therefore had no chance of becoming a top-ranking professional such as a physician. Instead he was apprenticed, first to an apothecary and then two surgeons, before enrolling as a pupil at St Thomas' Hospital under the redoubtable Astley Cooper.[6]

Wakley was a keen pupil and a quick learner. Like all the students before him, he adored Cooper and wanted nothing more than to emulate the celebrated surgeon. Diligent and gifted, he was appointed Cooper's dresser – responsible for the surgical instruments and bandages – but was forced to stand aside as Cooper's mediocre nephews were eased into jobs at the hospital. This unjust treatment left a deep scar. With only a slender allowance from his frugal father, Wakley supplemented his income by playing billiards and challenging boxers in the notorious Southwark taverns, making a name for himself as a force to be reckoned with. In the holidays he walked home to Devon.

His prospects improved considerably when he was sent with another student to visit a wealthy Southwark merchant, Joseph Goodchild, to appeal for funds for St Thomas'. Showing typical pluck, he had come back with not only a £100 donation, but an introduction to Goodchild's youngest daughter, Elizabeth, whom he subsequently married. After passing his exams to qualify as a surgeon in 1817, he hoped to prosper as one of the new breed of general practitioners plying their trade in London. The arson attack and swirling suspicions dashed those hopes to the ground. But if nothing else, Wakley was a fighter – in life, as well as in the ring.

On the ropes but not beaten, Wakley had hit on a radical plan. He decided to give up practising medicine altogether and launch a pioneering medical journal. He was encouraged by William Cobbett, the political agitator who had founded the radical newspaper, the *Political Register*, twenty years earlier.[7] Rallying a handful of jobbing writers and medical enthusiasts to his cause, Wakley launched *The Lancet* from one room in a printer's shop in the Strand on 5 October 1823. It was a bold move, and would transform not only Wakley's life but also change the face of medicine – and journalism – for ever.

From the first issue, *The Lancet* sent shockwaves through London's hospitals – but nowhere more so than at St Thomas' and Guy's. The magazine was not only the first weekly medical publication in the UK, it was the first to publish independent reports of clinical cases and medical developments. Priced at just 6d an issue, it was targeted at rank-and-file practitioners and students, not only in London but in the provinces, colonies and services, while also providing lay readers with vital insight into health matters. But what marked out *The Lancet* most strikingly was its combative editorial stance. While other medical journals offered long, late and tedious reviews of clinical works, *The Lancet* was brash, abrasive and bang up to date.

Wakley had laid out his ambitious aims from the first issue. In his leading article – an innovation copied from Cobbett – he vowed to 'fearlessly discharge' his duties to end 'mystery and concealment' in medicine.[8] Not only did he promise to denounce charlatans and quacks, he would 'detect and expose the impositions of ignorant practitioners' within the profession itself. And he lost no time in doing so.

Readers opening the first issue were astounded to find graphic details of a hospital operation that had gone fatally wrong, a column revealing the ingredients of popular patent medicines, and – most controversially of all – a verbatim report of the first lecture on surgery of the autumn term delivered by Astley Cooper, now Sir Astley, at St Thomas'. For medical students, who could now read the wise words of the country's top surgeon for the weekly sum of 6d instead of the usual £5 per term fee, this was a huge boon – and a shrewd marketing ploy. For lecturers such as Cooper and his cronies, who stood to lose both their audiences and their lucrative fees, it was a flagrant assault. Furthermore, Wakley announced his intention to publish in full the entire winter-long course of lectures in succeeding editions.

Not surprisingly, Cooper's first response was to threaten to sue the upstart journal for breach of copyright unless it refrained from publishing his lectures. Wakley, who initially kept his identity as editor secret, simply ignored the warning.[9] A few weeks later, when he called at the house of his former student by chance, Cooper was astonished to find Wakley correcting the proofs of the lecture that Cooper had delivered the previous night. Graciously deciding to view this imposition in the manner in which it was intended – as a homage by a young admirer to a brilliant orator – Cooper agreed his lectures could continue to be published, as long as he could correct the proofs himself and his name was removed. But if Cooper treated the new weekly journal with amused indulgence – at least, at first – his peers did not find *The Lancet* a laughing matter.

Having recruited a team of undercover reporters, most of them medical students, *The Lancet* now printed excoriating details of bungled operations, clinical mishaps and administrative abuses across the metropolitan hospitals, alongside strident editorials attacking the medical establishment and its elitist institutions. Nothing and nobody was immune. Wakley attacked the Royal College of Physicians, the Royal College of Surgeons and the Society of Apothecaries, the medical school professors and the hospital officials, quack healers and incompetent doctors alike, all in the snide satirical voice which would become the magazine's trademark, and enlivened by inventive nicknames. The RCS was dubbed the 'Bats' Cave' and the Society of Apothecaries 'Rhubarb Hall'; one pompous doctor was 'the cock sparrow' while a rival editor became 'the Yellow Goth'.

The magazine's intrepid exposures and rousing campaigns split the medical profession down the middle. Students and provincial practitioners valued its information and rejoiced at its irreverence. Members of the professional elite were outraged by its insolence and terrified of becoming its next target. Many more disparaged the journal in public but devoured its columns in private. Within eighteen months *The Lancet*'s circulation topped 4,000 a week – and Wakley was facing his first lawsuit.

Less forgiving than Cooper, John Abernethy, senior surgeon at St Bartholomew's Hospital, applied for an injunction to stop *The Lancet* publishing his lectures. Abernethy had already tried ordering the undercover 'hireling' to reveal himself in the lecture theatre and had even extinguished the lamps to prevent students taking notes, unaware that the person supplying Wakley with copy was his own, trusted assistant. Although Abernethy lost his first suit he won on appeal, but Wakley simply ignored the ruling and continued regardless, eventually overturning the decision.

During its first ten years *The Lancet* would fight ten legal battles including six libel cases. Although Wakley lost several suits, he generally won the moral high ground and recouped his costs through public donations. These were heady times for editor and staff alike. 'In the earlier days there was a good deal of adventure and excitement,' said one student-reporter. Although Wakley could be 'abusive, unscrupulous, bold', staff agreed that, whatever his faults, 'he was brave, determined, and manly'. Yet despite his veneration for his former tutor, Wakley reserved his fiercest attacks for St Thomas' and Guy's. Week after week, *The Lancet* lambasted the corrupt appointments system at the United Hospitals. Wakley neither acknowledged nor appeared to care that patronage and palm-greasing pervaded every aspect of early nineteenth-century society – from the Court and government, to the church and the law courts. Britain was run by an oligarchy of moneyed and propertied men who handed out favours and decided fortunes with a nod or a wink. From the penchant of the Royal Family for marrying their own cousins to the sealing of business contracts in gentlemen's clubs, nepotism and jobbery ruled. Yet Wakley was determined to stamp out such practices – in medicine, at least.

The nepotistic system was 'foul and stinks to heaven', he stormed.[10] 'Human life is sacrificed to it; medical science is sacrificed to it; the character and respect of the profession are sacrificed to it.' He even hoisted Cooper by his own petard, gleefully quoting him explaining that a comment he had made about indiscriminate dosing with mercury could not have been intended to cast aspersions on the surgeons at Guy's since,

'Mr Travers was my apprentice, Mr Green is my godson, Mr Tyrrell is my nephew, Mr Key is my nephew, Mr Morgan was my apprentice'. Wakley duly nicknamed Travers, Green and Tyrrell 'the Three Ninny-hammers' and detailed their botched operations in a column with the incendiary title 'Hole-and-Corner Surgery'.[11] In his most brazen attack, he published a blow-by-blow account of an abominably bungled operation to remove a bladder stone undertaken by Cooper's favourite nephew and heir apparent, Bransby Cooper, which ended with the patient's death, under the headline 'The Operation of Lithotomy, by Mr Bransby Cooper, which lasted nearly one hour!!'[12] Bransby Cooper won the inevitable libel suit but Wakley's supporters cheerfully paid the £100 compensation, and far from being deterred, Wakley only stepped up his campaign against the 'neveys and noodles' who dominated hospital positions.

Enraged by this relentlessly hostile spotlight, surgeons at St Thomas' slammed their doors in Wakley's face. Eight months after the launch of *The Lancet*, Wakley was banned from the operating theatre. Having paid his fees to become a perpetual student, Wakley simply brushed aside the edict and continued to turn up at lectures and operations like Banquo's ghost. With his reputation as a prize-fighter going before him, he strode through the wards and demanded to view the casebooks, on the principle that the hospitals were public charities and should therefore be subject to public scrutiny. By 1824, the United Hospitals had become a battleground, with Wakley and his young allies pitched against the senior staff and governing body. John Elliotson found himself smack in the middle of this war zone.

Having won his long-awaited post as senior physician in the same year *The Lancet* first appeared, Elliotson was now effectively part of the cabal that ruled the United Hospitals. Wakley's attacks on individual practitioners could be viewed as an attack on the entire hospital, while his insistence on roaming the wards to winkle out further scandals represented a threat to them all. There was a spy in their midst – a spymaster and his team of spies, no less – and the place bristled with suspicion and distrust.

Elliotson's best interest lay in loyally supporting the hospital establishment. Yet Elliotson had himself suffered from the corrupt and nepotistic regime Wakley was striving to end and had likewise made powerful enemies among the 'Southwark Junto', as *The Lancet* dubbed 'King Harrison' and his cronies. He was still incensed by the continuing ban on St Thomas' physicians lecturing in their own hospital to the extent that he boycotted the annual dinner for ex-pupils in early 1824.[13] More importantly, Elliotson found himself in tune with Wakley's radical ideals and ambitions not only to revolutionise the medical profession and promote scientific advances, but also to bring about a fairer, more equal society with greater rights for working people. At a time of widespread social unrest fuelled by high food prices, mass unemployment and wage cuts, Wakley used his journal not only to highlight medical corruption but also to campaign for reform of the poor law system to provide better help for the worst off, an end to the Corn Laws which artificially inflated the price of wheat, and the repeal of the Stamp Act on newspapers and pamphlets which he viewed as a tax on information.

So Elliotson faced a stark choice. He could align himself with the dinosaurs of the medical establishment such as Cooper and Abernethy – and he would very likely rise fast in reputation and earnings – or he could throw in his lot with daring young radicals such as Wakley and his student acolytes in the hope of effecting change. Ever attracted to rebellion and novelty, Elliotson chose to set his face towards the future.

It is not known precisely when Elliotson and Wakley first met but before long they had become friends and allies. Since Wakley had enrolled at St Thomas' in 1815 and spent the next eighteen months 'walking the wards', it is likely he met Elliotson then. Wakley had lodged just off Tooley Street, not far from the Elliotson chemist shop, and had attended the Webb Street school where Elliotson later taught. Indeed they shared a passion for forensic medicine; Wakley campaigned for coroners to be medically qualified and would later become only the second doctor to hold such a post. Moreover, Wakley was impossible to miss. At five feet ten inches, with his muscular frame and striding gait, he cut a flamboyant figure strolling around Southwark. His golden curls framed a handsome, intelligent face with penetrating blue eyes and, like Elliotson, he was something of a dandy, sporting nankeen trousers, frilled white shirts and brightly coloured waistcoats. He must have made a striking sight as he squared up to bare-knuckled boxers in the local alehouses. As one friend later said, he could 'smooth a curl or crack a pate with equal facility'.[14] Later on, when he substituted his fists for his pen, another said he 'could crush an enemy as he would a wasp'.

Elliotson and Wakley were a natural fit. Both were clever, ambitious, self-confident and pugnacious. Both perceived themselves to be self-made men who had struggled against the disadvantages of birth and circumstance. Elliotson had been born on the wrong side of the river and bridled at his family's association with trade. He told one friend he was proud that he was 'not driven to practice as a trader'.[15] Wakley had been born at the wrong end of the family and had had to use his wits and fists to make ends meet. 'I came to this town unknowing and unknown,' he later said. 'I fought my own battle, not always an easy one.'[16] Together they made an eye-catching pair: Wakley tall, flaxen-haired and youthful; Elliotson short, dark and whiskered – both decked out in the latest fashions. United by their shared experiences and a mutual passion to improve the deplorable state of the medical profession, they forged a formidable alliance.

As a surgeon, Wakley reserved his greatest contempt for the Royal College of Surgeons. He denounced its self-elected council, which not only excluded ordinary members from decision-making, but even insisted they enter the building via a back door in a dingy side street instead of the neoclassical portico fronting Lincoln's Inn Fields. At one point he orchestrated a demonstration of more than 300 college members who invaded the council chamber, stamping and jeering until they drowned out proceedings.[17] As the protest descended into a brawl, Wakley was ejected by Bow Street police officers and struck on the shoulder with a truncheon; true to form he sued the offending constable.

Elliotson became a vocal supporter of *The Lancet* campaign to open up access to the Hunterian Museum, the magnificent anatomy collection of the late surgeon John Hunter, which had been entrusted to the RCS with a government grant but was kept under lock and key most of the time. At one fiery meeting, gloatingly reported in *The Lancet*, Elliotson – who was a museum trustee – urged that the museum be open four times a week to members of both colleges in common with museums he had visited abroad.[18] Elliotson was just as vehement in supporting Wakley's campaign to modernise the Royal College of Physicians. He was one of the most outspoken supporters of demands to give full status to RCP licentiates – those second-class members with Scottish degrees – despite being a full fellow himself. The system of self-election among the officers was 'not at all calculated for the present age', Elliotson told a parliamentary select committee, while discriminating 'simply on account of the difference of latitude of the places of study, I think would be most barbarous, not to say unjust'.[19]

At the same time, Wakley and Elliotson made common cause to dispel the prevailing ignorance in medical practice through the rigorous investigation of potential new remedies and dissemination of the most up-to-date scientific knowledge. Now he was a senior physician, Elliotson had free rein to test his ideas on patients at St Thomas' and he did not hold back. Throughout the 1820s he conducted scores of experiments and was eager to broadcast the results. With its high circulation and wide influence, *The Lancet* was the ideal vehicle. As he told Combe in early 1824: 'The work sells prodigiously out of the profession as well as in & has great power.'[20] Wakley was happy to oblige. He published the results of Elliotson's research in *The Lancet* and lauded his achievements.

Having already shown the efficacy of iodine for goitre, Elliotson had moved on to investigate quinine.[21] In 1819 two French chemists had isolated quinine, the active ingredient in cinchona or Peruvian bark, a native South American remedy for fever, which had been used to treat malaria in the West since the seventeenth century. In 1822 Elliotson began the first trials on quinine in the British Isles. Keen to compare pure quinine with the traditional bark, Elliotson had pills prepared in the St Thomas' laboratory and gave them to patients suffering malaria, which was still prevalent in low-lying areas of England, as well as other illnesses. He carefully recorded the results. In passing he provided poignant snapshots of the desperate people who filled the wards, such as the 'poor Irishwoman, half-starved and flooding' who was admitted with typhus fever. Prescribed a course of quinine, along with a daily pint of porter and the 'full diet', she was discharged 'perfectly strong and well' – and no doubt proclaiming Elliotson a saint.

Elliotson's trials showed that pure quinine or sulphate of quinine cured malaria in every one of eleven cases, even when the bark had failed. Furthermore, the tablets were easier to swallow than the nauseating powdered bark. Delighted with his success he announced his findings in July 1823 to the Medical and Chirurgical Society (MCS) and his paper was later published in the society's *Transactions*. He admitted: 'It is very true that Quinina and Cinchonina cannot strictly be called new medicines, because they exist, one or both, in the Cinchona which we have all been prescribing.' Unable to resist showing off his intellectual prowess, he added: 'We are in the situation of M. Jourdain, in Molière's *Bourgeois Gentilhomme*, who had been speaking prose all his life without knowing it.' Rather less usefully, he conducted trials on sub-carbonate of iron, sulphate of copper and creosote, and claimed positive results for each – though any benefits these may have had were doubtless outweighed by their toxic qualities.[22]

Elliotson was more successful in demonstrating that the horse infection glanders could be transmitted to humans when he investigated three cases of patients who had died at St Thomas' after contact with diseased horses.[23] Previously it was thought that only rabies and cowpox were communicable from animals to humans. The scale of his detective work was remarkable. Discovering that one patient, the son of a blacksmith, had symptoms akin to glanders, he had visited Lambeth to interview the family. The parents were adamant that the boy had not been near a horse with glanders, but his brother eventually revealed that a diseased horse in a neighbouring stables had collapsed one day and the boy had 'patted it about the head as it lay' before it died in his arms. Now Elliotson determined to trace the family of an earlier patient, a stable boy from Woolwich. Travelling to Woolwich, he scoured the district's inns and even recruited some students to help with the quest. When finally tracked down, the family denied that the boy had been in contact with a diseased horse, but Elliotson refused to give up. At last an uncle confessed that the youth occasionally helped to harness a neighbour's horse, 'a miserable worn-out poney, covered with sores' which had been 'sent to the knackers a few months after his death'. There was no cure for human glanders, but at least practical precautions could now be taken.

Likewise, Elliotson was the first to argue that hay fever was caused by grass pollen. Hay fever had first been described by John Bostock, a chemistry lecturer at Guy's, who had given a paper on his own 'summer catarrh' to the MCS in 1819. Bostock did not believe the affliction was caused by grass, since he still suffered when no grass was in sight. Despite having met with only one case – the condition was still rare – Elliotson told his students: 'I believe certainly that it does not depend upon the hay, and therefore ought not to be called hay-fever, but upon the *flower* of the grass, and probably upon the pollen.'[24] He argued that 'a minute quantity of the emanation from the flower of grass is sufficient to produce it – so minute that you can be in few parts of the country at all without the chance of its reaching you through the atmosphere'.

Elliotson was just as eager to investigate commonly used therapies which were plainly not effective. So he tested the patent medicine Dr James's Powder, one of the most popular remedies since the middle of the eighteenth century (and no doubt a best-seller in his father's shop).[25] Favoured by George III and Samuel Johnson, along with thousands of others, the medicine had been shown in 1791 to be comprised of antimony and calcium phosphate. Despite the toxic effects of the first ingredient and the completely useless inclusion of the second, the powder remained as popular as ever. After testing the medicine on several patients at St Thomas', as well as on his father's footman, Elliotson triumphantly declared that Dr James's Powder 'serves no other purpose than to amuse the patient and the practitioner'.

Most of Elliotson's discoveries were first reported to the MCS and published in its *Transactions*, then subsequently broadcast in *The Lancet* with lavish praise. Reporting Elliotson's trials on quinine, the journal enthused: 'One of the most valuable medicines which modern chemistry has given to us, is the sulphate of quinine.'[26] Describing Elliotson's tests on copper sulphate, *The Lancet* announced, 'we are enabled to say with confidence that it is a valuable remedy in such cases'. While most of the capital's practitioners opened *The Lancet* with trembling fingers each week, for fear they should prove its latest target, Elliotson could seemingly do no wrong.

At first Elliotson confessed himself baffled by this apparent favouritism. Just a few months after the launch of *The Lancet* he told Combe he had been 'spontaneously appraised' by the magazine's proprietors – presumably Wakley – that 'while I preserve my present line of conduct & my present character, I . . . shall be held sound & be untouched, while all others . . . are cut & hacked without mercy'.[27] Why the normally ruthless journal should accord him such respect he was 'utterly unable to imagine'. Before long, however, he accepted this charmed existence as of right.

From the first edition of *The Lancet*, Wakley had declared his determination to denounce quackery and he was doggedly faithful to his word – for the most part. He ridiculed the German physician Samuel

Hahnemann for his homoeopathy doctrine and described the English Homeopathic Association as 'an audacious set of quacks' supported by 'noodles and knaves'.[28] He was even more vehement against John St John Long, the son of an Irish basket weaver who had set up business in London's Harley Street and had amassed a fortune by selling an ointment he claimed could cure all ills.[29] Long's trick was to diagnose an incurable illness in a healthy client, apply his caustic ointment to produce ulcers then allow the sores to heal and thus proclaim a miraculous cure. When a young Irish woman died in agony as a result of her treatment, Wakley represented the family at the subsequent inquest. Although Long was found guilty of manslaughter, he was only fined a paltry £250.

Wakley reserved his most flamboyant campaign, however, for a French showman named Monsieur Chabert who styled himself the 'Fire King' and claimed he could enter searing hot ovens and swallow caustic acids.[30] Wakley turned up at one of Chabert's shows – he made a habit of turning up where he was least wanted – and challenged the man to drink a vial of prussic acid which he helpfully produced from a pocket. As the crowd bayed in support, the Fire King turned tail and bolted through a window. Other unconventional doctrines, however, were enthusiastically acclaimed in *The Lancet* – especially when backed by Elliotson.

From its earliest days *The Lancet* had endorsed phrenology as 'this beautiful and useful branch of philosophy'.[31] The journal described the London Phrenological Society – Elliotson's new organisation – as 'one of the most respectable [societies] in the metropolis' and earnestly detailed its debates as members studied the casts of murderers for telltale signs of evil intent. Indeed Wakley himself joined in 1824, the same year Elliotson assured Combe *The Lancet* 'will advocate phrenology most warmly'.[32] The following year the journal welcomed the arrival of Johann Spurzheim in London – even if Elliotson did not – and published all eighteen lectures he delivered. Over the succeeding years *The Lancet* would award more than 600 pages to the intricacies of phrenological debate.

At the same time, Wakley supported experiments by Elliotson on galvanism – treatment with electric shocks – and acupuncture. Introduced into the West in 1810 by a Parisian professor, Louis Berlioz, acupuncture was first promoted in Britain by James Churchill in 1821. Elliotson began testing acupuncture on both his hospital and private patients in 1824 and was impressed by the results. 'The effects are often magical,' he wrote.[33] 'The pain sometimes ceases while the needle is in the flesh, but generally three or four applications to each painful part are required.' He reported that acupuncture cured thirty out of forty-two cases of rheumatic pain during three years of trials at St Thomas'. He was mystified as to how the needles worked, but was convinced it was not through 'any effect of the mind'. He said: 'I have seen as much benefit where people have laughed at acupuncture as where they had faith in it.'

Wakley eagerly reported Elliotson's 'cures' with acupuncture and only occasionally inserted a note of caution at his friend's fixation with novelty and 'excess of zeal' in administering large doses.[34] He jested: 'At one time we find him *boring* every patient in the Hospital with acupuncturation needles, another time *ironing* his patients, whilst at the present period, he is on the *coppering* plan.'

At the same time, of course, both Elliotson and Wakley – along with hundreds of contemporaries – continued to recommend the utterly useless and frequently harmful therapies of bloodletting, cupping, purging and blistering. Given their commitment to scientific investigation, it seems almost inexplicable that such intelligent and questioning men still clung to such practices despite the plain evidence that they hastened, if not caused, the deaths of numerous patients. When the Duke of Kent died in 1820 after being relentlessly bled, blistered and cupped in a vain effort to beat a fever, his wife lambasted the 'cruel doctors' and wailed 'there is hardly a spot on his dear body that has not been touched by cupping, blisters or bleeding'.[35] Even when patients were already fading from blood loss due to injuries or internal haemorrhaging, doctors brandished their lancets or produced leeches to remove more blood. As the poet John Keats coughed up blood in the final stages of consumption in 1821, his doctor slashed a vein to bleed him further; he promptly expired.[36]

Bloodletting, blistering and cupping stubbornly persisted due to the absence of rigorous scientific method, such as comparing one remedy with a dummy or placebo. When patients recovered from illness after the standard tortures, this was seen as proof of the method's efficacy – though in reality they had simply survived *despite* their doctors' attentions. Conversely, when patients died, it was surmised that the therapies had not gone far enough, or were not applied sufficiently early or in the correct formulation. In fairness, many patients demanded such treatments and suspected they were being short-changed if they were not provided.

So Elliotson urged his pupils to bleed patients suffering from inflammation until they fainted. Equally Wakley blamed the death of a patient from dysentery on the failure of a country doctor to follow the orthodox procedure. Describing the post-mortem he noted incredulously that 'although inflammation must for days have been raging violently, yet his arms bore not the smallest trace of a lancet puncture, nor his body the mark of a leech-bite or cupping glass!'[37] Yet both desperately desired a more rigorous scientific base. When testing creosote drops, Elliotson wisely remarked that he avoided reading other trials on the substance in order not to bias his observations.

Despite his unorthodox ideas and outspoken views, Elliotson's star was rising fast. In 1824 he delivered the prestigious Gulstonian lectures at the RCP and the following year he was elected one of the college's censors, a member of the elite board which examined applicants for membership and judged disciplinary matters. At the same time, he was becoming a popular figure in fashionable society and his house in Grafton Street was a magnet for intellectual gatherings and musical entertainment.

Still in his early thirties, a good-looking and urbane man about town, Elliotson was every inch the eligible bachelor. But he would never marry. All his closest friendships were with men – men of his own age with kindred interests, senior figures who fostered his prospects, and bright, young students who idolised him. His letters to Combe mention a raft of young men for whom he sought phrenological readings but never any young women, apart from his sisters. At one point he enthuses over the 'extraordinary . . . beauties' of one young friend who is 'sadly addicted to women'; another time he refers to 'one of the dearest of my friends' who was unmarried and 'as pure as before puberty'.[38] Just as he did with Combe, Elliotson would repeatedly throw himself into a fervent relationship with a new male friend only to find himself disappointed again all too soon. It is conceivable that he may have been homosexual, but this was a period when sex with men was not only utterly taboo but punishable by death. Nevertheless Elliotson was living life to the full under the bright lights of London's West End.

Meanwhile, beside the filthy Thames in gloomy Southwark, the simmering tensions were about to erupt. In 1825, Astley Cooper announced his retirement in the full expectation that his nephew Bransby would automatically succeed him as anatomy lecturer at St Thomas'.[39] But in a rare rejection of the customary system the board refused to appoint Bransby. In revenge, Cooper persuaded Guy's to establish a separate anatomy school jointly run by his nephews, Bransby and Aston Key. Soon afterwards St Thomas' pupils were refused entry to the Guy's operating theatre and police had to break up the ensuing riot at which six students were arrested. The United Hospitals were united no more.

Elliotson seized his chance. He took advantage of the split by immediately renewing his request to give lectures at St Thomas'. Since there was no longer any reason to protect Guy's' monopoly the governors agreed.[40] Wakley heartily applauded his victory in *The Lancet*, remarking that '*he* is never deficient in activity at least, and, I hope, will do credit to the school'.[41] Elliotson gleefully reported the news to Combe with the promise that he would promote phrenology 'to your hearts content'. Finally free to lecture on medicine within his own hospital, he entered the lecture theatre triumphantly in October 1825.

Over the course of sixty-two lectures, delivered three times a week throughout the winter, Elliotson provided a clear, methodical and comprehensive description of the symptoms, causes and treatment of all known diseases.[42] Although he advocated the traditional diagnostic methods of examining stools and urine, as well as the age-old therapies of bloodletting, blistering and purging, he also urged his students to use the stethoscope and thermometer, promoted quinine for malaria and iodine for goitre, and stressed the importance of post-mortem examinations. He illustrated his talks with stunning visual aids in the shape of skilfully dissected organs, both healthy and diseased. In one lecture, on hypertrophy – enlargement – of the heart, for example, he placed a normal heart side by side with that of a diseased patient, which was four times the size.

Most significantly, Elliotson supplemented his lectures with practical clinical instruction. He had learned the importance of bedside teaching on his Continental visits and was adamant about its value. On ward rounds Elliotson progressed from bed to bed without hurry, patiently encouraging his students to describe each patient's symptoms, attempt percussion and auscultation to hazard a diagnosis, and then suggest appropriate treatment before he weighed in with his own conclusions. Then once a week he delivered a 'clinical lecture' when he discussed the salient points of interesting cases admitted during the week.

Explaining his approach in *The Lancet,* Elliotson said it was 'impossible to teach the symptoms and history of diseases, with accuracy and minuteness, without the aid of living illustrations'.[43] His pupils were besotted with him and in awe of his kindly approach, so different to the aggressive, dismissive, baffling style of his predecessors. 'It may well be supposed that this system of clinical instruction was all but perfect,' enthused one.[44] Elliotson *taught* rather than lectured, he said, and added: 'Elliotson was the greatest clinical teacher of his time.'

It was a pivotal point in Elliotson's career and Wakley's support was critical to his success. From 1827 *The Lancet* regularly published clinical cases detailed by Elliotson and two years later the journal began serialising his lectures and clinical instruction week-by-week throughout the winter. Lauding his friend's innovative style, Wakley condemned other courses as 'ill-arranged, miserable compilations from medical and surgical dictionaries' while Elliotson's lectures 'contain all the evidences of acute and active observation'.[45] Almost overnight his reputation soared. Private patients flocked to his door and his income increased tenfold to £5,000 a year.[46] In twelve months, said one pupil, Elliotson became 'the talk of the town'. Elliotson himself admitted that from 1818 to 1828 his income had been static, not even covering his expenses.[47] He had treated more than 20,000 poor patients both at St Thomas' and in the Southwark area free of charge and his income from private fees had been minimal.[48] Yet as soon as his lectures appeared in *The Lancet* his private practice burgeoned as general practitioners referred their patients to him in droves. Buoyed up by this popularity, in 1829 he was elected a fellow of the Royal Society.[49] His success vindicated his bitter campaign against the vested interests at St Thomas'. But it was already too late.

Since the loss of its most famous surgeon, Cooper, St Thomas' had undergone a sharp decline. By 1831 student numbers had plummeted and the board considered closing the medical school. In desperation the governors appealed to the staff for ideas. But unlike the organs he displayed in the lecture theatre, Elliotson's heart was no longer in St Thomas'. At last he was presented with his chance to escape. In spring 1831 a vacancy arose at the new London University and rumours immediately circulated – courtesy of *The Lancet* – that Elliotson would win the post.

*

The idea of a university to provide an affordable, liberal and modern education for the sons of London's growing middle classes had first been floated by a Scottish poet, Thomas Campbell, in 1820.[50] The gauntlet was picked up by Henry Brougham, a charismatic lawyer and fiery Whig MP. A friend and backer of Thomas Wakley, Brougham – pronounced 'Broom' – often devoted his legal talents to defending *The Lancet*'s never-ending lawsuits. Organising a calves' head dinner in early 1825, Brougham rallied his supporters to raise funds by selling shares in a joint stock company that would allow the creation of an entirely new style of university. Unlike Oxford or Cambridge, it would be open to anyone who could pay the fees – all men, at least – regardless of religion, and would offer a range of modern subjects including astronomy, engineering and oriental languages alongside traditional subjects such as medicine. There would be no degrees in theology, indeed no religious instruction whatsoever. Uniting Whigs, radicals and dissenters to his cause, Brougham garnered sufficient subscriptions to buy eight acres of land on a former rubbish dump beside Gower Street in Bloomsbury. Out of this fetid mud rose a stately neoclassical edifice, designed by William Wilkins who would go on to create the National Gallery, and modelled on the Olympeum in Athens. The university opened its doors to students in 1828. Yet for all its idealistic aims, it was beset by problems from the start.

London University was attacked, as one contemporary put it, in 'Parliament, press and pulpit'.[51] Anglican leaders were appalled by its open-door policy and secular curriculum. Brougham was branded an 'infidel' and the university denounced as 'the Godless institution in Gower Street'. Tory party supporters were angered by its Whig leanings and immediately began fundraising for a rival university to represent king, church and state; King's College duly opened in the Strand in 1831. And the Tory press had a field day. The magazine *John Bull* dubbed London University 'Stinkomalee' on account of its swampy site, while the *Morning Chronicle* ridiculed its efforts to extend education with a poem which wailed: 'Tis a terrible crisis for Cam and for Isis!/Fat butchers are learning dissection.' In addition, the university was bedevilled by financial problems, arguments among staff and static student numbers – not least because until it received a royal charter in 1836, it had no right to grant degrees.

A medical school to rival those in Edinburgh and the Continent was always central to the vision for this new university. To that end the university council assembled a faculty comprising some of the most forward-thinking and innovative medical men of the age. Since Oxford and Cambridge admitted only Anglicans, London University became the only institution in England where Catholics, Quakers, Jews and those of other faiths – or none – could study medicine. Initially students flocked to enrol for the classes in surgery, medicine, anatomy and midwifery. But there were two rather tricky problems: the inability to award degrees and the complete lack of a hospital. Determined to maintain their duopoly, Oxford and Cambridge lobbied the government to prevent London University conferring medical degrees. And although ambitious plans were laid to build a two-winged hospital with 230 beds, they remained a blueprint since there were no funds left for bricks and mortar. In the meantime a dispensary for outpatients opened in a poky terraced house in George Street, north Bloomsbury.

As student numbers fell and the financial problems worsened, the future of London University seemed precarious. Rows and rivalry blighted the faculties and the medical school was no exception. In an atmosphere of open warfare, two lecturers, Charles Bell, the Professor of Surgery, and John Conolly, the Professor of Medicine, resigned in early 1831. A third, Granville Sharp Pattison, Professor of Anatomy, was expelled after students protested at his incompetent teaching and cavalier manner; he came to classes wearing a hunting jacket and riding boots. The turbulence made St Thomas' seem like a tea party and by May few expected the university to survive. Nonetheless, Elliotson decided to throw himself into this maelstrom.

Elliotson was appointed Professor of the Theory and Practice of Medicine in May 1831, replacing Conolly, with the unanimous backing of the medical faculty.[52] Writing to Brougham – now Lord Brougham – to apply for the post, he detailed his research and qualifications and – 'what I esteem a real honour' – his membership of the council of the Society for the Diffusion of Useful Knowledge, the organisation Brougham had founded in order to bring scientific texts to working-class readers. (Elliotson could fawn and crouch when occasion required.) Commending Elliotson for the post in preference to some dozen others, David Davis, the Professor of Midwifery, declared: 'He has, indeed, already created for himself a reputation both as a physician and a teacher that extends to the most distant districts of the kingdom.' Elliotson would later say that London University was 'the only university in England founded upon principles which I approve'. Wakley, of course, was jubilant, applauding the university's choice in *The Lancet* and insisting that Elliotson 'is not surpassed by any physician in the metropolis'.

The next three years were fraught as Elliotson shuttled back and forth across London Bridge giving lectures three evenings a week in Bloomsbury as well as a clinical lecture every Saturday at St Thomas', attending patients at St Thomas', while also being 'almost overwhelmed with private practice'.[53] Yet there was never any question where his loyalties lay. In his introductory lecture at the university in October, Elliotson railed against the 'dark persecution' and 'secret insinuations' he had endured at St Thomas' while saluting the 'fresh and young' London University, which was 'unincumbered by monkish habits and antique fashions'.[54]

Bolstered by Elliotson's reputation and dedication, the medical school thrived. As he galvanised the professors into a rare show of unity, a fragile peace descended and the medical faculty became known as 'the school of all the talents'.[55] Student numbers soared, bringing much-needed funds. At the same time, Elliotson devoted much of his time, energy and money to establishing a hospital. There was a desperate need. The tiny George Street dispensary was wholly inadequate for the hordes of poor who flocked from the sprawling slums of Camden Town, Somers Town and St Pancras. The population of these mushrooming north London suburbs had almost doubled in the previous twenty years, to 340,000 – despite the infectious diseases, including the new scourge of cholera, that naturally kept the numbers down. John Hogg, the devoted resident apothecary at the dispensary, said that infant mortality among the poor was so high that to rear children at all 'was a task of difficulty, and is not infrequently impracticable'.[56]

Elliotson fervently agreed with the urgent need for a hospital – even if he was thinking more of his students' education than the local population's welfare. Establishing a hospital was 'imperiously necessary' to the medical school, and the dispensary 'a miserable substitute' for teaching the students, he said, but hastily added, 'to say nothing of the advantages of an hospital to the University, one is absolutely wanted in this situation'.[57] He tirelessly lobbied the university council to raise funds, donated money himself and rallied friends and family to the cause; Thomas,

Eliza and Emma all stumped up funds.[58] Led by Elliotson, the medical school professors donated their fees to the hospital fund, yet time still passed without a brick being laid.

With a mutiny of professors and students threatening, at last the council provided part of the university's own site, directly opposite its colonnaded façade in Gower Street, and a public appeal was launched to finance the building. Princess Victoria was among the first subscribers. The foundation stone was laid in 1832 for a modest, plain building with just 130 beds. Yet still the work stalled as funds faltered. Finally, exasperated by the delays, in July 1834 Elliotson – now Dean of the faculty – persuaded the council to raise a £2,000 loan to finish the hospital in time for the autumn term.[59] North London Hospital opened on 1 November 1834.

It had been a long wait. Ragged and filthy, ill-shod and barefoot, the inhabitants of north London flocked to the hospital's doors. Many of them were starving and destitute; all were poor and sick. Stooped men arrived with chronic coughs caused by industrial diseases made worse by the London smog. Painters and lead factory workers complained of nausea due to lead poisoning – or 'painter's colic' – while labourers digging tunnels for the new railways snaking out from Bloomsbury were carried in unconscious after accidents. Pale young women in service presented with headaches and nervous conditions due to the gruelling hours and a starvation diet. Women in their forties and fifties came to give birth for the tenth, twelfth and fourteenth time. And they brought their children too: listless, sunken-eyed infants laid low by fever and mewling, flame-cheeked babies too weak to suckle.

Climbing the steps to the front entrance, patients arrived in a narrow hall with corridors leading left and right to a ward on either side.[60] Continuing straight on, they reached a windowless 180-foot corridor running the entire length of the building. Double doors straight ahead concealed the operating theatre – conveniently next to the mortuary and the post-mortem room. Turning left led to the casualty room, the outpatients' waiting room and the dispensary where medicines were provided free of charge. Turning right led to an eye department, with its own surgery and outpatients' room, and an examination room for pregnant women. And hidden from public view, at the front corners of the building, sat a boardroom, where the medical committee met, and a lecture room, where the professors taught. There were four more wards on the first floor – making a total of six – providing less than a third of the beds available at St Thomas' or Guy's.

Yet for all its modest provision and simple functionality, the hospital represented a significant achievement, made plain by the agreement of the fifteen-year-old Princess Victoria, now first in line to the throne, to become its patron. It was the only hospital in England attached to a university, with all the talents of the faculty focused on curing the sick – at least until King's College caught up by annexing Charing Cross Hospital.

It had been a long wait for the professors and for the students too. Now he was finally embedded in a brand new hospital, Elliotson resigned from St Thomas'.[61] Throwing himself into his job, he badgered the council to change the new hospital's name to University College Hospital (UCH) in line with the university's own change to University College London (UCL). Such a title would not only be 'more respectable & academical' than that of North London – 'which reminds of the South London Waterworks' – but would 'show that it is in connection with, nay, a very part of, the School of University College'.[62] The name was duly changed in 1837. From its humble beginnings UCH would become one of the leading teaching hospitals and medical centres in the world.

More than any of his colleagues, Elliotson tirelessly championed UCL's medical school and worked unstintingly for UCH. Acutely aware of their mutual dependence, he viewed the twin institutions as his personal fiefdom and their success as a matter of personal pride. He was one of the most active members of the university senate, the body representing all the faculties' professors, and he frequently took the lead on medical matters. Never forgetting the importance of clinical observation, he awarded two gold medals annually to the students who presented the best patient case studies.[63]

Now in his early forties, Elliotson was at the height of his reputation. He commanded one of the biggest medical classes in London while his private practice was among the largest in the capital. He was 'one of the most popular teachers that ever existed', said one student. 'He was at the zenith of his fame, in the prime of life.'[64] His income now soaring, in 1832 Elliotson moved into an elegant house at 37 Conduit Street, just off Regent Street, in the most fashionable quarter of the West End.[65] Formerly the home of the late prime minister, George Canning, the house boasted a 'splendid suite of rooms' with a coach house and stables at the rear. It was staffed by half a dozen servants, including a butler, housekeeper and coachman.

In his new home, Elliotson played host to grand dinner parties, where guests ate from china decorated with his coat of arms, and musical soirees featuring the celebrated musicians of the day. A keen advocate of the arts, Elliotson was elected an honorary officer of the Royal Society of Musicians in 1833 and a few years later he would sit at the chief table with the Duchess of Richmond at the society's centenary festival.[66] Soon after joining UCL he invited the university secretary, Thomas Coates, to an impromptu recital, informing him, 'I expect some beautiful music at my house tomorrow evening, & probably some Italian improvisation.' Favoured students were also invited; one such was Edmond Sheppard Symes, a former pupil from St Thomas', now in his late twenties, who visited Elliotson's home most days and would remain his most devoted disciple. According to an effusive sketch in *The Lancet* in 1833, Elliotson was 'a very delightful fellow in general society who holds interesting Medical conversaziones, gives splendid musical parties which are attended by the best medical professors in London'.[67]

That same year, Elliotson was elected president of the Medical and Chirurgical Society, by now the most prestigious medical society in the land. Under his leadership, over the next two years the society not only moved into smart West End premises but gained a royal charter from William IV, becoming the forerunner of today's Royal Society of Medicine.[68] During the five months the society was effectively homeless, its council met in Elliotson's house and it was there that the seal was affixed to the royal charter.

Now that he was hobnobbing with high society, in March 1835 Elliotson was presented to William IV at a royal levee in St James's Palace and, five months later, he was invited to a summer ball hosted by the Duchess of Kent and her daughter, Princess Victoria.[69] Recording Elliotson among the guests in her diary, the sixteen-year-old princess danced five quadrilles and declared herself – contrary to the later stereotype – '*very* much amused'.

A portrait of Elliotson, painted during the 1830s by the artist James Ramsay, depicts a serious, handsome man, with curling black hair and thoughtful dark eyes, in the stiff, tall collar and tight, black stock of the period against the dark red background traditionally associated with physicians.[70] He seems lost in thought, perhaps contemplating a thorny medical issue or lamenting an unfortunate patient.

Yet for all his prestige he had lost none of his fiery temper or peevish vanity. Before leaving St Thomas', Elliotson had fallen out with his fellow lecturer Robert Williams after discovering that his views were 'diametrically opposite upon almost every single subject'.[71] Then in 1832 he quarrelled with the *London Medical Gazette*, a weekly journal launched by Abernethy and his cronies as a Tory alternative to *The Lancet*. From the start the *LMG* had attacked Wakley, denouncing him as a 'literary plunderer' for publishing lectures without permission, even as it aped *The Lancet*'s style and content. Since its backers hailed from the traditional medical schools, the journal treated UCL and its new hospital with unbridled disdain. At first Elliotson escaped this treatment. Taking its cue from *The Lancet*, the *LMG* reported Elliotson's clinical cases and, with his consent, published his lectures. But in 1832 the journal took exception to the professor's rapturous assertions of the superiority of UCL and leapt to the defence of the older medical schools.[72] Elliotson responded with characteristic speed and temper. He immediately withdrew consent for his lectures to be published and made the printers add a notice on the journal's wrapper stating that he was not answerable for its content. The spat gave the *LMG* the excuse it had been waiting for. Now it bracketed Elliotson with Wakley and treated him as fair game for an all-out assault. An editorial stormed, 'the truth is, the Doctor has long been the pet of *The Lancet*, and is as sensitive and easily offended as a spoilt child'. He had made a powerful enemy.

More sensationally, Elliotson became embroiled in a ridiculous row with a Frenchman, Francesco Moscati, who was a complete fantasist and outright fraud. Moscati claimed he was a marquis who had served under Napoleon but, being down on his luck, had resorted to teaching Italian and lecturing on science.[73] Having met Moscati in 1831, Elliotson paraded him at dinner parties and introduced him into London society. Spinning ludicrous tales of global adventures, which included crossing the desert on an elephant and visiting the Great Wall of China, Moscati hoodwinked dinner guests and fleeced them for funds. He pretended he worked for *The Times* while incidentally claiming to have two stomachs and a bullet lodged in his head. Gullibly sucked in, Elliotson successfully appealed to the writers' charity, the Royal Literary Fund, for a £20 grant to help his 'destitute' friend. As Moscati's lies ballooned out of control, the Frenchman even claimed he had written the notes to Elliotson's translation of Blumenbach. Furious at this outrage, Elliotson now accused Moscati of lying, exposed him to friends and denounced him to *The Times*; he even repaid the £20 donation to the Royal Literary Fund 'to make complete reparation for the loss which I innocently associated'. In revenge, in 1834, Moscati published a forty-page pamphlet viciously attacking Elliotson and the following year he sued *The Times* in a libel case, in which Elliotson was a prominent witness. He ended the year in debtors' prison.

Moscati was a pathetic imposter and a pathological liar yet some of his criticisms of Elliotson contained the ring of truth. Although Elliotson 'worked very hard', he was 'not very generous', Moscati wrote and added, 'every one who enters his house must think him *vain*, – that his arms are to be seen on every dish, and even on his wooden chairs'. Elliotson had 'called himself *my best, and most sincere friend*' and 'monopolised me as a Lion' for two years, said Moscati, before they quarrelled and he 'became *my bitterest enemy*'. The relationship with Moscati followed that old cycle of effusive friendship followed by disillusion leading to total enmity. Inevitably this same pattern would lead to trouble at UCL too.

Even if he had soured relations with the *LMG*, Elliotson felt secure in the continued patronage of *The Lancet*. But Wakley had changed: he was no longer the reckless young pugilist who had gambled everything on founding his journal. Now in his forties, a family man with three sons, Thomas, Henry and James, and a daughter, Elizabeth, all under the age of fourteen, he had bought a splendid house in Bloomsbury's Bedford Square where he played host to both radical activists and liberal-minded aristocrats. Fiercely proud of his children, he would encourage his sons to follow him into public life – two would later co-edit *The Lancet* and a third would go into law – though his wife, Elizabeth, would always remain in the background. Just as he grew in stature, so he was expanding in girth – a consequence of the lavish entertainments he threw which stretched family funds to breaking point. Yet even if his days in the ring were behind him, Wakley pursued his causes with as much vigour as ever.

True to his democratic principles, Wakley had campaigned tirelessly in support of the Reform Bill to increase representation for working people.[74] When the country was teetering on the brink of civil war between 1830 and 1832, Wakley chaired protest meetings, spoke at public demonstrations and had even founded a newspaper, *The Ballot*, which he edited for two years, in support of popular demands. When the bill became law in 1832, Wakley stood for parliament and on his third attempt, in February 1835, he was elected MP for Finsbury, a new constituency representing some 330,000 people across a swathe of north London. On the day he won his seat, Bedford Square was crammed with 10,000 supporters who cheered as he gave a victory speech from the balcony of his first-floor drawing room. The poor patients who thronged UCH were now his constituents – even if they were mostly still denied the vote.

Characteristically, Wakley's maiden speech in parliament called for a pardon for the six Dorset farm labourers, known as the Tolpuddle Martyrs, who had been transported to Australia for attempting to form a trade union in protest at wage cuts. Although his motion was lost, the point was made; the following year the men were pardoned and came home. Wakley would represent Finsbury for almost the rest of his life but he never attached himself to any party nor allied himself with any group; he was an independent through and through. In parliament he campaigned for wider electoral reform, greater workers' rights, the abolition of slavery, a free Ireland and, of course, medical reform.

As a radical MP and campaigning journalist, Wakley was more determined than ever to maintain the independence of his journal. He still admired Elliotson's talents and enjoyed his company, but unlike during the continual battles at St Thomas', he was less willing to take sides. A fervent supporter of UCL – he became a shareholder in 1837 – he tirelessly promoted its new hospital. In particular he was delighted that every junior position – the posts of house pupils, clinical clerks and dressers – was awarded to students entirely on merit, through a viva test called a 'concours', instead of the usual patronage system. But when the precarious peace within the medical school began to crumble, Wakley would have to decide where his loyalties lay.

Meanwhile Elliotson was growing increasingly frustrated at his impotence to stem the onslaught of ailments that overwhelmed the wards of UCH. He was testing new medicines in ever-increasing quantities, yet there was still no sign of a breakthrough. According to one contemporary, he would try 'every new remedy' initially with caution, but 'would occasionally carry his doses to such an extent that his pupils were astonished and alarmed'.[75] He still placed his faith in phrenology, yet for all its supposed revelations bump-reading had failed to yield any real benefits to medicine. Even so, Elliotson remained convinced that the mind held the key to many bodily ills. He was searching for a miracle cure, a medicine or therapy that could beat the conditions with which he battled every day. It would make his name, establish his reputation on an international stage, maybe even secure his place in history.

And then, in June 1837, hope arrived in the form of a diminutive Frenchman who introduced himself under the flamboyant title of Baron Jules Denis Dupotet de Sennevoy.

4

A New Power is Revealed to the World

Maddox Street, London, June 1837

Baron Dupotet was a short, compact man with a pale face, dark cropped hair, close-cut sideburns and large, compelling brown eyes.[1] The baron arrived in England on 5 June, rented a house in Maddox Street in London's West End and placed an advertisement in *The Times* announcing a series of daily lectures and demonstrations on 'Animal Magnetism'. Then he waited for the crowds to arrive. By July he was still waiting.

In France Dupotet had been celebrated and revered. Born in 1796 in Burgundy into an aristocratic family which lost its fortune in the Revolution, Dupotet had trained in medicine and established a successful practice in Paris. Before long, however, he had become interested in the doctrine of animal magnetism, or mesmerism, and after mastering the technique had set up a 'school of magnetism' which had attracted nearly 100 pupils. Now he was keen to try his luck – and no doubt make his fortune – in Britain. But the baron spoke not a word of English and was entirely unknown in London. Furthermore he soon encountered the widespread post-war prejudice of the British towards France and all things French. Only a handful of visitors straggled along to his rooms to watch his demonstrations. He would have had more success, he lamented, if he had brought with him a strange beast, such as an 'orang-outang', or taken to the stage to sing and dance.[2]

Undeterred, the baron wrote to every hospital in London, offering to demonstrate the marvels of his craft. He had one reply: from Herbert Mayo, senior surgeon at the Middlesex Hospital and Professor of Physiology and Pathological Anatomy at King's College London. An intelligent man and skilled anatomist, Mayo had made his name as a young physiologist by announcing some important discoveries about the facial nerves but his promising career had been marred by an ugly row with his former teacher, Charles Bell, erstwhile Professor of Surgery at UCL, who claimed – wrongly – that the discovery was his.[3] Now in his early forties, Mayo had twice been passed over for a post as Professor of Anatomy at UCL. This was no doubt snobbishness. Nicknamed 'the Owl' in *The Lancet* because he lectured with his eyes half-shut, Mayo spoke with a lisp and – what was worse – a cockney accent. As one member of the UCL selection committee put it, his intonation in lectures was 'peculiarly unpleasant'. Nonetheless, he was a respected member of the Royal Society as well as the Royal Medical and Chirurgical Society. Convinced the nervous system was responsible for many physical ailments, Mayo was keen to discover whether mesmerism might have therapeutic benefits.

When he arrived at the Middlesex Hospital, Dupotet was delighted to find Mayo had assembled a selection of patients as well as a crowd of medical men. It soon became clear, however, that the spectators were not taking him seriously. One jested that if the baron's technique failed to work on a patient he would find him a donkey instead, while others made no effort to hide their laughter. Much to Dupotet's chagrin it took several attempts before his methods took effect. Although Mayo was impressed – and would remain a fervent advocate of mesmerism all his life – interest in the baron's demonstrations at the Middlesex soon waned. Abandoned on a ward with only his interpreter for company, Dupotet left in humiliation. What he needed was a more progressive, open-minded patron with a solid reputation within London's scientific community. It was then that one of the Middlesex physicians, John Wilson, directed him to John Elliotson.

Elliotson was intrigued when he first heard reports of the baron's demonstrations but he approached the subject with due caution. He had been fooled once already by a charismatic Frenchman with a plausible patter, and he did not want to be subjected to such public humiliation again. Furthermore, he was no stranger to mesmerism. For he had already encountered the phenomenon eight years previously and was well aware of its controversial history.

Mesmerism was named after a German physician, Franz Anton Mesmer, who had studied medicine in Vienna and had established himself there as a respected practitioner during the second half of the eighteenth century.[4] Growing disillusioned with conventional therapies, Mesmer was keen to try new methods. Then in 1774, a Hungarian Jesuit priest with the memorable name of Father Maximilian Hell, who was Professor of Astronomy at Vienna, told Mesmer he had cured his own heartburn by applying steel magnets to his body. Mesmer was fascinated and immediately trialled the method on his own patients. Convinced that magnets could manipulate an invisible fluid, which he named 'animal magnetism', circulating within the human body – and through all animate and inanimate objects – Mesmer published his theory and soon attracted a queue of patients.

Mesmer's success was cut short three years later when he was forced to flee Vienna due to a scandal involving a celebrated eighteen-year-old pianist, Maria Theresia von Paradis, who had been blind since infancy. According to one story, Mesmer was denounced as a fraud for claiming to have cured the girl even though an eminent eye specialist insisted she was still blind. Another tale suggested the girl's parents had threatened to sue Mesmer because when he cured her blindness, she promptly lost her musical talent. Undaunted, Mesmer had taken to the road and travelled Europe, touting his new therapy as a cure for all ills. At first he used iron rods to direct the invisible force but before long he gave up the rods and used only his hands to touch and stroke his patients or simply make movements, known as 'passes', close to the face and body while looking intently into their eyes.

What Mesmer had stumbled upon was a method of inducing a sleep-like trance through repetitive motions and suggestion. He found that once they were lulled into this state, people would often respond slavishly to commands, act out wild behaviour and exhibit insensitivity to pain. Much later, of course, this effect would be named hypnotism; though mesmerism achieved its ends chiefly through repetitive hand movements, the outcome was essentially the same.

Mesmer was not the first to use hypnotic methods. The 'sleep temples' popular in Ancient Egypt and Greece, where people seeking a cure imbibed herbal concoctions before being led by priests intoning religious incantations through dimly lit passages, are thought to have worked through similar means. Other cultures around the world had developed their own ways of inducing sleep-like states in order to perform rituals and healing through repetitive touch, sounds, movements and scents.[5] Although opinions still differ on how hypnosis actually works, it is likely that the combination of sensory overload along with the subjects' expectations and the healers' suggestions could trigger a behavioural response; in the case of the sleep temples, the potent herbal cocktails probably helped as well. But Mesmer was the first, systematically and consciously, to harness the technique for medical purposes. It was through Mesmer and his belief in an invisible magnetic fluid that hypnotism as we know it today would eventually spread throughout the world.

Settling in Paris in 1778, Mesmer had attracted large numbers of followers as well as many detractors. People flocked to his salons where they would sit in a darkened room walled with mirrors while Mesmer, dressed in a long lilac robe embroidered with gold flowers, performed his curious hand movements to the accompaniment of a glass harmonica. In order to treat more people at once, he introduced a magnetic tub or 'baquet' – an oval bath packed with bottles filled with water and iron filings covered with an iron lid. The vessel was supposed to concentrate the magnetic force. His clients, many of them wealthy ladies, would sit around the tub with their knees touching to form a human circuit and grasp one of the iron rods that protruded at intervals from the lid. Then handsome young male assistants would sit behind the patients and clasp them between their knees while rubbing their spines and applying 'gentle pressure upon the breasts of the ladies'. It was scarcely surprisingly that, before long, 'the cheeks of the ladies began to glow, their imaginations to become inflamed; and off they went, one after the other, in convulsive fits'.[6] For those too poor to afford such thrills, Mesmer 'magnetised' certain trees so that peasants could touch the bark. Feted by fashionable Parisian society, not least Marie Antoinette, Mesmer amassed a fortune which was further enlarged as he sold his 'secret' to eager disciples for the sizeable sum of 100 Louis-d'or each. Eventually Mesmer's erotic exhibitions brought down the scorn of the French medical establishment who persuaded Louis XVI to set up a royal commission in 1784 to investigate the phenomenon.

The team of inquiry comprised some of the most eminent scientific thinkers of the age, including the chemist Antoine-Laurent Lavoisier, who had identified and isolated oxygen, the physician Joseph-Ignace Guillotin, who later proposed the instrument of capital punishment that would earn him a dubious fame, and the American polymath Benjamin Franklin who had escaped British persecution for exile in France.[7] Their inquiry concluded that there was no such thing as an invisible magnetic fluid flowing through the human body and insisted that any benefit people might perceive from Mesmer's methods was entirely due to the 'imagination'. Yet rather than seek to investigate this powerful effect further and exploit its use for the public good, the inquiry emphatically denounced Mesmer and all his works. Mesmer left Paris in disgrace and spent the next thirty years wandering Europe, treating patients and teaching his techniques until his death in 1815.

Mesmerism, as it came to be called, had enjoyed a brief spell of popularity in Britain in the late 1780s, promoted by some of Mesmer's pupils, but was soon tainted by the unfolding terror of the French Revolution and the ensuing Napoleonic Wars. On the Continent, however, the doctrine spread through France, Switzerland, Germany, Holland and Scandinavia as Mesmer's growing band of devotees developed their individual schools of practice. Particularly influential was Armand-Marie-Jacques de Chastenet, Marquis de Puységur, who discovered he could use mesmeric passes to induce a state akin to sleepwalking in which the subject could walk and talk as well as perform more unusual acts. He named this state 'magnetic sleep' or 'mesmeric somnambulism'.[8] Another disciple, the Abbé José Custódio de Faria, a Catholic priest born in Portuguese-governed Goa, was the first to argue that mesmerism worked through suggestion. By the 1820s mesmerism was once again attracting large numbers of enthusiasts across Continental Europe while also drawing serious interest from the medical profession.

In 1826, the French Royal Academy of Medicine launched a new inquiry into the phenomenon.[9] As before, the investigating committee included some of the most respected scientists of the era. Over the next five years the panel witnessed an exhaustive series of demonstrations by practitioners who had learned their techniques from Mesmer or his pupils. Prominent among them was Baron Dupotet, who not only demonstrated his skills on patients but even mesmerised one of the committee members, a physician named Jean Itard, who had suffered rheumatism for eight years. Put to sleep in seven minutes, Itard awoke to declare that his pain had entirely disappeared. As the committee was quick to point out, Itard was a 'man of reason' and therefore could not possibly have imagined his response.

Finally, in 1831, the committee concluded that mesmerism was a genuine phenomenon which worked through the use of repeated hand movements and 'fixed looks' on people of all ages and both sexes, though not on everyone. The inquiry even substantiated reports that a sixty-four-year-old woman, one Madame Plantin, had undergone an operation on 12 April 1829 to remove her cancerous right breast in the Hôtel-Dieu hospital in Paris while in a mesmeric sleep.[10] Throughout the operation the woman had conversed calmly with her surgeon and had remained asleep for forty-eight hours. Even more remarkably, the patient's daughter was mesmerised and had predicted that her mother would die sixteen days after the operation, as indeed she did – no doubt from a post-operative infection. However, the inquiry was unconvinced by the wilder assertions of some mesmerists, including Dupotet, who claimed that when mesmerised, certain people could predict the future, diagnose their own and other patients' ailments, read with their finger-tips and speak languages they had never learned.

Despite this feverish excitement on mainland Europe, mesmerism still prompted scant interest in Britain. Revelling in its recent military victory over France while remaining wary of anything that smacked of French radicalism, Britain responded to the latest news on mesmerism with a giant yawn. A few enthusiasts ventured across the Channel in an effort to spread the word to the British public but they were greeted either with suspicion or indifference. A handful of home-grown entrepreneurs set up as mesmerists in Britain, but their activities went largely unnoticed.[11] And some British intellectuals even tried the Continental craze for themselves. The poet Percy Bysshe Shelley was mesmerised several times in an effort to quell the pain from his kidney stones and wrote a poem inspired by his experience which began: 'Sleep on! sleep on! Forget thy pain,/My hand is on thy brow.'[12] But by and large the British populace did sleep on regardless.

Dismayed by this general apathy, a Scottish lawyer, John Campbell Colquhoun, who had encountered mesmerism while studying in Germany, published an English translation of the French inquiry report in 1833.[13] He concluded that the evidence in favour of mesmerism was 'almost irresistible' and urged the British medical profession to investigate. The methods mesmerists used, he argued, were far safer than many of the toxic drugs generally prescribed by orthodox doctors, and were probably just as effective. Colquhoun's appeal met with a deafening silence.

With his extensive reading of foreign medical journals and annual trips to Continental Europe, Elliotson had inevitably become familiar with the idea of mesmerism during the 1820s. In Germany he had seen lectures advertised in university medical schools and he had also come across a clinic devoted to mesmeric treatment in Berlin.[14] One eminent German physician, Arnold Wienholt, practising in Bremen, had been converted to mesmerism after his own six-year-old child had been apparently cured of a stomach complaint. In France, Elliotson knew, the revered naturalist Georges Cuvier had become convinced that mesmerism was 'real and independent of all imagination', while the mathematician and astronomer Pierre-Simon Laplace refused to dismiss the phenomenon. Yet without seeing sound scientific evidence for himself Elliotson had remained sceptical. Then, in early 1829, while he was still working at St Thomas', he had encountered an Irish chemist named Richard Chenevix, who had studied mesmerism in France and was keen to stage some demonstrations in London. Eager to see whether mesmerism might offer any benefits for medicine, Elliotson had been one of the first in line.

Elliotson had first watched Chenevix send to sleep two sisters, aged sixteen and nineteen, but since the girls had been mesmerised by Chenevix previously he was not convinced the effects were genuine. So he had invited Chenevix to St Thomas' and selected some female patients for a more neutral test.[15] This time, when Chenevix waved his hands in front of a girl being treated for epilepsy she had lapsed into a seizure, which he attempted, in vain, to end. Another woman with epilepsy appeared to fall asleep but denied she had been sleeping. A further six women felt no effect whatsoever, apart from one who professed a slight heaviness of the head. Elliotson was rapidly becoming disillusioned. But when Chenevix tried his skills on a ninth patient the effects were startling.

'She was an ignorant Irish girl, and unprepared to expect any thing,' Elliotson wrote. Yet within a minute of Chenevix starting his hand movements she felt faint, begged him to stop and began to exhibit some remarkable reactions. When Chenevix told her to raise her arm, she was powerless to do so until he 'unlocked' it with a wave of his hand. A waft of Chenevix's hand brought on a pain in her chest and another relieved it; a simple movement produced a pain in her abdomen and another banished it.

Determined to test the experiment to its limits, Elliotson had instructed Chenevix – in French so the patient would not understand – which part of the girl should be rendered powerless and which should be restored. Every order was performed exactly as he requested and the girl responded perfectly. 'Deception was impossible,' Elliotson said. 'Mr C. looked round at me, and asked, in French, if I was satisfied. I really felt ashamed to say no; and yet I could scarcely credit my senses enough to say yes. I remained silent.' With Elliotson rendered uncharacteristically speechless, Chenevix continued to inflict and relieve pain on the poor Irish girl until finally Elliotson admitted he was convinced. 'From this time I was satisfied that such a power as mesmerism exists, and hoped some day to inquire into it,' Elliotson said.

Chenevix performed demonstrations at several London hospitals during 1829 before prominent figures including Benjamin Brodie, then surgeon to George IV, Michael Faraday, director of the laboratory of the Royal Institution, and Elliotson's chum, the chemist William Prout. Later Chenevix published details of his experiments in the *London Medical and Physical Journal* with an addendum by Elliotson attesting to what he had witnessed.[16] Yet while Elliotson was never afraid to put his name to an unorthodox idea, many of his associates were less happy to risk their reputations on some mystical French import. Elliotson later said that both Brodie and Prout had declared themselves convinced by Chenevix's demonstrations but had been too 'proud and obstinate' to admit their belief.[17] Faraday, meanwhile, said 'he saw nothing which a paid actor could not play', although at least he agreed that the phenomenon warranted further investigation.

The medical press responded with equal disdain. When the *LMPJ* published Chenevix's account, its editors added: 'For our own parts, we candidly confess we are yet to be converted.'[18] Despite Elliotson's endorsement, *The Lancet* too was scathing. Wakley derided Chenevix as a quack and his ideas as 'a wretched and disgraceful piece of deception'. He added, 'we suppose that, like a dog with a tin kettle ... Mr C. will drag this "mesmerism" about, till one of the two, Mr C. or the subject ... gives up the ghost'.

That prediction came true sooner even than Wakley could have anticipated. Returning to Paris defeated, Chenevix died the following year and mesmerism in Britain quickly faded back into the obscurity in which it had previously languished. Yet Elliotson remained intrigued by the idea and was determined one day to investigate it further. That opportunity now arose with the arrival of Baron Dupotet in June 1837.

That same month, on 20 June, William IV died and his niece Victoria, who had just turned eighteen, ascended the British throne. The country was desperate for change. Sickened by the decadent lives of George IV and his brother William IV, with their openly paraded mistresses and large illegitimate families, and exhausted by decades of political turmoil and economic strife, the British people were looking to a new era. They embraced the demure young Queen Victoria as the symbol of a more sober, sensible, stable new age. Elliotson too was eager for change. The medical theories and practices of the past were not working. Perhaps the answer lay with Baron Dupotet.

Elliotson did not immediately embrace the baron with his usual enthusiasm for all things Gallic. There was too much at stake. It was six years since he had been appointed professor at UCL and physician to UCH and he was as popular within the university as he was admired at the hospital. He was now a more mature, cautious man than the young hothead who had locked horns with the authorities at St Thomas'. Admittedly, he was no less enthusiastic about phrenology – but so were half the medical men in London. In May Elliotson had been among a party of doctors who had watched as the cast was taken of the head of a notorious murderer, James Greenacre, immediately after he had been hanged for killing his fiancée. Giving his earnest opinion in *The Lancet*, Elliotson declared: 'Greenacre's head is so truly horrid, that I can believe every thing which has been asserted of him.'[19] It was not just human heads that interested him either. In June the British naturalist George Tradescant Lay, a missionary to China, sent him the head of a tapir from Malaysia; Elliotson donated the skull to the UCL museum.[20]

That same month Elliotson's beloved mother died, a year after his father, and he was therefore now the head of his little family with responsibility for Thomas, now working as a physician in Clapham, and his unmarried sisters Emma and Eliza, who lived in the family home nearby.[21] It was with guarded circumspection, therefore, that he invited

Dupotet to UCH on 4 July and introduced him to a twenty-four-year-old patient named Thomas Orton.

Orton was a carefree young man who enjoyed a few drinks and whatever they might lead to; he had twice been treated for syphilis in the past two years.[22] But his happy-go-lucky lifestyle had suffered a devastating blow the previous summer when he had suddenly felt a sharp pain in his head and numbness in his left arm. The next moment he had collapsed to the floor, foaming at the mouth and twitching. Orton had suffered an epileptic seizure. Worried about losing his job as a stable groom, he had ignored the attack, but ten days later another ensued. Forced to give up his job, he had sought medical help in the shape of Thomas Elliotson at his Clapham practice. The younger Elliotson had treated Orton in the customary manner – by bleeding him profusely and dosing him with toxic potions. To his bafflement these remedies had no effect and Orton suffered increasingly frequent seizures. At a loss for ideas, Thomas then sought his brother John's advice and Orton was duly admitted to UCH in December 1836. But John Elliotson had had no more success than his brother. After six months in UCH, being dosed with every caustic concoction Elliotson could throw down his throat, Orton still showed no signs of improvement – until he was presented to Baron Dupotet on 4 July.

That afternoon the students gathered on one of the male wards as their professor sat Orton in a chair and introduced Dupotet. The baron spoke no English, of course, but he didn't need to. He immediately fixed the groom with an unblinking stare and extended his hands towards his head.[23] As the bemused students watched, Dupotet moved his hands slowly up and down in front of Orton's face. Some thought the fact that Dupotet was missing a thumb on his right hand was a critical factor; others attributed his influence to his penetrating dark eyes. Whatever the secret, within ten minutes Orton's head had drooped and he seemed to be fast asleep. After allowing Orton to slumber for several minutes the baron began moving his hands in a horizontal direction in front of his face and the patient suddenly awoke.

From 4 July onwards Dupotet mesmerised Orton into a trance on an almost daily basis. On each occasion he was 'charmed to sleep', as the ward casebooks put it, in a shorter time. Gradually Orton's seizures diminished and he was discharged three months later, apparently cured. Orton was the first patient to be mesmerised at UCH but many more would follow.

Encouraged by the baron's success with Orton, Elliotson selected three more patients for him to mesmerise.[24] All three were female and all were suffering from so-called 'nervous' complaints; two had been diagnosed with epilepsy, like Orton, and the third was said to be suffering from occasional 'fits' and 'hysteria' – a catch-all diagnosis for unexplained or inconvenient complaints in women.[25] Having treated each of them for several months with every medicine in his armoury, Elliotson had 'despaired' of any improvement. When the patients were introduced to the baron, however, the results were astounding.

Like Orton, the three female patients all fell into a trance and then exhibited a range of strange responses. 'Their breathing became heavy; and sometimes they changed from waking to sleeping in an instant,' recorded Elliotson. 'When they were asleep, the head nodded or fell in one direction or another, the arms fell, they breathed loud or even snored.' In this enchanted state, their arms, legs and fingers twitched. At times the girl with hysteria would roll her eyes from side to side and smack her lips. At other times she was unable to open her eyes at all until the baron made the requisite passes before her face. 'If we raised her eyelids, they instantly fell,' said a bewildered Elliotson. 'We begged her to open them; but, till the fingers of him who had mesmerised her made transverse movements, they remained closed, however long we waited.'

Elliotson was fascinated by these results. In the long tradition of medical men offering themselves up as experimental subjects, he now submitted to being mesmerised by the baron, along with several students and some male visitors. Although the effects were not as spectacular as with the patients, almost all the men confessed to feeling a tingling or twitching in their limbs and face combined with a heaviness in the chest and drowsiness. A few even felt as if they were 'under some strange influence', said Elliotson, yet none fell into the deep slumber produced in his patients. 'I was mesmerised frequently,' he wrote, 'and always but once with the effect of tingling and twitchings only.' He was quick to dismiss the idea that the men were influenced by what they expected to happen and therefore resisted any effect. Some had already witnessed patients being entranced and were convinced mesmerism worked yet 'none could be sent to sleep', although 'many, who sat down laughing at the whole as nonsense, honestly confessed they were affected by some influence'. Elliotson even went so far as to have his pet parrot mesmerised; after a few strokes on its back it fell obediently asleep on its perch.[26]

Throughout July and August Elliotson encouraged Dupotet to test mesmerism on more patients at UCH and also asked the baron to teach his methods. Elliotson's clinical clerk, a devoted student named William Wood, meticulously recorded their reactions in the casebooks. At first Elliotson limited mesmerism to a handful of patients, most of them young women and girls. Indeed, he would always favour female patients as subjects despite the fact that the first demonstration had been successfully performed on a man. Having noted the milder responses of himself and his male associates, Elliotson leapt to the conclusion that mesmerism was more effective on the female sex – and presumably parrots – and especially on poor young women of little education with 'nervous' conditions. The same tendency had been remarked in Mesmer's demonstrations and by the French investigating committee of 1831. This belief chimed perfectly with the dominant nineteenth-century view that women were the weaker, more sensitive sex and were therefore more susceptible to external influences. In reality, the tendency, if indeed there was any, was more likely due to the huge power imbalance between the wealthy, self-assured professor and his poor, uneducated female patients than any intrinsic gender difference.[27]

Treading carefully for the moment, Elliotson continued to treat the majority of his patients with the usual large doses of the metallic-based medicines he favoured, along with electricity and acupuncture – at least when patients allowed it; one woman with rheumatism discharged herself in July after refusing to submit to any further needles. Yet the effects of mesmerism were so striking that soon Elliotson was completely converted.

Although mesmerism had no effect on some patients, others seemed to recover from previously incurable ailments after only a few days or weeks. The 'hysterical' girl in the first batch of patients, an eighteen-year-old nursery maid named Caroline Shea, was discharged just a month after admission apparently cured.[28] The epileptic seizures suffered by one of the other female patients became less frequent.

Elliotson had no idea how mesmerism might work. But then, as he pertinently observed, he had no explanation either for the way infectious diseases spread, or how traits such as blue eyes were passed from a father to his offspring.[29] In time, he trusted, scientific research would unravel all these enigmas – as indeed it would. He thought, however, that there was nothing intrinsically surprising about people falling asleep and exhibiting strange behaviour in certain circumstances. Such responses were no different to the reactions he had seen in patients suffering epileptic seizures or mental derangement, nor were they dissimilar to sleepwalking. He speculated that the custom in some cultures of massaging children to help them sleep was really a form of mesmerism and even the religious act of laying on hands in blessing might work by a similar action.

Viewed from a modern perspective, it is possible to speculate that the apparently miraculous cures Elliotson was witnessing were really due to the influence exerted on his patients' minds. The combination of suggestion, expectation and relaxation caused by the baron's hypnotic hand movements and comments may well have benefited those with so-called 'nervous' conditions. Although true epilepsy does not have a psychological cause, it is possible that the 'seizures' described were due to a different condition with a psychological root. In addition to these 'miracle' cures, some patients exhibited other remarkable traits under mesmerism, such as insensitivity to pain.

Elliotson first noted this response in Shea, the nursery maid, who entered such a profound sleep under mesmerism that if she was pinched or pricked with pins she showed no reaction whatsoever.[30] Another patient, who was brought into UCH by one of the students, exhibited an even more dramatic insensibility to pain. Lucy Clarke, who was eighteen, was being treated privately for epilepsy by a doctor with whom the student, George Denton, lodged. After watching the baron's demonstrations at UCH, Denton had rushed home to try the new method on his landlord's patient. He found Lucy so susceptible to mesmerism that from that day onwards he brought her to the hospital three times a week to show her off to others. At these demonstrations, the obliging Lucy was rapidly sent to sleep by Dupotet. 'From this moment, we could do what we pleased without waking her, – halloo in her ears, dash her arms in any direction, pull her hair out, pinch her hand, put snuff up her nose,' said Elliotson. No matter what tortures the professor and his students dreamt up, the girl remained 'perfectly insensible' until the baron woke her with 'two or three transverse movements'.

Elliotson was quick to appreciate the extraordinary potential of this response. He was well aware of the reports from France describing the operation on Mme Plantin in 1829. Now he believed that mesmerism could be harnessed to perform operations without pain in Britain too. By September 1837 – a full nine years before the arrival of chemical anaesthesia – Elliotson was arguing that 'the perfect coma' he had seen induced in some of his patients could prove 'an inestimable blessing in the case of a surgical operation, which I am positive might have been performed without the slightest sensation on some of the female patients, exactly as took place at the Hotel-Dieu'.[31]

There was one patient, however, who seemed even more responsive to mesmerism than any other, and she exhibited the most profoundly strange behaviour under its influence. Her name was Elizabeth Okey. Elizabeth had been admitted to ward three of UCH earlier in 1837, on 4 April, suffering from frequent epileptic seizures and headaches. The casebooks describe her on admission as a sixteen-year-old housemaid of 'diminutive conformation' and note that her headaches began after a fall when she was twelve.[32] She was so slight she seemed almost childlike – she had only started menstruating in June, according to the casebooks, which routinely noted such details – but she was universally described as beguilingly pretty. She had a 'fair complexion' and was 'eminently handsome', wrote one rapt observer who watched the baron's demonstrations that summer.[33] He noted with approval her 'downcast eyes' and red hands – 'vouchers for honest labour' – and conjectured, somewhat romantically, that she was 'neither servant-girl nor sempstress, but the daughter of an artisan or small tradesman, who scrubbed her father's stairs, washed his linen and did the rest of the hard work of the house'. One of the students was equally smitten. He described her 'full dark eyes and long black lashes' whose 'jetty fringe' – lashes as black as jet – swept her cheeks. Because of the length of her eyelashes it was sometimes hard to tell, he noted, whether she was awake or asleep. All who met her were plainly bewitched. Even the professor was not unmoved. Although he passed over her physical attributes, he was impressed by her sharp intelligence and demure comportment.

At the time Elizabeth was first admitted her younger sister, Jane, who was fourteen, was already a patient at UCH, also being treated for epilepsy, although she was discharged again by June.[34] The casebooks record their surname as 'O'Key' and the newspapers, who soon took a fervent interest in the 'patient-sisters', repeated this error so that the girls would be routinely and lastingly characterised as poor, ignorant Irish girls and subjected to all the prejudice and bigotry that brought with it. At a time of widespread hardship, the Irish were widely despised for taking jobs the native English thought were theirs by right. Yet, the Okeys were not Irish at all, of course, but came from a long-established English family – the name Okey derives from the quintessentially English oak tree.

Elizabeth was the second eldest in a family of nine children – they would eventually number eleven – who lived in a ramshackle tenement building in the burgeoning district of Somers Town.[35] She was born on 9 December 1820 and baptised Elizabeth Arter (the curious middle name belonged to an uncle). Her father, George Talbot Okey, came from a long line of Okeys who had settled in London, while her mother, born Jane Mundell, hailed from the Isle of Wight. They were not desperately poor – George's father had been a writing tutor, while his wife, Jane, was described as 'respectable' though 'very uneducated' – but neither were they comfortably off. At the time of Elizabeth's birth the family had been living in Euston Crescent, a fine row of tall white stuccoed houses with iron railings and balconies just north of the New Road (now Euston Road), although the likelihood is they occupied a damp basement or cramped garret. Her sister Jane was born two years later, but by then the family had moved to less salubrious lodgings. Their father, George, had trained as a goldsmith, having been apprenticed as a youth by the City of London charity the Bridewell Hospital to a well-known gold- and silversmith, William Frisbee, who made silverware for the royal family. George made a living as a 'chaser', someone who crafted gold and silver chains. But the family had grown rapidly, work was in short supply and finances were strained by rising food prices so that by the time Elizabeth reached her teens she had to work as a housemaid to supplement the family's meagre income. So although she was indeed 'the daughter of an artisan', she had subsequently been reduced to a plain 'servant-girl'.

At the mercy of their fluctuating fortunes, the family had shifted from one rented lodging to another in the districts of Somers Town, St Pancras and Camden Town. Once quiet country villages beyond London's northern fringe, these were now overcrowded suburbs housing thousands of poor British labourers who lived cheek-by-jowl with foreign refugees in cheap boarding-houses and crumbling tenements surrounded by brickfields and dustheaps. The young Charles Dickens had lived with his family in lodgings in Somers Town after his father was released from the Marshalsea prison in the 1820s; he then walked two miles to and from his job in a boot-blacking factory in Covent

Garden every day.[36] By 1837 the Okey family was living in Denton's Buildings, a cheap rental block off Brill Row near St Pancras Road. The area of narrow, criss-crossing streets, filled with costermongers' barrows and stalls, was famous for the Brill Tavern, where hawkers gathered on Sunday mornings to sell cheap fish, meat and clothes. One contemporary described the district as 'dingy with smoke and deprived almost entirely of gardens and fields', while another said the courts and alleys were 'in a sad state of filth and dirt'.[37]

The Okey family's financial constraints were plainly not helped by the medical problems of the two eldest daughters. According to Uncle Arter, one Arter Frederick Randall, who ran a bookshop in Hampshire, both girls had suffered epileptic seizures for several years, which caused 'a great expense' to their parents.[38] Indeed, the two girls had spent much of their childhood living under Uncle Arter's roof, no doubt to give their exhausted parents a break, so that they regarded their 'uncle-papa' with a great deal of affection. The girls' parents were 'pious', according to Uncle Arter, although they had left the Church of England around 1830, since the next four children were baptised in a non-Conformist church.[39] And although one student at UCH later described Elizabeth as 'illiterate', both girls had evidently learned to read and write; they were frequently described as being clever, good-natured and hard-working. In Elliotson's opinion, Elizabeth was 'very intelligent' and 'of excellent behaviour'. According to another student, she possessed 'extraordinary cleverness and shrewdness'.[40] The Okeys were, in essence, the Victorian model of a decent, law-abiding, hard-working family.

Elizabeth's increasingly regular seizures must have made it difficult for her to maintain her position as a housemaid. Not long before her admission to UCH, her parents had taken her to see a local physician, Dr Theophilus Thompson, who specialised in 'nervous diseases' and who worked at the Northern Dispensary, a tiny clinic in Somers Place on the northern side of the New Road. A thoughtful and compassionate physician, Thompson had studied medicine at Edinburgh, like Elliotson, but lacking Elliotson's connections, he had never secured a hospital post.[41] Initially Elizabeth was brought to see him for 'phrenitis', inflammation of the brain or delirium, but this soon developed into epilepsy. It was Thompson who referred Elizabeth to Elliotson at UCH, where her sister was already being treated. A prolonged stay in hospital, with three meals provided daily, must have come as a boon to the girls as much as to their parents. The respite from her domestic service was no doubt welcome to Elizabeth too, not to mention the release from family chores; another baby brother was born in July. But there is also no doubt that her condition was painful, distressing and debilitating.

At the time of her admission, Elizabeth was suffering from seizures at least once a week. When these came on, she suddenly lost consciousness, her limbs became rigid then started to jerk uncontrollably, her face became contorted and her eyes rolled. Afterwards she experienced a throbbing headache, which often lasted several hours; indeed she was scarcely ever free of pain in her head. Her symptoms mirrored the classic pattern of what would now be termed a tonic clonic seizure, previously known as a 'grand mal'. Such seizures often begin in childhood and are sometimes triggered by a head injury or inflammation of the brain, such as meningitis, or may have no obvious cause. As with all forms of epilepsy, these seizures are now known to be caused by a disturbance in the electrical activity of the brain. Knowledge, however, was in short supply when it came to understanding epilepsy in the 1830s.

Surrounded by superstition and myth, epilepsy – derived from the Greek word meaning to 'seize' or 'possess' – has baffled and fascinated observers since earliest times.[42] People suffering epileptic seizures were often thought to be possessed by divine or, more often, evil spirits, and were frequently shunned or abused. In ancient Mesopotamia, epileptics were banned from marriage, while the Romans spat on anyone they saw having a seizure. Yet as long ago as 400 BC, disciples of the Greek physician Hippocrates argued that epilepsy was neither sacred nor evil but caused by a malfunction in the brain and should therefore be treated not by magic but through diet and drugs. Taking this sage advice to heart, later physicians prescribed a variety of medicinal concoctions including powdered human skull, burnt human bones, vulture's blood and mistletoe. By the early nineteenth century, these macabre remedies had given way to the more general – yet equally useless – therapies of bleeding, blistering and enemas. It would be 1857 before the first effective treatment was discovered – potassium bromide – although even at the end of the nineteenth century some patients were still being castrated or subjected to clitoridectomy in the belief that sexual excess was to blame.

Elliotson had taken an interest in epilepsy since his early days as a physician at St Thomas'. Lecturing on the topic, he vividly described the different kinds of seizures, explaining that they were caused by a problem in part of the brain and correctly asserting that when they began in childhood they often resolved of their own accord.[43] He accurately reasoned that epilepsy was probably hereditary in some cases and was well aware that seizures often began after a blow to the head or brain fever. Yet he had no more solution to the problem than the ancient Greeks or Romans, resorting by default to his favourite metallic-based compounds and copious bleeding. Ruefully he confessed: 'Of all diseases it is one of the most intractable to treat. We may alleviate – not cure.'

At first, when Elizabeth was admitted in April, Elliotson exposed her to his usual battery of remedies. She was bled repeatedly by the lancet and with leeches, cupped, blistered and administered a large daily dose of silver nitrate, copper sulphate and ammoniated copper, supplemented by creosote to quell the nausea caused by the first two drugs.[44] She often had as much as ten ounces of blood (roughly half a pint or 284 ml) removed at a time and this was repeated every two or three days. It is hardly surprising that she was often described as pale and tired nor that her seizures were now accompanied with nausea and delirium when she was 'wandering and confused'.

Then, on 4 August, Elizabeth was 'magnetised' for the first time by Baron Dupotet. The effects were both immediate and astonishing. After a few minutes her ravings ceased and she fell into a peaceful sleep. When she was brought out of her trance a few minutes later she seemed perfectly recovered from her mania until at length she relapsed again and had to be mesmerised anew. As Elizabeth was mesmerised on an almost daily basis – and sometimes twice a day – by the baron or one of the ward clerks, her seizures disappeared. From 4 August she suffered no further attacks, apart from two lapses in October, although she continued to be delirious in between the bouts of mesmerism. Yet this seemingly remarkable recovery was almost completely eclipsed by the other bizarre traits that Elizabeth now began to exhibit.

In common with most of the patients at UCH who were subjected to mesmerism, at first Elizabeth simply dropped into a trance. But after a few weeks, a strange transformation came over her. One day, while in her entranced state, she suddenly opened her eyes and began to chatter, sing, dance and perform a host of other entertaining antics. As Elliotson and his astonished students turned to watch, Elizabeth regaled them with animated stories, mimicked the conversations of fellow patients, copied the baron's elaborate flourishes, whistled comic tunes and sang with professional aplomb.[45] She was seemingly both asleep and awake at the same time or 'sleep-waking' as Elliotson termed it. 'All at once she would become perfectly insensible, but her eyes would remain wide open, but perfectly insensible to the effect of light: pulling her hair produced no impression on her,' he recorded. 'Her sense of hearing was lost to all ordinary sound. Though her eyes were open yet she was perfectly blind; when you dashed the fingers suddenly towards her eyes there was no winking.'

In this state, Elizabeth would sometimes fly into a rage and remonstrate at being mesmerised or swear at the shocked spectators; then, just as suddenly, she would begin to entertain them with witty ribaldry or amorous remarks. When she was returned to her normal state she had no recollection of any of this behaviour. 'She would become suddenly still, look wild for an instant, rub her eyes, be sensible of everything around her, and resume her natural character, which was that of a quiet, modest girl,' said Elliotson.

Everyone who came to view Elizabeth agreed that this strange behaviour was completely at odds with her usual meek demeanour. 'This girl, when in her natural state, has great intelligence and sound sense,' said one observer, 'her temper is of remarkable sweetness, her disposition singularly affectionate, and her countenance is characterised by a corresponding expression.'[46] Indeed, when she was informed of her behaviour while in a mesmeric trance, Elizabeth was always ashamed and humbly begged her spectators' pardon. At the same time, her delirium diminished so that she would seem quite well for days at a time and when she did lapse back she was quickly recovered through mesmerism.

Elliotson was enthralled. At last he was witnessing some of the wilder manifestations the baron had predicted. To watch Elizabeth 'talking incoherently, now whistling aloud, now singing in the ward, cross, miserable, rude, dancing about' and then two or three seconds later see her 'completely herself, smiling, perfectly rational, amiable, well behaved, with an expression of great intelligence, was one of the most extraordinary changes I ever witnessed,' he wrote. This ability of the brain to switch so completely from utter derangement to complete sanity 'made an impression upon me never to be effaced'.

Eager to share news of these developments, Elliotson invited some medical friends and selected guests to a demonstration at UCH on 17 August. More than twenty doctors, students and visitors crowded into ward three to watch the baron perform. One of the spectators, a seasoned traveller named Lieutenant-Colonel Thomas Perronet Thompson, who had previously dismissed snake charming in India and magic tricks in Egypt with a shrug, was determined to remain a sceptic.[47] A veteran of several naval and army campaigns, Thompson had been captured by the Spanish in South America, fought the French in the Peninsular War and tackled Arab pirates off the coast of Bombay. When Dupotet made no impression on the first patient, a twenty-year-old woman with epilepsy, Thompson's cynicism was confirmed. Then Elizabeth sat down. She wore a dress with *gigot* or 'leg-of-mutton' sleeves – the elaborately puffed-up sleeves which were the height of fashion – and a shawl with which she played nervously, he recalled. The comely effect was rather marred, however, by a seton – a thread of silk or horsehair – which had been inserted into the back of her neck. Another common medical torture favoured by doctors of the period, this was meant to maintain a weeping wound. From the excitement Elizabeth drew from the assembled crowd, Thompson discerned she was 'the patient *par excellence*, the *prima donna* of the "magnetic" stage'.

The baron now made a few 'passes' with his hands and Elizabeth's eyes obediently closed. Asked by one of the guests to open them, she declared she could not. Yet when the baron rubbed her eye sockets with his thumbs her eyelids sprang open. Attempting to rise from her seat, she gave a deep breath 'between a sigh and a sob' then slumped over the arm of the chair 'as if dead'. At this point she was laid out on the floor, motionless, with all the appearance 'of a recent corpse'. The guests now took turns to pinch her hands, 'each harder than his predecessor', and force snuff up her nose 'at an unmerciful rate' while Elizabeth slept soundly like a fairy tale princess surrounded by a bevy of sadistic suitors. Shaking her and shouting in her ear produced no response either until suddenly she jumped into life with the exclamation: 'I won't be turned out, as I was before, for the servants to laugh at.' Now she was in full spate. 'There was a man went mad, and he jumped out of bed without his clothes and ran into the street,' she declared. Another shake produced: 'I thought how droll it would have been, if he had run into a meeting of old quakers.' In between these ribald comments, she berated the clerk, cuffed an impertinent questioner, and described the hospital apothecary as 'an old gallipot-scraper'.

By the end of this exhibition the cynical scorner of Indian snake charming and Egyptian necromancy was convinced mesmerism was genuine. 'I entirely gave up the idea of collusion on the part of the patient,' Thompson wrote in a long letter to *The Lancet*, which he coyly signed 'T'. 'She was much too pretty and light-hearted to be the instrument of a cold-blooded and painful fraud.' He added: 'To say no more of the pinching and the snuff, it would have required a long drilling to teach a girl the symptoms to be counterfeited.' Astutely, Thompson suggested that the baron's hand-waving triggered a response in the brain similar to the dizziness produced by looking at running water. He appealed for the medical community to investigate the phenomenon and determine its true cause rather than be swayed by any supernatural explanation. This, of course, was exactly what Elliotson intended to do.

As news of the surprising scenes unfolding at UCH spread through London medical circles, and beyond, Elliotson was bombarded with requests to witness the mesmeric performances. Happy to accommodate them all, he invited parties of doctors, scientists, writers and assorted friends and associates to gather at his patients' bedsides throughout the summer of 1837. Soon the corridors, staircases and wards were thronged with visitors marvelling at what they saw. It was scarcely surprising that his fellow professors should grow weary of this unseemly crush. But when Elliotson announced he was going to deliver a lecture on his discoveries, they could ignore the spectacle no longer.

In the first week of September, students filed into the UCH lecture theatre in anticipation of Elliotson's address. The theatre had been the source of much contention over the past few months.[48] Although the room had been built with 250 seats in three ascending rows, the school now boasted some 350 medical students – partly thanks to Elliotson's reputation – so many had to sit or stand on the steps. Since the theatre was shared by all the medical school professors, with no interval between lectures, mayhem erupted in the scramble for seats when one lecture ended and another began. Amid this havoc, the professors themselves did battle, as one set up an illustration for a lecture on medicine while a colleague removed pickled body parts after a lecture on anatomy. In the chaos, bottles containing precious specimens were broken and valuable drawings torn. Furthermore the students complained that the theatre was cold and that the nearby dissecting room exuded a stench which permeated theatre, corridors and stairs. Yet the cold, the crush and the odour were quickly forgotten as Elliotson took the lectern.

For the next hour, Elliotson held the students in thrall as he detailed the 'remarkable' events taking place on the wards. After describing the history and Continental interest in mesmerism, he triumphantly related Dupotet's experiments on Elizabeth Okey and his success in curing not only Elizabeth but 'a great number of female patients', as well as one male. Nevertheless, Elliotson insisted he remained deeply sceptical of the more preposterous claims emerging from the Continent. Stories of patients being able to see with their eyes bandaged, to describe items placed on their skin, even to read the contents of a sealed letter placed on the stomach, were flooding in from France, Italy, Germany and America, he said. A doctor in America had related the case of a sixteen-year-old girl who, in a mesmeric trance, could beat an expert player at backgammon having never played the game before. Two patients in Boulogne were said not only to have seen but tasted food placed on their stomachs. The baron had assured Elliotson that it was only a matter of time before Elizabeth Okey would exhibit similar traits. Whether such outlandish claims were true, Elliotson did not know, but he insisted on seeing for himself before passing judgement.

Putting the finishing touches that month to his latest version of Blumenbach's translation – or *Human Physiology* as it was now titled – Elliotson devoted thirty-seven pages to mesmerism and the recent occurrences at UCH.[49] 'I have witnessed its power at least three times a week for two months: and should despise myself if I hesitated to declare my decided conviction of the truth of mesmerism,' he wrote. Just as he had been laughed at for advocating the stethoscope and promoting quinine, now he was ready to endure ridicule again until 'the truth of mesmerism [is] also admitted and the world forget that it was ever doubted'.

Although a handful of medical men in Britain had also come out in favour of mesmerism – including Herbert Mayo and his Middlesex colleague, John Wilson – Elliotson was by far the most prominent. It was his backing which gave Dupotet his entry into British society; it was his endorsement which gave mesmerism the toehold it needed in the British medical world. He had even asked the baron to teach his method to himself and his students. But to convince the profession at large, Elliotson knew he needed the support of the nation's leading medical journal.

Thomas Wakley's first reaction to mesmerism – in his mocking account of Chenevix's experiments in *The Lancet* in 1829 – did not bode well. Since then, however, *The Lancet* had reported the French inquiry's conclusions with more muted scepticism. Reviewing Colquhoun's translation of the inquiry's report in 1833, the journal declined to dispute the conclusions drawn by 'men of known respectability and veracity' even though it was impossible to explain 'such apparently incomprehensible phenomena'.[50] Yet now that mesmerism had again breached British shores and taken root in the hospital which was not only within his parliamentary constituency but on his very doorstep, Wakley approached the subject with caution. He was a shareholder in UCL, as well as a friend and political ally of its president, Lord Brougham. Close as he was to Elliotson, he had other friends in the medical school too. And although he was as ready as ever to face down his detractors – an ever-burgeoning group – he now had a solid political following to consider.

At the general election in July following the death of William IV, Wakley had topped the poll and now represented Finsbury for a second term.[51] While continuing the demanding job of editing *The Lancet*, he was busier than ever with his political missions. When Queen Victoria gave her first queen's speech at the state opening of parliament that month – essentially a ceremonial event – Wakley hijacked the occasion by trying to present a petition which not only attacked the poverty of the young monarch's subjects but also called for the abolition of the House of Lords and separation of church and state. Never one to be cowed by protocol – he would later complain about the cost of plumbing at Buckingham Palace compared to the deprivations of the poor – he proclaimed himself 'a representative of Labour'. Having been re-elected with a larger mandate, Wakley was determined to build on the victories of the Reform Act and so devoted his energies to campaigning for universal suffrage, annual elections and a secret ballot – demands which would form major planks in the fledgling Chartist movement. He was just as zealous in pursuing other social reforms. Wakley had led demands for an end to flogging in the army following the death of a soldier at Woolwich Barracks in 1836. The man, William Saundry, had received 200 lashes from the notorious 'cat o' nine tails' and his screams had been heard more than a mile away. At the same time, Wakley ruthlessly exposed the cruel extremes of the workhouses.

Yet most of all he was committed to continuing his crusade for medical reform. Keeping up his attack on the vested interests of the elite, Wakley spearheaded moves to create a single body to regulate the medical profession. Instead of the seventeen organisations which could currently license apothecaries, surgeons and physicians, he argued for a single organisation to oversee a general register for all doctors. Fundamental to this aim was his determination to hound all unorthodox practitioners out of business and banish quackery from British shores.

In the meantime, Wakley worked a sixteen-hour day – often eating and writing in his carriage as he travelled up to seventy miles daily. He had also overstretched himself financially, through his myriad interests and the hefty costs of maintaining his lavish household in Bedford Square. And his only daughter, Elizabeth, now fifteen, was seriously ill. It would have been perfectly understandable if Wakley had given his friend's latest obsession short shrift.

Nevertheless, Wakley published Thompson's eyewitness account of Dupotet's demonstration in *The Lancet* on 9 September, along with Elliotson's lecture, without editorial comment. A week later he printed a letter from the baron himself who had taken umbrage at the perceived humorous tone of the report by 'T'.[52] While praising Elliotson for his openness to new ideas, Dupotet made it clear that *he* was the expert on mesmerism and had come to England specifically to teach the art to the benighted medical profession. 'I invite all the world to become auditors of my precepts,' he declared and grandly announced: 'Yes, Mr Editor, a new power is revealed to the world.' Still, anxious not to heap further criticism on the embattled UCL and its fledgling hospital, Mr Editor withheld his thoughts on the subject.

Shortly after delivering his lecture on mesmerism, Elliotson left for the Continent on his usual annual holiday. This yearly break was 'absolutely necessary' for his health, he insisted; Dupotet would later snipe that Elliotson was 'too grand a doctor' to remain in London during the holidays.[53] Before leaving for his tour of the Swiss Alps, however, the professor gave the baron permission to continue his experiments on 'three or four' of the female patients at UCH. With hindsight it was not the most opportune moment to leave the country. For it was now that Elliotson's enemies saw their chance.

5

Daggers Drawn

University College Hospital, London, 19 September 1837

The students and visitors shoved and pushed as they tried to find a vantage point for the start of Baron Dupotet's daily demonstration in the lecture theatre. They were soon disappointed. For, as Dupotet sheepishly explained, all exhibitions of mesmerism had been abruptly suspended by the university medical committee.[1] Mesmerism was banned from the hospital wards, demonstrations were forbidden in the lecture theatre, and Dupotet was now banished from the hospital. For the second time in two months, Baron Dupotet had to leave a London hospital with his tail between his legs.

It was scarcely surprising that Elliotson's colleagues had seized this moment to act. While Elliotson was merrily hiking in the Alps, his fellow professors had become increasingly fed up with the mobs of visitors thronging the lecture theatre and wards in order to see Dupotet's daily pantomimes. Although Elliotson had left the baron with strict instructions to continue his experiments on only 'three or four' named patients, Dupotet had far exceeded his remit. As soon as his patron was out of sight, Dupotet had assumed control of the wards, issuing orders to staff like a triumphant Napoleon planting his standard on British soil. Not only had he enrolled several more in-patients in his experiments, he had also flung open the doors of UCH with the invitation that 'all the poor people who wished to be mesmerised might apply to him at the hospital'.[2] And even more disturbing than the queues of patients jostling to consult the Frenchman, was the fact that Dupotet had extended the scope of his experiments. Determined to demonstrate to the doubting British public that mesmerism could produce the supernatural phenomena he had predicted, he had launched a raft of bizarre new experiments. According to one observer, the scenes on the wards had become 'most absurd' and even 'bordered on the disgusting'. Yet this only served to draw larger crowds to his performances.

As before, the baron had concentrated his efforts on the sixteen-year-old patient who was now routinely hailed as 'the prima donna of the magnetic stage'. He had tried mesmerising more male patients to no avail and had worked on several other female patients with little success. Yet Elizabeth Okey could always be relied upon to obey his commands. No longer satisfied, however, with her crazed babbling or insensibility to pain, Dupotet was determined to take mesmerism to the next level. Impatient to broadcast fresh wonders, he set out to prove that Elizabeth could predict the future, diagnose other patients' illnesses and see with her eyes shut.

As guests had crowded round her bed or watched her in the theatre, Elizabeth had been mesmerised by the baron and then asked to predict when she would be cured of her epilepsy. But the dates she had volunteered varied wildly. She was likewise asked to diagnose other patients' ailments and recommend suitable treatment; these responses were equally changeable and unenlightening. Undeterred, the baron asked her to tell the time with her eyes closed. At one point he had even placed a gold watch and chain in her hand and promised she could keep them if she gave the correct time. As the daughter of a goldchaser, Elizabeth well knew the value of a gold watch and chain. Once or twice she even came close to the right answer but when the spectators' watches were altered to different times she failed to answer correctly. Furthermore, when anyone voiced doubts about her ability to see with her eyes shut, she grew angry and vituperative, shouting 'gross and offensive' abuse at them. All in all the baron's new experiments were a joke.

One observer wrote indignantly to *The Lancet* to express his outrage.[3] Apart from demonstrating the ability of mesmerism to induce sleep, the baron had completely failed to prove his predictions, said the correspondent, who described himself only as 'An Eye-Witness'. Although he held back from directly accusing the baron of being a charlatan, the writer had no such qualms regarding Elizabeth Okey. He did not believe Elizabeth was 'too pretty and light-hearted' to be a fraud. Yet rather than bluntly accusing her of deceit, 'Eye-Witness' suggested she had been indirectly coerced into collusion. Her vanity was 'flattered' at being consulted on other patients' ailments, he said; then becoming more ambitious she 'wished to seem to accomplish things which the Baron constantly promised she should perform'. This was an astute summary of what is now known as the placebo effect, by which patients unconsciously try to 'please' their medical practitioner by conforming to their suggestions. All in all, 'Eye-Witness' concluded, the notion of mesmerism producing any effect beyond mere sleep was a 'fallacy'.

The tide of public opinion was beginning to turn. Although Wakley published the letter condemning Dupotet's extravagant displays in *The Lancet*, he declined to express a view on mesmerism himself. Other publications were less reticent. Wakley's arch-rival, the *London Medical Gazette*, fairly leapt at the opportunity to attack both the infidel university and its absent professor in an article headlined 'Fallacy of Animal Magnetism'.[4] Poking fun at Elliotson's reported success in mesmerising his pet parrot, the *LMG* argued that he was just as likely to induce sleep if he stroked his cat's head or rocked a child's cradle. Although the journal admitted mesmerism might produce a sleep-like condition in some people, it denounced the idea of a magnetic fluid circulating inside the human body. So far, said the *LMG*, none of the baron's demonstrations suggested the effects produced by mesmerism were anything other than 'the result of an impression made on the imagination', though, in common with most sceptics, the editors saw no value in investigating this powerful response any further. Mesmerism, it stormed, should be completely rejected by all 'except the credulous and the idle'.

The baron's exhibitions at UCH had excited attention in the mainstream press too. *The Times* condemned the experiments as 'examples of the revolting imposture, which is called "Animal Magnetism"'.[5] If the demonstrations had been staged with any motive other than to warn pupils against the outrages of quackery, then the hospital should be denounced as 'a seminary for mountebankery', the newspaper thundered. The *Patriot* argued that the demonstrations were 'all a system of imposture from beginning to end', while the *Satirist* lived up to its name by ridiculing such 'highly intellectual beings' as Dupotet and Elliotson for espousing a cause supported only by 'charlatans and hypocrites'. Going one step further, *Blackwood's Edinburgh Magazine* lampooned the whole subject with a spoof story relating how the baron had mesmerised an Irish hod-carrier who had had both legs amputated after falling from a four-storey building. Not only had the man's legs regrown, but he had managed to read an inscription from the Rosetta Stone using only his elbow and the tip of his ear.

In the light of this increasingly hostile press and the precarious position of both the university and the hospital, the decision by the medical authorities to ban mesmerism from the premises seemed wholly understandable.[6] Yet the motive behind this action had little to do with reputation or the growing scepticism around mesmerism; in reality, the move was almost entirely due to professional rivalry and personal enmity. And there is little doubt that it was engineered by one man – UCL's Professor of Clinical Surgery, Robert Liston. His aim was simple: to take revenge on his sworn enemy and rival. He had been waiting a long time for this chance and mesmerism had come along at the right moment.

Ever since Liston had arrived in London at the end of 1834 he had clashed loudly and furiously with Elliotson. Arguments between the two men regularly erupted into ugly scenes in the hospital boardroom when the rows sometimes grew so fierce that onlookers expected the pair to resort to violence.[7] In many ways they were just too similar. They shared a determination to improve medicine, a desire to help the poor and an unremitting confidence in their own talents. Although Liston was three years younger and, at six feet two inches, roughly six inches taller than Elliotson, they even bore a striking resemblance to each other: with his receding, dark curly hair, thick eyebrows and bushy side-whiskers Liston could have passed for Elliotson's younger brother.

Born in Scotland in 1794, the son of a minister, Liston had studied medicine at Edinburgh University just a few years after Elliotson, and had then secured a post as a junior surgeon at Edinburgh Royal Infirmary.[8] He spent two years 'walking the wards' in London, training under two of the best regarded surgeons of the time, John Abernethy at St Bartholomew's and William Blizard at the London Hospital. Returning to Edinburgh in 1818, Liston had established a reputation as a skilled surgeon and a brilliant anatomist – boosted by his talent for procuring fresh corpses in his nocturnal forays to the city's graveyards. He was equally renowned for his vaulting ambition and fiery temper.

Indeed Liston had become so unpopular with hospital staff that he was expelled from the Infirmary for five years; it was said he boasted of saving patients the Infirmary had discharged as untreatable and sent an assistant around the wards to entice patients to defect to his care. On one occasion he knocked a fellow anatomist to the ground in front of a class of students because he was convinced the pupils had taken liberties with the embalmed body of a young woman.[9] Another time, when a visitor interrupted him at home while he was dissecting, he had threatened the guest with his scalpel. Despite the quarrels, Liston had secured a permanent post at the Infirmary in 1827 and became its chief surgeon a year later. But when, in 1833, he was passed over for the post of Professor of Surgery at Edinburgh University in favour of a more junior colleague, Liston was unforgiving. He turned his back on Scotland and accepted the post of surgeon at UCH just as it opened its doors in November 1834. A month later he was elected Professor of Clinical Surgery at UCL. Yet while he was frequently abrasive and argumentative with his peers, Liston was idolised by his students and his patients – and with good reason.

Liston was a superb surgeon who operated with speed, precision and – generally – success. Tall, powerful and muscular, he arrived for an operation dressed in a green frockcoat and wellington boots. Having checked the position of the operating table, he arranged his instruments with the 'sang froid' of a waiter preparing for a dinner party, said one contemporary.[10] Once the patient had given consent and been firmly secured to the table, Liston ordered his students to time him. Their pocket watches duly recorded that he could amputate a leg in less than thirty seconds, sparing his patient much pain and blood loss. According to one observer, 'the gleam of his knife was followed so instantaneously by the sound of sawing as to make the two actions almost simultaneous'.[11] When he needed to have both hands free to tie an artery or probe a wound, he gripped his knife between his teeth. Indeed at times Liston's dexterity was rather too rapid. In his hurry to amputate a leg on one occasion he removed a patient's left testicle as well.[12] Another operation was even more drastic. Although he amputated the patient's leg in two-and-a-half minutes, he also sliced off his assistant's fingers and slashed through the coat-tails of a spectator. Since the spectator dropped dead from the shock and the patient and assistant both died later from infection, the event went down in history as the only operation with a 300 per cent mortality.

Yet Liston was also regarded as a compassionate man. An assistant reported that he lost many hours sleep in anticipation of an operation, while his daughter said he always travelled to the hospital in silence on operating days. Liston showed no sentimentality, however, with cowering patients. When he heard that one patient who was scheduled for an operation was hiding in the lavatory, Liston slipped the bolt, grabbed the man by the seat of his breeches and hauled him onto the operating table where he promptly performed the surgery.[13]

Despite his swashbuckling approach, Liston was meticulous about hygiene – considered something of an eccentricity many decades before the discovery of bacteria – and insisted that wounds should be dressed with clean bandages soaked in water rather than applying the caustic poultices and greasy plasters more commonly used. He invented a transparent sticking plaster made from fish bladders (isinglass) so he could monitor wounds as they healed, devised a splint for fractured femurs which is still in use today and wrote a classic textbook, *Practical Surgery*, which would become the students' standard, indeed a companion volume to Elliotson's *Human Physiology*.

Luring the celebrated surgeon to UCH was a major coup for the university. Now that Astley Cooper had all but retired, and Abernethy and Blizard were approaching their dotage, Liston was regarded as the best surgeon of his time. Shortly after his appointment, *The Lancet* remarked that his fame 'extended throughout Europe'.[14] As Professor of Clinical Surgery, Liston was assigned to give clinical lectures – now established in most London medical schools following Elliotson's example – while his colleague, senior surgeon Samuel Cooper, gave lectures on the theory of surgery (since Cooper was a 'slow and somewhat clumsy' surgeon his lectures were certainly more use in theory than practice).[15] Students flocked to hear Liston describe the novel and daring operations he performed each week. The Scotsman's appointment therefore boded well for the future success of both university and hospital.

Yet far from bringing stability to the medical school, Liston's arrival had brought discord. The fragile harmony that had reigned since Elliotson's appointment in 1831 was shattered as rows and resentment divided the faculty. At the time of Liston's arrival, Elliotson was the university's golden boy, the undisputed star of the medical school. He had poured his energies into founding the hospital, striven to secure the university's right to award degrees, and united the staff in promoting the medical school's best interests. Nobody had worked harder for the good of the university and hospital than Elliotson. Summing up his commitment to UCL in 1835, Elliotson said that he 'considered his life cannot be better spent than in making [his] exertions all tend directly or indirectly, as much as possible, to its welfare'.[16] Yet Elliotson was only completely happy when his colleagues bowed to his greater talents and submitted to his will. This was decidedly not Liston's style – as he had patently demonstrated in Edinburgh. Just as Elliotson was determined to rule the roost, so Liston was adamant to have his own way. It was a recipe for disaster.

From the beginning there were ructions. The medical faculty comprised eleven professors, including three physicians and three surgeons, but now they divided sharply into two factions. With his seniority and experience, Elliotson always commanded the bigger faction and was able to outvote his rival at committee meetings. To Liston's fury, Elliotson repeatedly won the backing of the two other surgeons, Cooper and Richard Quain, while Liston could count on support only from his fellow Scot, the physician Anthony Todd Thomson. Both outspoken, both hot-tempered, both bloody-minded, Liston and Elliotson squared up to each other in the boardroom like two fighting cocks whose sole purpose was to annihilate each other. 'They were constantly at daggers drawn,' said a student.[17] Because of their antagonism the medical committee was 'always quarrelling'. Yet both were equally popular with the students – and therein lay the problem. 'I think there can be no doubt that jealousy was the mainspring of this unfortunate condition of things,' the student wrote. 'Elliotson and Liston were both supreme favourites with the pupils, and neither could bear "a brother near the throne".'

While professional rivalry was undeniably at the root of the two men's animosity, many of the arguments, at least at first, were triggered by Liston's determination to put his own interests before those of the university.

Just a few months after joining UCL and beginning his clinical lectures, Liston wangled a job lecturing on surgery at a rival medical school linked with St George's Hospital. With a wife and six children to look after he obviously needed the fees, but he also believed the competing role would strengthen his hand at UCL. Liston's ties with his former teachers from the traditional London medical schools and his Scottish background meant that he simply did not share the loyalty to UCL that Elliotson and most of his colleagues felt. Liston confessed to a friend, his former assistant James Miller, in Edinburgh, that the university council was 'alarmed' by his move and the medical faculty even demanded he resign as Professor of Surgery. But Liston defiantly declared: 'This I won't do, though I don't value the title a straw.'[18] It was clear that Elliotson was behind the calls for him to resign since Liston told Miller that 'Cantab' – as he had dubbed him – 'looked rather shy when last intercepted'. Liston refused to back down. 'They begin to find I am not a musical instrument,' he said, and he proved his case when the UCL council reluctantly conceded that he was contractually within his rights.

Shortly afterwards, no doubt in retaliation, Elliotson summoned a special meeting of the medical committee to complain that Liston had performed surgery during his own visiting hours.[19] Liston had probably performed some minor operations on the ward itself – a not uncommon practice – but Elliotson plainly thought the screams of patients as they felt the Scotsman's knife were not conducive to a civilised ward round. The medical committee sided with Elliotson – as usual – and stipulated that surgeons should stick to the set hours. But war had been declared. 'I'll get the better of the enemy at the Stinkomalee School,' Liston told Miller. 'The prime mover is Cantab. & I think he is ashamed of himself. I laid it into him (pitched it in) at a meeting he called the other day to censure me for operating at the hospital at his hour.'

Not long afterwards, a vacancy arose for a new Professor of Anatomy. Liston and two colleagues backed Richard Grainger, who had inherited the Webb Street School, where Elliotson had first lectured, when his brother Edward died. But Elliotson and his coterie supported a Scottish candidate, William Sharpey, who was duly elected by the council by nine votes to two.[20] As with Mayo, the decision was almost certainly prompted by snobbery since Grainger, who was born in Birmingham, was also said to have a 'peculiarly unpleasant' intonation when lecturing.

As time went by the rivalry intensified. Liston's operations and lectures drew large crowds of students – as he repeatedly boasted to his friend Miller. His lectures were 'impartially looked on as the best at the University', he said, but did not volunteer the identity of this impartial judge.[21] 'I now stand capitally not only with the students, but with all & sundry,' he wrote, though he had to add, 'except Cantab & he be damned'. Yet far from wanting to resolve their differences for the good of the institution, Liston relished the battle. 'I have been tickling them rather hard of late,' he told Miller at the beginning of 1837. 'They are jealous as the devil of my popularity with the pupils.'

As Liston and Elliotson vied for supremacy, the rows in the board-room spilled over into the wider arena.[22] Ward rounds and lectures were punctuated by contemptuous comments levelled by one man at the other's practices and views. Students and junior staff found themselves forced to choose sides. Liston's house surgeon was barely on speaking terms with Elliotson's house physician, and at one point the two students almost came to blows in defence of their respective teachers. While most of the pupils regarded the hostilities with 'curiosity and amusement', others grew concerned at the threat they posed to the university's reputation.

One student who was watching events transpire with particular interest was James Fernandez Clarke, the latest recruit to *The Lancet* staff. Clarke, the son of a Buckinghamshire lace merchant who had been apprenticed to a London police surgeon, had enrolled at UCL in 1833 at the age of twenty.[23] He had declared Elliotson 'the most accomplished physician of the period', but a year later, when Liston joined, he was equally in awe of the Scotsman's skills. At first Clarke reported cases for the quarterly *Medico-Chirurgical Review* to help pay his fees, but in 1834 he switched loyalties to Wakley and from that point on he duti-fully filed weekly reports on lectures, operations and clinical cases to *The Lancet*. While still admiring of Elliotson, Clarke became a close friend and confidante to Liston, accompanying him on ward rounds and visits to private patients while listening patiently to his grouses about 'Cantab'.

'He complained to me constantly of the indignations to which he was subjected,' Clarke later wrote. 'He said "Cantab has attacked me again. It's too much for my temper; I cannot long endure it".'[24] At one point Liston was so infuriated by his rival that he threatened to quit the hospi-tal. On another occasion Clarke grew so alarmed at Liston's temper that he begged his teacher to restrain himself. As Clarke admitted, 'Liston's impetuous temperament urged him to say very uncivil and very bitter things.' For now Liston was prepared to bide his time. Furthermore he knew he had a secret weapon: his friendship with Thomas Wakley.

As a trained surgeon, Wakley naturally admired Liston's talents in the operating theatre and had enthusiastically welcomed the Scotsman's appointment to UCH in *The Lancet*. The pair met soon afterwards and immediately became friends. Indeed it was Liston who introduced the student Clarke to Wakley as a potential journalist. Despite Liston's coarse manners and volatile temper, Wakley applauded the surgeon's refusal to kowtow to authority and his zeal for medical reform. Just as he had nurtured Elliotson's career a decade earlier, now Wakley helped his new friend by publishing details of his innovative operations and serialising his clinical lectures in *The Lancet*.

Readers were enthralled by the grisly details of Liston's heroic procedures – all performed, of course, without any pain relief for his patients. In one operation he carefully reconstructed the nose of a nineteen-year-old girl by cutting a flap of skin from her forehead then twisting and grafting the section in place; the procedure had been imported from India forty years earlier but was still rarely attempted.[25] In another, he removed a large bladder stone from an eighty-year-old man using the standard method which entailed tying the patient up like a trussed chicken, cutting through the perineum and withdrawing the stone with forceps. Scarcely two tablespoonfuls of blood were lost, Liston boasted, though admittedly the patient died five days later, most probably from infection. In a third operation, he removed a tumour from the face of a two-year-old child; the infant was wrapped in a sheet to keep him from squirming and went home a month later with only a small scar as proof of his ordeal. Step-by-step reports of these complicated operations were interspersed with glowing descriptions of Liston's skills as a teacher. When Liston refused a belated offer of a chair in surgery from Edinburgh at the end of 1835, Wakley declared that, had he left UCL, the students 'would have incurred an irreparable loss'.[26] When Liston's textbook, *Practical Surgery*, was published, it was acclaimed in *The Lancet* for its faithful depiction of the many operations its author had perfected in his 'long and brilliant practice of the art'.

Bragging about his growing celebrity to Miller in Edinburgh, Liston crowed that *The Lancet* was 'pretty favourable to me'.[27] Although the *LMG* reported Liston's career with the same disdain it accorded all UCL professors, Liston took for granted *The Lancet*'s approval – just as Elliotson had done. He met regularly with Wakley to apprise him of his clinical initiatives as well as confiding the squabbles taking place at UCH. At one point the pair discussed a quarrel which had arisen between Elliotson and Wakley in late 1835 over an item in *The Lancet*. It probably concerned a letter from a Glaswegian doctor, John Walker, who disputed Elliotson's recommendation of creosote to quell vomiting, arguing that it had the opposite effect.[28] Elliotson had no doubt taken umbrage at Wakley's decision to print the letter. Clearly relishing his enemy's predicament, Liston told Miller: 'Old Wakley chuckled when I went over the matter with him. He [Elliotson] has behaved unjustifiably and ill to W & will not be forgiven.'[29]

At the same time, Liston proved an ally in Wakley's crusade for change in the medical world. Both Wakley and Liston had addressed a mass meeting of London students in early 1836, demanding an end to the Society of Apothecaries' corrupt examination system. Liston told the cheering students: 'I am a mere tyro in medical politics, but you will find in me a staunch supporter of medical reform.'[30] When Liston was attacked in the *LMG* for supporting the campaign, Wakley leapt to his defence. Liston's fame 'already extended throughout Europe' and no misrepresentation could check 'the course of his brilliant and successful career'. But Liston also had a more personal and poignant relationship with Wakley. For in January that same year Liston was called in, along with the elderly Astley Cooper, to treat Wakley's daughter Elizabeth who was now gravely ill with an undisclosed complaint.[31] Since they were both family men with daughters of a similar age Liston must have shared Wakley's distress.

As the rivalry between Elliotson and Liston intensified, Wakley remained impeccably neutral. Kept abreast of the growing tensions by his spy in the camp, Clarke, Wakley watched developments with growing concern but declined to take sides. Eager to support the struggling medical school and its brave attempt at meritocracy, he kept all mention of the quarrels out of *The Lancet*. Wakley reported operations by Liston which ended fatally with the same studied impartiality that he detailed Elliotson's controversial experiments with mesmerism.

By the summer of 1837 – just as Dupotet introduced mesmerism into UCH – the arguments between the two were coming to a head. Earlier in the year Liston had been ticked off by the medical committee for demonstrating operations on a dead body which he had obtained by nefarious means. He had presumably bought the corpse from one of the body-snatchers still in business instead of applying to the Inspector of Anatomy according to the strictures of the new Anatomy Law.[32] He was also under investigation by the university council for squirrelling away specimens from post-mortems at UCH to his private collection rather than placing them in the hospital museum as required. And he had crossed swords with his colleague Samuel Cooper in a row over house surgeons. Still, Liston remained ebullient and even boasted of mastering his fury. 'I have learned the advantage of keeping my temper at the meetings & much to the annoyance of the others,' he wrote.[33] And then, in August, a spectacular row had erupted when Liston's new house surgeon, a student named Kearsey Cannan, had resigned in protest at his teacher's conduct.

Cannan initially complained to the medical faculty that Liston had behaved towards him in 'so uncourteous & rude a character as to have excited general observation' but, since his three-month appointment had already elapsed, the committee resolved to do nothing.[34] Plainly scenting blood, however, at the end of August – shortly before he left for the Continent – Elliotson had called a special meeting to discuss more serious allegations lodged by Cannan. The complaint involved a sixty-one-year-old patient who had died on 30 June, four days after undergoing an operation by Liston to remove some bladder stones. Rather than performing a risky lithotomy, Liston had used an instrument called a lithotrite which was introduced through the urethra and into the bladder to crush and withdraw the stone in pieces. When he later lectured on the operation, Liston had placed the blame for the man's death squarely on the shoulders of young Cannan. A subsequent report in *The Lancet*, which Liston sanctioned, accused Cannan of misrepresenting the patient's health before the operation and perforating the patient's urethra with a catheter.

These were highly serious allegations to make against a junior surgeon, both before his peers and in print, and potentially jeopardised Cannan's career. At the faculty meeting, which Elliotson chaired, Liston brazenly insisted that *The Lancet* story was true. Then Elliotson called in Cannan who told the meeting quite humbly that he had inserted a catheter at Liston's request without using undue force and was sure he had not torn the urethra. Later another house surgeon had repeated the procedure. The evidence hinged on the anatomical parts which had been removed at the subsequent post-mortem. Elliotson demanded that Liston produce these parts to settle the dispute, but Liston, who had whisked the specimens home according to his usual custom, refused on the grounds that he was 'not on trial'. Neither man would back down: Elliotson refused to allow a decision without seeing the specimens and Liston refused to fetch them. It was a perfect stalemate which would have been comical had it not been so tragic. Finally Elliotson stormed out. It was evidently one of those meetings at which the two men almost came to blows. With the more placatory Sharpey in the chair, Liston agreed a compromise. Although he still refused to admit any failing on his part, he accepted that Cannan was not to blame for the death and even sent to his house to retrieve the disputed specimens.

Although peace was restored, Liston had been forced into a humiliating climbdown. Not only had the incident called into question his celebrated surgical skills, his attempt to shift the blame for a patient's death onto his pupil smacked of ungentlemanly conduct. It was a lesson for Wakley too. He had allowed Liston to amend the proof of the article in question but perhaps the surgeon's word was not as trustworthy as he had assumed. Liston knew he needed to tread carefully; he must keep that famous temper in check. Yet he was determined to exact his revenge. Elliotson's absence during September gave him the perfect opportunity, and Baron Dupotet's experiments the ideal weapon.

When Elliotson returned to London at the end of September it was to a quieter, calmer and significantly emptier hospital. All traces of mesmerism had been erased; not a whiff of garlic lingered to suggest that Dupotet had ever been there. The medical staff bustled around as busily as ever, applying leeches, slicing veins and administering enemas. Elliotson knew he had been defeated – for the moment – and he knew exactly by whom. He had no choice but to submit to the medical committee's decision. And in truth, the baron's banishment came as something of a blessing. With his Gallic theatricality and preposterous claims, Dupotet had become rather an embarrassment. In his final edition of *Human Physiology*, which was just about to emerge from the press, Elliotson described the baron as 'credulous'.[35] He would later accuse Dupotet of 'great weakness and want of propriety' in the liberties he had taken at UCH, and said he 'highly approved' of the medical faculty's steps to remove him.

At first Dupotet survived his expulsion relatively unscathed. He continued to advertise demonstrations and medical consultations in a succession of rented houses in London's West End, and began to draw substantial crowds. Charging spectators 2s 6d, the baron mesmerised volunteers from the audience with varying success, but his favourite and most responsive subject was his own servant, a stout, middle-aged peasant named Julie, who issued medical diagnoses whilst in a trance and suffered pins to be stuck into her flesh without complaint. One journalist, who attended a show that September, told the entranced Julie he had a headache. She prescribed castor oil and chicken broth and even provided a recipe.[36] The reporter declared that 'if there is not something extraordinary in mesmerism itself, there is something very wonderful indeed in Julie's acting'. Dupotet went on to publish a series of articles on mesmerism in the *LMG* despite the journal's previous attack on the 'fallacy of animal magnetism'.

But before long Dupotet's fortunes would begin to wane. Running seriously into debt, he turned to his former patron, but Elliotson refused to help and Dupotet returned to Paris impoverished after less than two years in London. The baron would later publish a book in which he looked back ruefully on his English sojourn and attacked Elliotson for his lack of understanding of mesmerism.[37] It was yet another example of a brief and heady friendship that soon turned sour. Elliotson later dismissed the baron with the verdict: 'In truth, he was an innocent sort of man, very weak and of little information, and he knew no more of mesmerism than the most superficial facts.'[38]

If Elliotson's colleagues believed that by sending Dupotet packing they had seen the last of mesmerism, however, they were very much mistaken. Now the baron was out of the way the path was clear for Elliotson to take full charge of the investigations. As Clarke shrewdly noted, Elliotson had never enjoyed sharing a crown. Potential allies were almost always seen as rivals. Elliotson also attacked Colquhoun, the lawyer who had translated the French inquiry report, describing his views as 'fit only for old divines and nursery maids'.[39] Plainly there was only one man in Britain fit to investigate mesmerism with scientific integrity, and he used his first lecture of the new academic year to make his intentions crystal clear.

For his introductory lecture at the beginning of October Elliotson chose the theme of experimentation.[40] It was a clever choice, guaranteed to appeal to the new students who saw themselves as the future of medicine. Throughout his life, Elliotson said, he had been denounced as 'an experimenter' by 'the idle, the ignorant, and the envious' but it was only by making 'judicious experiments' that he had discovered therapies for diseases which were previously considered untreatable. Now he was approaching mesmerism in exactly the same way. He had only begun his experiments at UCH after witnessing solid evidence that the method was worth investigating. Those trials had convinced him that mesmerism could induce sleep, coma and somnambulism. Being 'naturally very incredulous', he did not believe 'a ten-thousandth part' of what others had claimed respecting the practice. But he was determined, no matter the opposition he faced, to carry on with his research. It was going to be a fascinating academic year.

His message was clear: mesmerism was back. And there was nothing Elliotson's medical colleagues could do about it. It was one thing to ban a foreign interloper from the hospital, but to interfere with a fellow professor's autonomy in treating his patients or teaching his students was simply unconscionable. Liston could only seethe in silence.

Swiftly reasserting his authority within the medical school, Elliotson persuaded the medical committee to refer the dispute between Liston and his former house surgeon Cannan to the university council.[41] Even though a compromise had now been reached, Elliotson was determined not to let the matter drop. With his outside lecturing frowned upon and his private anatomy collection still under question, Liston was in trouble and he knew it. Licking his wounds, he took leave from the hospital in November – right at the busiest time in terms of the teaching, and with the onset of winter ailments. 'You have no notion how I am <u>beset</u> or rather have been,' he complained to his penpal Miller.[42] 'But they will find that they have dug a pit for themselves. I never can or shall put confidence in some of them again, & they shall feel this ere long.' He named no names but there could be little doubt who he meant when he referred to 'one Blackguard' who was trying to scupper his plans for advancement. 'I will bide my time,' he wrote, adding ominously: 'I'll diddle him or I am a Dutchman.'

Refreshed and re-energised, Elliotson immediately reinstated his mesmeric experiments, only now he made sure that the trials were all performed by himself or his loyal assistants. And he was impatient to take his investigation further.

On the Continent mesmerism enthusiasts had roughly divided into two schools of thought: the 'fluidists' who clung to Mesmer's theory that the influence worked through the manipulation of an invisible physical fluid or force, and the 'animists' who believed the mesmerising effect was brought about purely by 'psychical principles' – in other words the power of the mind.[43]

Working with Dupotet, Elliotson had swallowed the theory that the mesmerising influence was an actual physical force which existed throughout the natural world but was invisible to the naked eye. The various phenomena he had witnessed 'must be ascribed to a peculiar power; to a power acting, I have no doubt, constantly in all living things, vegetable and animal, but shown in a peculiar manner by the processes of mesmerism', he wrote in autumn 1837.[44] For Elliotson, this made perfect sense – indeed it made far more sense at the time than the woolly notion of some mystical trick of the mind, given that fellow scientists were then investigating phenomena such as sound waves, magnetism and electricity, which had all been proven to exist despite being invisible. His friend Faraday, for example, was conducting experiments to determine the precise nature of different forms of electricity, such as electromagnetism. Charles Wheatstone, another friend and fellow phrenologist who was Professor of Experimental Physics at the rival KCL, had just devised a method of transmitting messages along electric wires which would soon come into general use as the electric telegraph. So if an invisible mesmeric power existed, then it too should operate according to definable scientific principles, Elliotson believed.

Beginning that autumn, Elliotson and two disciples, his clinical clerk William Wood and the hospital apothecary John Taylor, launched a series of tests designed to define and measure the powers of mesmerism. Yet for all his determination to proceed according to scientific principles, Elliotson concentrated his efforts exclusively on Elizabeth Okey. There was some logic in this too. Since Elizabeth responded more reliably, more rapidly and more dramatically to mesmerism than any other patient, it made sense to test the phenomenon on her. In retrospect this was clearly a basic error. Not only did his failure to compare the effects of mesmerism on other patients cast doubt on the validity of the tests, it gave Elizabeth a dangerous degree of control over the results and a manifest prestige within the wards. She was not just the prima donna, she was now the *only* donna. Expectations were high and she did not disappoint.

*

From 30 September onwards, Elizabeth was mesmerised into a trance almost every day, and sometimes several times a day, for the next three months. No longer satisfied with watching her lapse alternately into her trance and delirium, the three experimenters devised ingenious trials to try to pin down rules about the way mesmerism worked. The results were diligently recorded by Wood in the hospital casebooks.[45]

In one series of tests, the experimenters blindfolded Elizabeth to see whether she became mesmerised without being able to see their hand movements. Telling her they were going to play hide-and-seek, Wood pretended to leave the room but remained standing before her with his hand extended towards her face.[46] Five minutes later she emerged from her delirium as usual. The fun and games continued. Blindfolding her again, Wood stood silently and motionlessly beside her bed. After fifteen minutes she recovered as usual, thus proving, in Wood's mind at least, that mere proximity to the mesmerist had the same effect as the hand movements. Further experiments tested whether the mesmeric power increased when more than one mesmerist worked together, in just the same way electricity was multiplied when additional batteries were used.

Yet repeated tests produced conflicting results. Sometimes Elizabeth fell asleep in five minutes, while at other times it took as long as forty-five; sometimes she fell into a trance without any hand movements but at other times she did not. This was scarcely surprising. Elliotson and his team had been careful to follow the golden rule of scientific experiment: they first formulated a hypothesis and then devised experiments to test their theory. But beyond that, scientific principles had gone out the window. The conditions of each experiment varied, there was no 'control' subject to test what happened with other patients, and they failed to allow for their own or their subject's expectations. Whenever a trial produced the expected result this was greeted as a eureka moment that proved their theory right, but if a test failed or took an interminable time to work, they devised a justification for that failure. In one test, for example, Elizabeth was working at her needlework beside the fire while Wood stood motionless four feet away for thirty minutes. When her head finally drooped this was hailed as proof that his presence had induced a trance, rather than being due to the soporific effect of the embroidery or the fire.

In the meantime, Elizabeth's clinical symptoms were becoming increasingly marked. She lapsed into 'delirium' every day and sometimes remained in that state for days at a time. She complained of headaches, breathlessness and a pain in her side. In October she had two epileptic seizures for the first time since July. And at the end of November her delirium took a new form in which she had difficulty recognising people she knew. Whether these symptoms were the result of her peculiar form of epilepsy – if indeed that is what she had – or were a new problem, perhaps exacerbated by her daily bouts of mesmerism, was never considered. So intent were the experimenters on testing mesmerism to its limits that they never questioned whether they might be harming their subject. Nor did Elliotson and his team seem to consider whether Elizabeth might be feigning any of her behaviour – even when one violent 'fit' resolved spontaneously the moment staff suggested giving her an enema.

Yet for all her erratic responses and strange ailments, the sixteen-year-old housemaid was consuming an increasing proportion of Elliotson's time. Other patients were admitted and treated with the usual stock remedies, then discharged as cured, unrelieved or dead. None merited more than a paragraph or two in the casebooks while the details concerning Elizabeth meandered over fifteen pages. Elliotson's house in Conduit Street was as thickly thronged with the carriages of his private patients as ever, yet he was spending more and more time in Gower Street. He was just as passionate about reading bumps as before. At the November meeting of the Phrenological Society of London he railed against the naivety of some fellow enthusiasts for supposing a direct link between the size of a subject's 'organs of generation' and their sexual appetite.[47] He even found the time to launch a business venture. In partnership with his former pupil and trusty friend Edmond Sheppard Symes, Elliotson launched a life insurance company, the National Loan Fund, for which the pair were medical advisors.[48] Yet none of these interests were as enthralling as the events taking place on ward three. Indeed, as Elliotson and his staff stood like petrified statues with their arms outstretched, staring at Elizabeth Okey for half an hour at a time while ward life bustled around them, it seemed that they were the ones who were truly entranced.

Regardless of the conflicting results of his research, by the end of the year Elliotson had concluded beyond doubt that mesmerism represented a powerful therapy, which he was ready to extend to more patients at

UCH. Having learned his lesson from the debacle over Dupotet, he was more circumspect about broadcasting mesmerism's merits to the wider public. There had been no more demonstrations in the lecture theatres, no large crowds mobbing the wards. But as a steady trickle of guests gravitated towards Elizabeth Okey's bed, he was garnering some influential support.

As the New Year approached, Elliotson had won backing for his work from several esteemed scientists. They included Herbert Mayo, Professor of Anatomy at KCL, who was following Elliotson's experiments with zeal, and Lord Philip Henry Stanhope, president of the Royal Medico-Botanical Society, who was now an ardent disciple of mesmerism.[49] Even more enthusiastic was the physician George Sigmond, Professor of *Materia Medica* to the same society, who had taught himself the technique and tested it on nearly 100 people including, he told *The Lancet*, the daughter of a wealthy family at a dinner party.[50] When mesmerism had come up in conversation – as it not infrequently did at such fashionable gatherings – one of the young women had laughingly proposed herself as the subject of an experiment and Sigmond 'very willingly assented'.

Sigmond had begun by making the usual 'passes', much to the 'laughter and incredulity' of the guests, but after five minutes the young woman's eyelids had closed and she was 'in the most complete trance I had ever yet witnessed'. Wonder soon turned to concern as Sigmond's attempts to rouse the slumbering belle proved in vain. Her hands were icy cold, her breathing had slowed and her face wore such a 'deathly cast' that her family became quite alarmed. Despite Sigmond's efforts to 'apply warmth and friction to the extremities', she slept soundly for the next four hours. Helped back to her room, looking for all the world like a sleepwalker from a gothic novel, she did not awake until morning. Sigmond was chastened by his experience; mesmerism was plainly not to be trifled with. However, this did not deter him from continuing to practise it on patients and friends alike, nor from encouraging his fellow professionals to 'try the same process'.

As controversy over mesmerism simmered, Wakley remained inscrutably neutral. Reporting Elliotson's research in detail, he published letters from supporters and sceptics alike without taking sides. But the stakes were now imperatively high. Ever since he had launched *The Lancet* fifteen years earlier, Wakley had taken up the standard to fight quackery and establish orthodox medical professionals as the unquestioned arbiters of medical practice. In parliament Wakley was actively pursuing attempts to outlaw quackery by setting up a register of qualified medical practitioners. And in his first editorial of 1838, he called on the medical profession to unite in order to banish quackery from British shores.[51]

Wakley condemned the 'deplorable ignorance' of the public in favouring quack remedies over established therapies but he blamed the medical profession too, for veiling medicine in 'mystery and secretness'. Ever the democrat, Wakley felt sure that improved schooling for the poor would help them see the light. 'Remove ignorance from the people, and mysticism from the practice of medicine, and the quack's avocation will soon be gone.'

Having staked his colours so firmly to the mast, Wakley could therefore not avoid the 'much-agitated subject' of mesmerism. Giving his views on the experiments at UCH for the first time, he said he had been delighted when he heard his friend Elliotson was investigating the subject. Now that mesmerism was attracting growing public attention, he urged his friend to put the phenomenon to scientific test with 'the utmost vigour' so he could ultimately avow whether mesmerism was 'a mere illusion of disordered imaginations and an instrument of fraud in the hands of charlatans, or whether it has any existence in a natural cause'. Determined to resist making a premature judgement, Wakley insisted that 'for the present, at least, *criticism*, whether speculative or philosophical, on the subject of animal magnetism, shall not advance a single inch in our columns'. Yet the warning bells rang out clearly in his final paragraph. 'With regard to our own belief in the existence or the non-existence of "ANIMAL MAGNETISM," we still scrupulously refrain from offering any exposition.' There was no doubt in his message: mesmerism was on trial.

Elliotson was unperturbed. For as 1838 dawned, he attracted an ally to the cause who was already a household name.

6

I am a Believer

University College Hospital, London, 4 January 1838

From Charles Dickens's new home in Doughty Street, on the eastern edge of Bloomsbury, it was a brisk twenty-minute walk to the hospital in Gower Street. Dickens arrived on Thursday 4 January with his friend, the artist George Cruikshank, anticipating a pleasant diversion from his busy working day.[1] What he witnessed had a profound effect on both his life and his writing.

Although he was yet only twenty-five, Dickens had already earned widespread fame and critical acclaim as the author of *Sketches by Boz*, which were illustrated by Cruikshank, and his serialised *Pickwick Papers*, which had concluded the previous October.[2] He was currently working simultaneously on writing monthly instalments of *Oliver Twist*, beginning research for *Nicholas Nickleby* and sketching out a further novel which would become *Barnaby Rudge*, while editing the magazine *Bentley's Miscellany* and polishing the memoirs of the celebrated clown Grimaldi. Thankfully, since he was newly married with a son about to turn one and another child due shortly, Dickens's industry had brought him relative prosperity. The terraced house in Doughty Street, where he had moved with his small family the previous year, boasted three storeys with a neat back garden and stables. But Dickens was not the sort of man to forget his impoverished past.

Just like the wretched patients he saw as he walked through the wards of UCH, Dickens had spent much of his childhood flitting from one cramped lodging house to another in the dingy north London suburbs. After moving from Kent to London when Dickens was ten, his family had lived in progressively meaner lodgings in Camden Town, Somers Town and St Pancras as his father's debts mounted. A small, delicate and sensitive boy, unable to continue his schooling because his parents could not afford the fees, Charles had roamed the local streets where barefoot orphans begged for crusts and child prostitutes solicited for customers. As the family's circumstances worsened, he had taken furniture and books to the pawnbrokers to raise money for the rent. And when his father was committed to the Marshalsea, the debtors' prison in Southwark, the twelve-year-old Dickens had been sent to work in a blacking factory beside the river. While the rest of his family joined his father in prison, Dickens walked each day, an 'ill-clad, ill-fed' child, from the room he shared with two other boys in a Camden Town boarding house to his tedious job pasting labels on pots of boot-blacking. Worse, though, than the hunger, cold and exhaustion, Dickens would never forget the humiliation and loneliness of that period. He knew the pale, emaciated, sickly faces of the north London poor as well as he knew those of his own family, and he would people his novels with such characters. So when he met Elizabeth Okey, the pretty, intelligent housemaid whose life had been blighted by poverty and ill health, he saw how his own life might so easily have turned out.

Elliotson had invited Dickens and Cruikshank to ward three to watch his prize patient being mesmerised. It is not known who suggested the visit, but it was almost certainly the first time the author and the physician had met and it was a momentous occasion for them both.[3] James Fernandez Clarke, the medical student who was filing reports to *The Lancet*, described seeing the author with his 'smooth reflecting face', 'noble forehead' and 'fine expressive eyes'.[4] Something of a dandy at the time, Dickens sported flamboyant waistcoats and styled his dark brown hair in loose curls. Though he had outgrown his youthful lack of stature, he was still a slight figure with boyish looks, in contrast to Cruikshank who was approaching fifty. Although Cruikshank's career had faltered of late, he was currently enjoying a new wave of popularity through his collaboration with Dickens. Both of them known for their acute powers of observation, Dickens and Cruikshank were undoubtedly paying close attention as Elliotson signalled he was about to begin.

As his guests watched expectantly, Elliotson put Elizabeth through her paces. The display she gave on 4 January was one of her bravura performances.

When Dickens arrived on the ward, Elizabeth, now seventeen, had been in her delirious state; she had relapsed the previous night, according to the casebooks. It had become difficult, however, to distinguish this delirium from her behaviour under mesmerism. She was insensible to pain, just as she was when mesmerised, as Elliotson proceeded to demonstrate by pricking and pinching her skin then pulling her head backwards by her hair and ears. It is likely he encouraged his guests to do the same since this had become part of the routine. Next he showed that even though her eyes were open her vision was disturbed. When one finger was held before her face she insisted there were two, and when two fingers were held up she said there were 'such a many'. All the time, she kept spouting gibberish, uttering odd phrases such as 'it is such a big' and 'when is was just now' and 'when it is presently', which Wood, Elliotson's ever-present assistant, studiously recorded in the notes. She also expressed ludicrous fantasies, claiming to have no memory of her family or home and insisting that the hospital was her home and always had been, and that Elliotson was her father, Wood her mother and the medical students her brothers. But as Elliotson stood behind her chair and solemnly extended one hand towards her head a dramatic transformation came over her.

As Dickens and Cruikshank watched, Elizabeth's ramblings quietened then ceased altogether. The colour returned to her cheeks and her hands felt warmer. Then suddenly her eyelids fell and she appeared to be sound asleep. After a minute in this trance she gave a deep sigh and said: 'Oh dear!', then miraculously returned to her senses. All the babbling nonsense, crackpot ideas and obliviousness to pain were gone; she was a demure, sweet-natured, polite young woman again. Dickens was enthralled. He did not record his thoughts on the demonstration at UCH but the visit left a lasting impression. It was the beginning of a lifelong friendship with Elliotson, and a lifetime's fascination with mesmerism.

Soon after the visit, Elliotson became the Dickens family doctor. He would treat the author for his frequent colds and bouts of indigestion – no doubt brought on by overwork and anxiety – and his wife and children for their various ailments as well as coming to the aid, without charge, of a succession of impoverished acquaintances Dickens sent his way. A few years later, in 1841, Elliotson would become godfather to Dickens's second son, Walter, although he first made sure to extract a promise that he would be absolved 'from religious duties & every thing vulgar'.[5] Admiring Elliotson both for his congenial good humour and humanitarian ideals, Dickens would describe the doctor as 'one of my most intimate and valued friends'.

As the years progressed, they would become increasingly close companions. Within three years of that first meeting, Dickens wrote that whenever he was in town he met with Elliotson 'almost every day', and when he was away they kept up a 'very frequent correspondence'. They dined at each other's houses, enjoyed long, rowdy suppers with male friends in taverns, and toasted worthy causes with hock and punch in their private clubs. As their friendship grew, they also travelled together. Meeting the pair crossing the Channel from Boulogne to Folkestone on one occasion, an acquaintance recalled that both were 'awfully seasick' despite Dickens having consumed homoeopathic pills and Elliotson binding his stomach with bandages.[6] When Dickens moved his ever-growing family to Switzerland for a period, he invited Elliotson to join him for drinking sessions and hiking expeditions. Inspired by Elliotson, Dickens would also become an enthusiast for phrenology; they would even attend two public hangings together to compare notes on the murderers' bumps.

Trying to sum up their friendship, Dickens told one acquaintance: 'If I were to tell you what I know of his skill, patience, and humanity, you would love and honor him as much as I do. If my own life, or my wife's, or that of either of my children were in peril tomorrow I would trust it to him, implicitly.' To another he said simply, he 'is a good, as well as a clever man'. As a measure of his affection, Dickens dubbed Elliotson 'Blue Beard' – presumably in honour of his luxuriant black whiskers rather than any suspicion of murderous tendencies. And unlike so many of his other relationships, past and future, Elliotson would never quarrel with Dickens. They would always remain mutual friends.

Through Dickens, Elliotson became an integral member of an intimate circle of writers, artists and actors including the novelists William Makepeace Thackeray, Edward Bulwer-Lytton, William Harrison Ainsworth and Wilkie Collins, the actor William Macready, the artist Daniel Maclise and the literary critic John Forster. Elliotson would in turn become doctor to many of these friends, along with their families and their charitable cases too.

Yet almost as life-changing as this fortuitous meeting of minds was Dickens's sudden and complete conversion to the cause of mesmerism. Only the previous year Dickens had poked fun at the subject in a sketch for *Bentley's Miscellany* depicting the 'Mudfog Association for the Advancement of Everything', a parody of the recently founded British Association for the Advancement of Science. In Dickens's spoof report, the vice-president of the section for anatomy and medicine, Professor Nogo, describes 'an extraordinary case of animal magnetism' in which a watchman – who were notorious for falling asleep at their posts – had descended into a 'very drowsy and languid state' after merely being looked at by a mesmerist from across the street.[7] Dickens later confessed that before visiting UCH, he had been an outright sceptic. Yet now that he had witnessed the effects for himself, he was utterly convinced. 'With regard to my opinion on the subject of Mesmerism,' he would later write, 'I have no hesitation in saying that I have closely watched Dr Elliotson's experiments from the first . . . and that after what I have seen with my own eyes and observed with my own senses, I should be untrue both to him and myself, if I should shrink for a moment from saying that I am a believer, and that I became so against all my preconceived opinions.'[8]

From this first spark of interest, Dickens greedily consumed articles and books on mesmerism including Elliotson's *Human Physiology*, with its long chapter on the subject, and Dupotet's book, *An Introduction to the Study of Animal Magnetism*, which was published in English in 1838.[9] He even asked Elliotson to teach him how to perform mesmerism and in future years would practise with noted success on his wife, sister-in-law and several friends, although he would always resist becoming a subject himself. More significantly, perhaps, Dickens wove mesmerism into his writing.

Feverishly working to produce monthly instalments of *Oliver Twist* and *Nicholas Nickleby* throughout 1838, Dickens introduced mesmerism into both novels.[10] In chapter thirty-four of *Oliver Twist*, first published in June 1838, Oliver falls asleep but sees, or dreams that he sees, a vision of Fagin and his accomplice watching him through the window. Dickens's description of the boy's sleep as a kind of 'overpowering heaviness, a prostration of strength, and an utter inability to control our thoughts or power of motion' while he maintained 'a consciousness of all that is going on' smacks of a mesmeric trance, while Oliver's ability to see events occurring in another place conjures up the idea of clairvoyance, reported by enthusiasts such as Dupotet. More compellingly, Cruikshank's accompanying illustration depicts Oliver in a chair with his head slumped, his eyes closed and his arms hanging by his side in perfect imitation of a mesmeric trance. Dickens was even more explicit in chapter seven of *Nicholas Nickleby*, published in September, when the eponymous hero reads a book 'with as much thought or consciousness of what he was doing, as if he had been in a magnetic slumber'.

Dickens's fascination with mesmerism would remain a constant to the end of his writing days. In *Bleak House*, Lady Dedlock flees in a trance-like state – 'with eyes like almost as if she was blind'. Many of Dickens's villains, such as Quilp in *The Old Curiosity Shop* and Carker in *Dombey and Son*, appear to possess a mesmerising power over their victims. And Dickens's fascination with mesmerism would reach its apogee in his final, unfinished novel, *The Mystery of Edwin Drood*. In this story the evil John Jasper bewitches the object of his lust, Rosa Budd, with his hypnotic eyes – 'he has made a slave of me with his looks' – and commits his foul deeds in a trance, albeit one induced by opium rather than mesmerism. The idea of a 'twin' personality, or repressed alter ego, which might perform sinister or criminal deeds unknown to the conscious self, also became a recurring theme in Dickens's fiction.

Entranced by what he had seen, Dickens returned at least twice more to watch Elliotson's demonstrations at UCH in 1838, and he probably attended one or more of the major public exhibitions that summer. He introduced his friends and acquaintances to the powers of mesmerism too. In April he brought William Harrison Ainsworth to watch the experiments. Ainsworth, a rakish, good-looking playboy who lived with his cousin's widow after separating from his wife, had made his name writing gothic melodramas featuring swashbuckling heroes in the manner of Walter Scott.[11] It was Ainsworth who created the myth of the highwayman Dick Turpin's reckless ride from London to York in his first novel, *Rockwood*, and likewise made a folk hero of the notorious thief Jack Sheppard, who habitually escaped from Newgate in the early 1700s, in his eponymous second novel.

The dramatic effect of mesmerism had an inevitable appeal for Ainsworth. 'The other day I accompanied my friend Dickens to see some girls magnetised by Dr Eliotson [sic], and a more curious exhibition

I never beheld,' he wrote. 'Unless there was some collusion, which I can scarcely imagine, the effects of the magnetizer were truly surprising – almost magical . . .'

Another visitor that same month was William Macready, the leading actor of the day who had recently taken over management of the struggling Covent Garden Theatre while appearing in as many as four different roles a week. The versatile Macready had first met Dickens the previous year but he already knew Elliotson, who had become his family doctor a year earlier when Elliotson treated his sister Letitia. Elliotson had hectored Macready on the 'absurdity' of homoeopathy at the time. He had stayed for tea and Macready noted in his diary: 'I liked him very much.'[12]

Dickens called on Macready at the theatre with his friend Forster on 23 April, fittingly Shakespeare's birthday. The next day Macready went to UCH with a friend, the comic actor George Bartley, to watch 'Dr Elliotson's exhibition of his epileptic patients under a course of animal magnetism'. Macready was intrigued but unconvinced. 'It is very extraordinary, and I cannot help thinking that they are partly under a morbid influence and partly lend themselves to a delusion,' he wrote astutely. He would remain a sceptic. Later the same year, when Elliotson pressed him to attend a mesmerism demonstration in his own home, Macready would complain, 'he is infatuated on this subject', and many years later, after attending a lecture by Elliotson, he would write in disbelief, 'I was amazed to hear him declare the power of mesmerism, and insist upon its truth.' Yet if Macready was unimpressed by the theatrical efforts of Elizabeth Okey, many more people were becoming converts as word spread of the remarkable cures at UCH.

Emboldened by his growing support in the arts world and beyond, Elliotson abandoned the discretion he had cultivated since despatching Dupotet. He had convinced both the country's favourite novelist and its best-loved illustrator that mesmerism worked; he was not going to give up his research now for the sake of a few backbiting grumbles from the press. Throwing caution to the wind, he extended his experiments to increasing numbers of patients as they were admitted to UCH.[13] The results were quite astounding.

Most of Elliotson's subjects were admitted with neurological conditions such as epilepsy or with mysterious symptoms classified as 'hysteria'.

The vast majority were young and female. Although some patients exhibited little or no response to his efforts, others reacted dramatically and their conditions showed startling improvements.

One patient, a twenty-six-year-old Frenchwoman named Palmire Bosch was admitted with 'hysteria' and gastritis at the end of January 1838. It transpired she had a prolapsed womb after giving birth nine months earlier – it was no wonder she felt hysterical. She was first treated with the usual battery of orthodox therapies but after several months with no improvement Elliotson mesmerised her on 5 May. The effects were immediate and dramatic. She fell into a trance within minutes and proved so responsive that all other therapies were abandoned. A few weeks later she could walk unaided and in June she was discharged 'very much relieved'.

Another patient, Charlotte Cook, an eighteen-year-old 'servant of all work', was admitted in April with 'delirium and hysteria'. She had begun acting strangely three weeks earlier when she started following her mistress around the house and pulling at her clothes. A week later she had become so violent and demented that several people were required to hold her down. After being admitted to UCH, she spent most of her time crying in bed or wandering around the ward muttering to herself. Elliotson tried the usual remedies – bleeding, purging and mercury – to no effect. Then he decided to 'trust the case entirely to mesmerism'. She was first mesmerised on 9 April and a day later was 'very much improved'. After daily treatment she was discharged at the end of May 'quite well'. Delighted with this success, Elliotson declared: 'No cure was ever effected in a hospital more successfully. There was no expense beyond the patient's food, except for one pill and one draught before mesmerism was begun.'[14]

Another housemaid, seventeen-year-old Henrietta Power, was admitted at the end of April with St Vitus's dance (Sydenham's chorea), the neurological condition which causes involuntary jerking movements. Her symptoms had appeared a fortnight earlier when she had dropped a tea tray. By the time she was admitted, her limbs were twitching constantly, her eyes rolled and she was dragging one leg. She had to be strapped into bed to prevent her falling out. Elliotson prescribed mesmerism for half an hour a day. After the first treatment she slept for six hours and no longer needed to be confined to bed. A week later she could carry a saucepan of water across the ward without spilling a drop and by the end of May she was plying a needle with the deftness of an accomplished seamstress. In July she left the hospital 'cured'. As Elliotson wrote triumphantly: 'Here was another admirable cure without any expense for drugs.'

But the most outstanding cure was that of a twelve-year-old girl named Hannah Hunter who had been admitted on 1 January.[15] She had been sent to UCH from Dover, where she lived, by a surgeon, a Mr Hannan Thomson, who had read of Elliotson's work. A small and delicate girl, Hannah had lost the use of her legs when she was five and also suffered from chorea, epileptic seizures, headaches and asthma. Elliotson considered her condition to be a 'nervous' disease – he suspected it had a psychological root, which it quite possibly did – but confessed he did not understand what caused such symptoms. Thomson, in Dover, had subjected her to leeches, mercury and warm baths – with predictably little effect. At UCH she was treated with electric shocks, carbonate of iron and more warm baths – with an equal lack of success. 'She has now complete paralysis of the lower extremities; she cannot stand, and can only just move her legs in bed,' the casebooks noted. After four days of being mesmerised there was 'a *very striking improvement* in her *symptoms*' and at the end of the first week she could walk with help for the first time in seven years. Leaving off all other treatment, Hannah was mesmerised daily and on 18 April, three months after the start of her mesmeric treatment, she walked out of UCH 'quite well'. Thrilled with her recovery, Elliotson wrote: 'I saw clearly that the astonishing benefit could be ascribed to mesmerism only.'

The seemingly miraculous cure of patients such as Hannah Hunter provided powerful evidence of the potential benefits of mesmerism. Indeed, such cases are testament still to the extraordinary potential of hypnotism to treat a range of illnesses with a psychological or psychosomatic cause.

Encouraged by his success, Elliotson extended this new therapy to more patients arriving at UCH. And as he exhibited his patients on the wards and in the lecture theatre, his students and fellow medical men were inspired to test the remedy for themselves. By March, mesmerism had become so well established on Elliotson's wards at UCH that it was almost routine. Observing experiments on Hannah Hunter and Elizabeth Okey, a reporter from the *Morning Post* declared: 'This treatment is, it appears, no longer looked upon as a matter of experiment or curiosity in the hospital, but as a portion of a regular (though very peculiar) medical course, which has been found in these two cases to be productive of decidedly good results.'[16]

Had Elliotson confined his efforts to pursuing the 'decidedly good results' that mesmerism could produce in treating certain illnesses he might have saved himself a lot of trouble. Yet despite his success in relieving pain and distress, he was driven by an obsession to test the more outlandish claims that still clung to the practice. The casebooks make clear that patients were often kept in hospital after they had recovered so that Elliotson could conduct further experiments. Hannah Hunter, for example, was mesmerised for several weeks after recovering the use of her legs so that theories could be tested and the results exhibited to visitors. Another patient, a nine-year-old girl named Charlotte Dewberry, was even brought into the hospital purely because she showed an unusually strong response to mesmerism. She had been treated privately for a pain in her neck and bladder by William Hering, a surgeon-apothecary and phrenologist based near UCH.[17] Having heard of Elliotson's work, Hering had tried his hand at mesmerising Charlotte and found after just a few weeks that 'all her symptoms disappeared'. Yet despite her recovery, on 19 April Charlotte was admitted to UCH 'in order to have mesmerism continued and its powerful influence exhibited to the students and professors'. She was mesmerised daily on the wards and twice exhibited in the lecture theatre until, not surprisingly, her parents fetched her home ten days later, 'She being quite well'.

Still convinced mesmerism was an invisible physical force, Elliotson was eager to chart its characteristics. Could it be made to bend around corners – like light waves? Could it be harnessed and magnified – like electricity? Could it be reflected in mirrors or penetrate through doors and walls? Visitors to the wards were bemused, and frequently amused, when they chanced upon the professor's peculiar experiments. Clarke, *The Lancet*'s roving reporter, arrived one day to find Elliotson and two friends huddled at one end of the hospital's 180-foot main corridor making 'passes' into a mirror which was angled towards Elizabeth Okey, who sat on a chair with her back turned at the far end.[18] When she lapsed into her usual sleep, the experimenters jubilantly recorded that the 'mesmeric rays' could indeed be reflected.

In other experiments, designed to test whether the mesmeric force could be magnified by being channelled through several operators at once, Elliotson formed long chains of staff, students and visitors. At one point as many as twenty people joined hands and snaked through the ward in an effort to mesmerise a patient.[19] The patients themselves scarcely had any say in their involvement, of course. All of them poor, powerless, working-class servants or labourers from the grim suburbs, most of them female and some of them children, they meekly submitted to the trials – even if occasionally their parents would insist on taking them home.

Yet even though Elliotson drew more patients into his research, his efforts still focused primarily on Elizabeth Okey. Patients were admitted and discharged, shown to visitors and exhibited in the theatre, but none proved to be as fascinating as she did. Elizabeth reigned supreme as the indisputable star of the mesmeric stage, until – in early 1838 – a rival appeared. It was her sister.

Jane Okey, now fifteen, was readmitted to UCH on 27 February in a delirious state.[20] Since being discharged the previous June, her seizures had returned and gradually increased so that by February they were occurring on a daily basis – up to thirty times a day – accompanied, as with her sister, by frequent headaches. Jane had been hard of hearing since infancy, the casebooks noted, and had never had a sense of smell. Her first seizure had apparently been prompted when she was frightened by a rat – she must have been a sensitive soul since rats were undoubtedly a common sight amid the tenements of Somers Town. During her episodes she went rigid and lost consciousness, foamed at the mouth and seized the bedclothes between her teeth in a typical tonic clonic seizure. But, unlike classic cases of epilepsy, a week before her readmission Jane had lapsed into delirium, which had returned daily. In this delirious state, she was insensible to being pinched and her personality changed so that she became 'very spiteful and mischievous' and 'quite unmanageable'. During her delirium she too spoke a strange language, uttering phrases such as 'what's none when' and repeating the word 'little'. Asked whether she had a pain in her head, she said she had no head. The casebooks were careful to note that Jane had not visited the hospital in the previous two months and had only seen Elizabeth in delirium once. Yet all of her behaviour seemed to mirror her sister's exactly. Was their unusual mixture of epilepsy and delirium the result of an inherited family disorder? Or was something much stranger going on?

*

Although she was two years younger than her sister, Jane was taller and more robust than Elizabeth. She had a 'sanguineous temperament' – she was lively and cheerful, in medical terms – although she had not yet reached puberty, the casebooks noted. Like her sister, she was described as pretty and in her natural state she was 'bustling and hardworking'. Since being discharged from hospital she had worked as a housemaid until, presumably, her seizures and delirium had made that occupation impossible. The sisters were close; in their cramped family lodgings they would almost certainly have shared a room and most likely a bed. They had spent several years together when younger, of course, living with Uncle Arter, their 'uncle-papa', in Hampshire. Being removed from their parents and siblings to an unfamiliar rural environment must have created a strong bond. They had both developed seizures at a young age and these had become 'so frequent and troublesome', according to Elizabeth, that their mother had been 'driven to death with them'.[21] Yet these were plainly not typical epileptic seizures. For when she was 'out of her senses', in Elizabeth's words, she could produce skilled needlework, such as an embroidered sampler featuring the alphabet and a verse from the Bible, which she had no recollection of having made once she recovered. Jane, by contrast, developed a malevolent streak in her delirium. At one point their mother entered the room just in time to prevent Jane using a gridiron to 'warm the baby on the fire'. When they were not gripped by seizures or acting under the influence of their delirium, the two girls were said to be 'patterns of good conduct and good feeling'.

It is now known that some forms of epilepsy do have a genetic link so that the children of parents who developed epilepsy in childhood are at a slightly increased risk of developing epilepsy themselves.[22] If a child develops epilepsy there is also a higher chance that a sibling will develop the condition; the younger the age of onset, the higher the risk to the sibling. So it is feasible that both Elizabeth and Jane suffered from the same condition. Their father also apparently had 'fainting fits'. Yet the description of their symptoms, especially their delirious states, suggests there was a psychological element to their illness. It is possible that one sister mimicked the other, probably subconsciously, in a mutually dependent form of self-deception known medically as shared psychosis or 'folie à deux'.[23]

A rare and controversial diagnosis, 'folie à deux' was first named by two French psychologists in 1877. It occurs when two individuals, usually closely related, share identical delusions and exhibit similar behaviour. Usually the more passive partner mimics the symptoms of the dominant person who has a genuine psychotic condition. In this case when the pair are separated, the symptoms in the passive partner generally disappear. However, in some cases both people develop a psychosis independently and then mimic each other in a mutually dependent cycle. In certain cases, the symptoms may be shared among three or more people.

In the case of the Okey sisters, Elizabeth seemed to be the more dominant sibling and perhaps this would explain why Jane's seizures improved when she was first discharged from hospital. Yet they may have been equally dependent since it was Jane who had first been admitted to UCH, with Elizabeth only following later. No doubt Jane had missed her sister during the eight months they were apart. But it is also conceivable that she was jealous of the celebrity her older sibling was enjoying – being feted by famous authors and artists no less – and wanted to share in the limelight, whether consciously or not.

Yet there is another strange element lurking in the Okey sisters' past which may shed light on their behaviour. Clarke, *The Lancet* student-reporter, would later claim that, when she was younger, Elizabeth had 'spoken in tongues' at evangelical church services led by the firebrand Scottish preacher Edward Irving.[24] The allegation, which first surfaced in *The Lancet* in 1838, would haunt the Okey sisters all their lives.

Born in 1792, Edward Irving had been ordained into the Church of Scotland but, devoid of wealthy connections, had been forced to move to London and take charge of a virtually defunct church in Hatton Garden. A scholarly and eloquent man, who was good-looking and charismatic, he managed to build up a popular following. Indeed his powerful sermons attracted such a large and fashionable crowd that a new National Scotch Church was built in Regent Square, in Bloomsbury, to accommodate the 2,000 people who flocked to his services. But carried away by his success, Irving made wild prophecies – predicting the Second Coming of Christ in the year 1868 – and spurred his followers to frenzied contortions and incoherent ravings described as speaking in 'unknown tongues'. He was expelled from the Church of Scotland for heresy in 1833 but continued preaching to his followers in hired rooms in the West End and Islington Green for a further year before returning to Scotland where he died in 1834.

It was at Islington Green, Clarke would claim, that Elizabeth Okey had become 'one of the foremost actors in the farce of the "unknown tongues"'. As *The Lancet* later reported, she 'arose during the service, prophesied, and spoke the "unknown tongues" so clamourously that the deacons were induced to lead her out of the midst of the congregation'. Elliotson would later dismiss the story as 'a pure malicious invention of an unfeeling mind' and insist the Okey girls were never Irvingites.[25]

Yet the claim is not unreasonable. Elizabeth would have been thirteen at most when Irving was presiding over his services in London. The family lived near Islington at the time and they were dissenters from about 1830 onwards, so it is conceivable that they joined Irving's congregation. If that were the case, then the girls' nonsensical babble could well have been inspired by the Irvingites' 'unknown tongues' and it is possible they joined in. As *The Times* shrewdly remarked, 'these follies are contagious'.[26] Yet equally Clarke may have associated the sisters with the Irving church simply *because* they spoke gibberish. And whereas the Irvingites were described as speaking an unintelligible, foreign-sounding babble, the Okeys always jumbled, mangled or repeated English words and phrases. As Elliotson said: 'Their language was peculiar. Almost every word was spoiled, and always spoiled in the same way: but spoiled by each differently: and each had a strange mode of expressing herself and of introducing certain superfluous words between words and syllables. For example, for opportunity, one said opporwaytunywhatsty. Mr Wood was always Mr Waywood.'[27] In truth it sounded more like an invented adolescent language than speaking in tongues.

Whatever the history to their strange illness, Elliotson was naturally excited by the chance to study the two sisters together. In many ways ahead of his time, prefiguring Freudian psychoanalytical ideas, he posited that their delirious episodes were 'perfect specimens of double consciousness'. Like her sister, Jane adopted the notion that Elliotson was their father and Wood their mother, though it must be said that Elliotson and Wood did nothing to dispel – and often encouraged – these unwholesome ideas. 'If one of us disappeared, the elder began to cry,' Elliotson wrote, 'and on being told the other had swallowed him, firmly believed it, and entreated the other to pull him up again; and on pretending to do this and the absentee suddenly showing himself, would be overpowered with joy and thank the other.' Intrigued by Jane's strange symptoms, Elliotson could barely wait to mesmerise her.

*

The day after Jane was admitted Elliotson visited the ward to examine her for the first time. She had had a seizure earlier that day and was now delirious. Without contemplating any of the usual medicines, he immediately extended his hand towards her face. In less than two minutes her head slumped, her eyes closed and she could not be roused. When Elliotson rubbed her forehead she woke but was delirious again. After mesmerising her twice more and waking her again into delirium, he allowed her to stay in a trance and she remained in this state for the next twenty hours. Elliotson was ecstatic. Jane responded to mesmerism even more readily and profoundly than her sister. When she was in a trance Jane seemed 'petrified' as if turned to marble, he enthused, while her countenance became 'truly heavenly' like that which 'enraptures painters'.[28] Naturally he was impatient to share the news.

By now the stream of visitors trailing through the wards to witness the mesmeric experiments had grown again, to such an extent that Elliotson sometimes had to transfer his demonstrations to the lecture theatre or even the operating theatre. He was inundated with requests, he later said, from students, medical men, scientists, MPs, journalists and others, including 'the highest nobility and even royalty'.[29] Coyly he did not divulge which member of the royal family he meant, but the Duke of Sussex, Prince Augustus Frederick, who was Queen Victoria's uncle as well as president of the Royal Society, was certainly one visitor. In using the operating theatre to exhibit his patients, Elliotson reasoned he had as much right as any of the surgeons. At one point, therefore, Hannah Hunter was carried to the theatre in a mesmeric trance and laid out on the operating table completely comatose. She awoke in terror at seeing the rows of strange men ogling at her and had to be pacified by 'our shaking hands with her and laughing', Elliotson said.

On Saturday 3 March Elliotson duly requisitioned the operating theatre to present Jane to the scientific world for the first time. It was probably the largest demonstration of mesmerism to date and the benches were packed with medical practitioners, students and journalists. A journalist from the *Morning Post*, who had already seen Elizabeth and Hannah being mesmerised several times, reported excitedly: 'Another patient, a younger sister of epileptic O'Key, has been admitted, and proves to be more susceptible of mesmeric influence than either her sister or Hannah Hunter, but displays different phenomena.'[30] Jane more than fulfilled their expectations. On being mesmerised she fell into a trance within twenty seconds then woke up delirious when rubbed on her forehead. As Elliotson demonstrated Jane's alternating states over and again, the *Morning Post* reporter noted the expression on her face switched from 'wildness to lethargy' with astonishing speed so that she was 'momentarily mad, momentarily dead'. She dropped into a stupor in mid-sentence when Elliotson rubbed her forehead, then when he repeated the action picked up exactly where she had left off. Almost lost for words himself to describe the scene, the reporter urged: 'It must be seen; and even then it cannot be conceived.'

Over the ensuing months Elliotson concentrated his experiments on the Okey sisters and to a lesser extent on Hannah. While other patients were treated with mesmerism and sent home cured, these three remained in hospital as subjects for his research and exhibits for his spectators. On one occasion, for example, he made the three girls hold hands and sent them simultaneously to sleep.[31] In this trance they synchronised their movements in accordance with his actions. Like the players at one of his musical soirees, the girls responded to his commands as if obeying a conductor. At times it seemed as if Hannah too had been drawn into the Okeys' strange dependency. At one point, when a patient had her tonsils removed on the ward, the sight of blood so terrified all three that they developed seizures simultaneously.[32]

Yet Hannah could never match the Okey girls for sheer theatre. Jane could mesmerise herself if she extended her fingers towards her face and was sent to sleep simply by someone blowing on her eyelids from a yard away. Meanwhile her seizures declined and her general condition improved. She dropped her constant use of the word 'little' and became 'much quieter, less quarrelsome and more sensible' when delirious, although she displayed strong affection for certain people – her sister, Elliotson and Wood in particular – and equally strong dislike for others. For no apparent reason, Herbert Mayo aroused her scorn. As Elliotson recorded, 'she will tell him in the most angry tone, that she "cannot bear him," that she "likes him worse than the devil"'.[33]

Yet despite this improvement in her health there was no chance of Jane being sent home. She was far too interesting for that. The two 'sister-patients', as they were dubbed by the *Morning Post*, seemed to work in tandem. Like her sister, Jane sang, swore, joked, flirted, cavorted and insulted spectators, including the professor. Like Elizabeth,

Jane was a passive, sweet-natured young woman when returned to her normal senses. When they faced each other and pressed their palms together they both fell into a swoon. They were mirror images, perfectly reflecting each other; they were a compelling double act who kept their all-male audiences enthralled.

Evidently enjoying being the centre of attention as much as the Okeys did, Elliotson concocted ludicrous and even sadistic trials to astound the scientific world. 'At first the experiments on the O'Keys were quite legitimate and intelligible,' wrote Clarke, *The Lancet* journalist, 'but they soon became of a most objectionable character.'[34] Early in 1838 Elliotson's attention focused on the ability of mesmerism to banish pain. In February he invited guests to watch as Elizabeth had a seton threaded through the back of her neck while mesmerised. Throughout the process she chattered away and 'never altered a feature or a tone' as Wood inserted the needle and thread.[35] Elliotson would later describe the event as the 'first operation rendered painless in Great Britain by mesmerism'. No doubt he believed the seton was a useful therapeutic measure. But other experiments were designed purely to test their threshold of pain.

On 23 April Elliotson invited a large audience to one of the theatres at UCH.[36] He first demonstrated the standard phenomena in Hannah and the Okeys – but this was becoming routine. Then he produced a powerful galvanic battery. His friend, Charles Wheatstone, one of the country's foremost experts on electricity, gallantly agreed to operate the apparatus. At Elliotson's signal, Wheatstone connected Elizabeth to the machine and exposed her to the current for a full three minutes. Although her hands contracted, she showed no sign of pain or stress. Incredulous at what they had seen, several of the male spectators, including the MP Sir William Molesworth, gamely volunteered to test their strength. None could withstand the shock for more than thirty seconds. The experiment was repeated on Hannah, who showed 'no appearance of pain in the face', then Jane, who displayed 'perfect indifference, and seeming freedom from all pain'. Finally a Leyden jar, a device used to store static electricity, was charged and all three girls were exposed to the current in turn. Asked afterwards what she had felt, Elizabeth said she heard the galvanic machine 'go giggle, giggle, giggle' and added: 'I saw the light.'

Molesworth was so impressed by this spectacle that he donated 30 guineas to UCH for Elliotson to continue his research and 'extend the bounds of science'.[37] The reporter from the *Morning Post* was in no doubt of the significance of the phenomenon. 'If by this means painful operations may be performed without the knowledge of the patient, why do surgeons hesitate for one moment to put its efficacy more extensively to the test?' Why indeed?

Some experiments seemed more bent on testing the stoicism – or veracity – of the patients than extending the 'bounds of science'. Even Elliotson had to admit his trials sometimes went too far, especially in the case of Elizabeth. 'Some persons chose to doubt the reality of her anaesthesia, and stuck pins in her, and made various experiments which they thought would hurt her,' he later wrote.[38] *The Lancet* reporter Clarke witnessed spectators attempting tests 'of a very cruel kind' on the Okey girls without – he said – Elliotson's knowledge.[39] On one occasion, a needle was found embedded in Jane's arm. Another witness recalled seeing a sharp instrument being inserted under Elizabeth's fingernail.

Other experiments were more comical than cruel. On 24 April, the day after the electricity demonstration, Elliotson invited a small party of men to witness what was undoubtedly his most ridiculous exhibition so far. To the guests' astonishment, he introduced a cat which lived on the ward (presumably it served a vital role in keeping down vermin). Gravely he raised the animal up and down in front of Elizabeth to ascertain whether it could exert the same influence as a human mesmerist. Not surprisingly, the feline proved devoid of mesmerising power. He repeated the experiment substituting the cat for a 'small child' with similarly ineffectual results. The afternoon grew curiouser and curiouser. Elliotson next introduced a seven-year-old girl – there was plainly no shortage of juvenile subjects – and instructed her to mesmerise Elizabeth, with partial success. At that point he placed his hand on the young girl's shoulder and asked four of the observers to do the same to add their strength to the mesmeric force. Sure enough, 'the somnambulist dropt her head on her bosom insensible', according to Mayo, who was now furnishing weekly despatches to the *LMG*.[40] It was in one of these reports that he coined the term 'trance' to describe the mesmeric sleep.

Elliotson's feline experiment was part of a wider fascination with the reaction of animals to 'animal magnetism'. Even if the UCH mouser had proved unable to mesmerise Elizabeth, it was soon discovered that certain animals were just as susceptible to mesmerism as humans. Encouraged by Elliotson's experiments, some of the medical students decided to try their skills on a lapdog, whose owner was a regular visitor to UCH. Discovering they could easily mesmerise the pooch into a stupor, the pupils 'sought every opportunity to exercise their *magnetic* power over the little beast' – much to its owner's annoyance.[41] The dog always fell into such a deep trance that it could only be roused by 'pulling its ears, or swinging it about by the tail', *The Lancet* gleefully reported. The wards at UCH may have been crowded, but at least it was possible to swing a lapdog.

Elsewhere in the capital, one physician attempted to mesmerise two girls in his hospital. Not only did they succumb to the mesmeric influence, they now amused themselves by mesmerising their ward's cat. The animal 'exhibited all the phenomena of *catalepsy*', *The Lancet* archly noted. Not to be outdone, the *LMG* described historic tales of dogs, horses and birds being stupefied when stared at. An Irishman had become so adept at calming wild horses by fixing them with his gaze, the journal revealed, that he had earned the nickname the 'Whisperer' – perhaps the first to enjoy that sobriquet. One physician was determined to put such anecdotal stories to scientific test.

In spring 1838 John Wilson, the Middlesex Hospital physician who had introduced Dupotet to Elliotson, launched a series of experiments to test the effects of mesmerism on a variety of animals, ranging from cats to lions.[42] Having dragooned friends and family into letting him experiment on their pets and farmyard animals, Wilson found he could induce sleep in cats and dogs, including a tomcat that could be lifted by the nape of its neck and have its ears tickled without stirring, and a female terrier named Vick, who curled up happily with a cat named Fuzzy (Wilson gave the names of most of the animals, though not their owners). Three ducks and a drake proved harder to influence but eventually grew drowsy, though Wilson was disconcerted when two died from mysterious causes a month later. Moving quickly on, he tried his skills on a tubful of fish hauled from the Thames that proved so receptive they let him stroke their backs. Similar effects were produced in geese, turkeys, a calf, some pigs, three macaws – Laura, Mac and Carl – and a famous but unidentified racehorse.

Emboldened by his success, Wilson took his charming talents to Surrey Zoological Gardens, a menagerie near Vauxhall that specialised in staging re-enactments of the eruption of Mount Vesuvius and the

Fire of London. His experiments on two leopards proved unconvincing, since they spent most of the day sleeping anyway. Next he tried to mesmerise a lioness but although she ceased growling there was no further effect. Finally Wilson used his arts on two Ceylon elephants, Rajah and Hadgee. Angered by his hand motions, they lashed out at him with their trunks, but after repeated efforts the female became drowsy and the male dozed for several minutes. At this stage, Wilson thought it best to retire gracefully, reasoning that if any of the wild animals turned delirious havoc might ensue.

Fuelled by accounts of these strange experiments and remarkable cures – not to mention levitating cats and whirling lapdogs – mesmerism was now the main topic of conversation at every social gathering, from East End taverns to West End clubs. Butcher-boys and barristers argued over whether Elliotson's discoveries represented the greatest advance in medicine to date, or a prime example of quackery. Costermongers and countesses debated whether the Okey sisters were poor unfortunates or cunning frauds. The media was divided; the medical and scientific communities were split.

'This singular subject is daily attracting more attention, and the contest respecting the reality or deceptiveness of the resulting phenomena is becoming more and more interesting,' reported the *Morning Post*.[43] Having observed Elizabeth at close quarters on several occasions, the *Post* had no doubts. 'We have conversed with the poor child in her ordinary state as she sat by the fire in her ward, suffering from the headache, which persecutes her almost continuously when not under the soothing influence of the magnetic operation, and we confess we never beheld anybody less likely to prove an imposter.' In her natural senses she was 'an intelligent gentle little girl' without any defect in language, though 'very pale' from being repeatedly bled. Yet when mesmerised 'all good sense appears lost' and she 'chatters away her gipsy patois, free from head-ache, untroubled by prudential considerations, unconscious of any operations, however painful, which may be performed on her'. The reporter from the *Globe* was more circumspect.[44] After watching Hannah and the Okey girls run through their usual performances, he remarked, 'we cannot say how far training might have perfected the girls in the part they played.' However, he concluded on balance that it was unlikely they were acting.

Other journalists were adamant the demonstrations were blatant trickery and the Okey sisters conniving fakes, quite possibly in collusion with their doctor. The *Satirist*, a Sunday newspaper which specialised in publishing scandal about prominent members of society, launched a tirade against Elliotson headlined 'Another Mesmerian Mountebank'.[45] The newspaper had already attacked Dupotet, still hosting his salons at this point, not only denouncing him as a charlatan but also charging him with sexual impropriety. While expressing 'disgust' at the baron's overly familiar physical contact with his female subjects, the journal supplied titillating detail, and even went so far as to suggest that his subjects – including the former UCH patient Lucy Clarke – were really prostitutes trained to collaborate with his tricks. Branding Elliotson as a 'mountebank' along with Dupotet, it urged fathers to 'be warned against committing their sons to his tuition' and the public to steer clear of his care.

Furthermore, the newspaper denounced 'Miss Oky', Elizabeth, as not only a fraud but a minx. It claimed she had been selected by Dupotet from his 'well-trained Coventry-court squad' – Coventry Court being a notorious haunt of prostitutes – even though she was, of course, already a patient at UCH when the baron arrived there. If she did not actually suffer from nymphomania, the journal suggested, then she 'certainly knows at least how to imitate the symptoms of that malady'. It went on to describe Elizabeth's behaviour towards Elliotson in sexualised terms. At one demonstration she had wrapped 'her dear magnetised arms round his neck and kissed him' and 'hugged the Doctor vehemently'. It speculated that the rapt students watching the demonstration could barely wait to try mesmerism for themselves 'first upon all their female cousins, and afterwards upon as many of their friends' wives and daughters as they could persuade to let them'.

In the light of such diverse reports, the medical profession was in a quandary. While some practitioners scoffed at Elliotson's outlandish exhibitions and implausible cures, others were eager to try the therapy for themselves – if not on their cousins at least on their charity patients. One surgeon, Samuel Sandys, in Kentish Town, tried mesmerising a forty-two-year-old seamstress who had suffered for years from dyspepsia, vomiting, skin complaints and assorted other ailments, which he grouped under the catch-all diagnosis 'hysteria'.[46] After fifty minutes he found she was insensitive to pain – even when she was cupped, bled with a scarificator (a fiendish device with rotating blades), and had a catheter inserted. Mesmerised daily she woke 'quite sensible' and 'much refreshed', he told the *LMG*.

Likewise, a physician, Thomas Chandler, who was a former pupil of Elliotson's based in Rotherhithe, thought mesmerism might help an eighteen-year-old youth suffering from rheumatism and delirium. First he tried mesmerising his wife, who laughed at the idea but after fifteen minutes fell soundly asleep. Encouraged by this success, Chandler mesmerised his patient daily for ten days. Gradually the youth's dementia reduced and finally ceased altogether, Chandler told *The Lancet* in April, as the man's father and two medical men who had witnessed the treatment would happily confirm.[47]

Another practitioner, J. N. Bainbridge, who treated inmates at St Martin's workhouse in Covent Garden, tried mesmerism on a twenty-nine-year-old woman who had suffered epilepsy since she was two.[48] The poor woman had been forced to enter the workhouse because her seizures prevented her from earning a living. Despite having 'ransacked the Pharmacopaeia for medicines', nothing helped. In desperation Bainbridge instructed one of his pupils to try mesmerism. To their mutual amazement, the woman fell into a trance in five minutes and had suffered no return of her seizures since.

Most dramatically, when Hannah Hunter returned home to Dover in April her case created a sensation among the local medical men. Many had previously witnessed her paralysis and were now astounded to see her walk across a room. Reading out grateful letters from Hannah and her mother at one of his lectures, Elliotson said she had 'attracted great attention' since the 'remarkable influences of Mesmerism upon her [had] been demonstrated before almost, if not all the medical men in that town'.[49] As Clarke put it, 'Even sceptics shook their heads, and, whilst declaring their unbelief in many of the phenomena' had to concede 'there was something in it'.[50]

Outside the medical sphere, the wider scientific community was intrigued by Elliotson's findings. Dionysius Lardner, a former Professor of Natural Philosophy and Astronomy at UCL, helped Elliotson conduct his experiments using mirrors and published admiring accounts in the *Monthly Chronicle*.[51] The young naturalist Richard Owen, who would later coin the word 'dinosaur', put his unsung talents to work testing Elizabeth Okey's skills in mimicry by making 'certain grimaces with one side of his nose, which he only of the party could make'.[52] Naturally she copied his movements perfectly. And Michael Faraday, now dividing his time between the study of electricity and magnets, added his efforts by testing the veracity of mesmerism. Suspecting the UCH patients of acting, Faraday did his best to trick Hannah Hunter into waking from her trance. First he tried to bring a blush to her cheeks by making rude remarks and when this had no effect he loudly proposed bleeding her and cauterising the wound with a red-hot poker. Obligingly Elliotson bound the girl's arm in readiness yet still this 'produced not the slightest effect upon her countenance or pulse'.[53]

While the eminent scientists who queued up to pull faces and shout abuse at Elliotson's patients were almost exclusively male, at least one female spectator also attended his demonstrations. One of the first women elected an honorary fellow of the Royal Astronomical Society, Mary Somerville was described by one contemporary as 'the most extraordinary woman in Europe'.[54] Friendly with Faraday and others in the RS circle, she attended one of Elliotson's demonstrations in early 1838. The *LMG* was eager to discover what impression the exhibition had made 'on a woman of Mrs Somerville's acute and scientific mind' and asked: 'Was she as much astonished and as thoroughly satisfied as the gentlemen were?' Sadly she never recorded her views.

By the end of April 1838, Elliotson had entranced the arts world, intrigued the medical profession and captivated the scientific community with his discoveries. His investigations were being avidly followed in the medical journals and national press. They were the talk of high society and the chatter of the streets; he had even enthralled royalty. Yet his colleagues at the university remained stubbornly unmoved. Within the medical faculty only three men – Robert Grant, Professor of Comparative Anatomy, John Lindley, Professor of Botany, and Thomas Graham, Professor of Chemistry – had deigned to witness his demonstrations, and not one of his fellow medical practitioners had attended.[55] Even reports of Hannah Hunter lying comatose in the operating theatre had not lured Liston or his fellow surgeons to view this beguiling phenomenon for themselves – or ponder whether it might prove useful to their writhing victims. But the university could not continue to ignore the sensational events taking place across the road in Gower Street and Elliotson's enemies now seized the opportunity to act.

7

The Prophetess of St Pancras

University College Hospital, London, 1 May 1838

In a corner of the hospital three men huddled together. They were not, for once, visitors come to witness Elliotson's experiments, but fellow professors determined to stop them. Anthony Todd Thomson, one of the most senior members of the medical staff, wrote out the letter in his neat sloping hand and signed his name at the bottom.[1] The other two, Robert Liston and David Davis, added their signatures. The letter was short and succinct – a single sentence on a single page. But for all its brevity, there could be no doubt – it was an act of professional treachery.

Liston and Thomson had become allies through shared circumstances and interests. Both Scots, both outspoken, both tall and powerful men, they disliked Elliotson with a mutual intensity. Thomson, now sixty, had joined the university when it opened in 1828 as Professor of Materia Medica but once Elliotson arrived he had never been able to match his fellow physician for reputation or popularity.[2] Although his textbook on medicines, *Elements of Materia Medica and Therapeutics*, was regarded as the 'best work' on the subject, Thomson was considered a poor lecturer and an indecisive practitioner in contrast with his eloquent and charismatic colleague. One student, *The Lancet* reporter Clarke, put it bluntly: 'Thomson was deficient in most of the natural gifts which belonged to his colleague.'

Liston, still nursing his grudge against Elliotson, had been quick to spot an ally. Having learned through bitter experience to master his temper in meetings, Liston had been biding his time. At last the pair had managed to recruit Davis, UCL's Professor of Midwifery, to their cause. Welsh-born Davis, a few months older than Thomson, had joined the medical faculty at the same time. Davis had been drawn to obstetrics when his own son had died after a difficult birth. Having risen to become a favourite midwife to society, he had attended the birth of the future Queen Victoria. Although Davis had enthusiastically promoted Elliotson's appointment in 1831, now his support had waned. The continual flood of visitors in the wards and theatres, the sensational headlines in the newspapers and bizarre accounts in the medical press, the salacious gossip at dinner parties and knowing winks in private clubs, had become too much. All three were now convinced Elliotson's experiments were damaging the reputation of the university, and impeding the work of the hospital.

The storm clouds had been gathering for some time. In March, the university's management committee – responsible for running the hospital – had asked the medical faculty to investigate complaints that the crowds at Elliotson's experiments were causing 'inconvenience to patients' and 'injury to the property of the establishment'.[3] In April Elliotson had stoutly defended himself when he assured the medical committee that 'no inconvenience' had resulted to patients from mesmerism and the damage to the furniture in the operating theatre was 'insignificant' or 'such as is liable to occur when a large number is collected to witness the performance of a Surgical Operation'. The medical committee, chaired by Richard Quain, usually Elliotson's ally, had meekly accepted Elliotson's explanation.

Yet the complaints had not gone away. The clinical clerks had been grumbling at the hours they spent each day 'pawing' the patients in their efforts to mesmerise them. 'Some of the gentlemen so engaged were worn out by this really very serious labour,' said Clarke.[4] Other staff had been muttering about the fact that Elizabeth Okey had now spent more than a year in hospital when rule 104 plainly stipulated that no patient should stay longer than two months.[5] One professor protested that he was unable to find beds for his own patients because Elliotson kept his patients in hospital for so long in order to mesmerise them.[6] Finally Lord

Brougham, the university's co-founder and president, had come to find out what all the fuss was about.

Brougham had turned up to a demonstration in the lecture theatre at the end of March with two friends, the radical MPs Sir William Molesworth and Richard Sheil.[7] Although Molesworth was convinced by what he saw, Brougham and Sheil remained doubtful. Another observer that day, the former lawyer Henry Crabb Robinson, who was a member of UCL's council, said the Okey sisters – whom he insisted on describing as Irish – 'talked in a *strange* voice & with the naïf humour of Irish children calling students by their names'.[8] While Robinson reserved judgement, Sheil accused Elliotson outright of coaching the girls. According to Robinson, 'he tht. the Doctor talked too much & was intelligible to the children'. At length Sheil declared himself incredulous, while Brougham quarrelled with Elliotson about his experimental methods and stomped out.

There was one point, at least, on which everyone was agreed. The last thing the university and its hospital needed was more hostile publicity. Beset by constant criticism and deepening financial problems, UCL was already in a parlous state. Conservative forces were determined to discredit the liberal institution, while recent fluctuations in the financial markets had hit hard. Plans had been drawn up for a new wing at the hospital to provide much-needed beds, yet lack of funds had delayed the work, while the rising cost of medicines and supplies – most notably leeches – had exacerbated the problems.[9] Constraints on funds had also prompted the medical committee to cut patients' rations earlier in the year, while the fabric of the hospital was looking decidedly shabby. Henry Crabb Robinson thought UCH looked 'beggarly' compared with the ostentatious university building across the road.[10]

The question of whether mesmerism was a genuine therapy that might actually help or even heal patients was largely immaterial to most of the university's professors and council members. It was the damage that Elliotson's experiments were causing to the institutions' reputation which concerned them. Although the university still commanded the support of the Whig government and the hospital now boasted Queen Victoria as its patron, both institutions were on shaky ground. The letter, which Thomson, Liston and Davis put their names to on 1 May, seized on this anxiety.

Having failed so far to limit Elliotson's experiments, the three professors now asked Quain to convene a special meeting of the medical committee to determine whether 'the continued exhibitions of Animal Magnetism be not detrimental to the character and the interests both of the College and of the Hospital'. Given the circumstances, it was a valid concern. Yet there can be no doubt – in the case of Liston and Thomson, if not necessarily Davis – that their main motivation was to attack and undermine their detested rival Elliotson. They had thrown down the gauntlet; now they waited for battle to commence.

Eager to resolve the dispute quietly – and spare the university further embarrassing headlines – Quain tried to broker a peaceful solution. Since Elliotson still commanded the biggest class within the medical school – and never tired of reminding his colleagues of this fact – Quain knew he had to tread carefully.[11] At first, therefore, he met privately with Elliotson and urged him to halt his demonstrations at UCH. Quain pleaded that 'whether the wonderful facts were true or not, and whether great benefit in the treatment of diseases would result or not, we ought to consider the interests of the school'.[12] Both Davis and Samuel Cooper, the Professor of Surgery, also made informal appeals, suggesting that Elliotson should hold the exhibitions at his own house instead. Elliotson, however, was in no mood for compromise.

In characteristically pompous style, Elliotson replied that the university had been created for 'the dissemination and discovery of truth' and that 'if the public were ignorant, we should enlighten them'. Yet it was his own colleagues, he plainly thought, that were in need of enlightenment. Elliotson was incredulous that his fellows had refused to witness – let alone acknowledge – the value of his work. Even though the wards contained 'cases innumerable, of diseases physicked and tormented to no purpose', mesmerism was 'as little thought of as steam carriages, electro-telegraphs, the penny post, or Handel or Beethoven's music, among the Caffres or Calmucks'.[13]

His fury was understandable. The medical profession was still enslaved to bleeding patients until they fainted for conditions ranging from typhus fever to typhoid – often fatally weakening the body's natural defences. In 1837–38 the *LMG* published a series of fifteen lectures devoted to the benefits of bloodletting in which the esteemed physician Henry Clutterbuck advised there were few diseases for which bloodletting was not advantageous.[14] Elliotson could bleed, purge and blister with the best of them – but when he saw even a glimmer of hope in an alternative remedy he was at least prepared to give it a go. At the same time, of course, he was not known for his persuasive skills and did not waste his breath attempting to mollify his colleagues. As he had shown time and time again, whenever he felt himself opposed, he simply dug in his heels and refused to give way. Far from encouraging him to scale down his investigations, therefore, the opposition of his colleagues made him determined to continue. Refusing to heed the warning signs, he believed he was invincible.

And so, just two days after Thomson, Liston and Davis had signed their demand for an inquiry, on 3 May Elliotson paraded the Okey sisters before another large assembly in the UCH lecture theatre. A journalist from the *Morning Post*, who devoted two successive columns to the demonstration, reported that the 'sister-patients' could be mesmerised from as far away as twelve feet, by holding hands with each other and even – 'start not, most sceptical reader!' – through a door.[15] 'Never was anything so ludicrously convincing!' the writer proclaimed. Not everyone was as impressed. The diarist Henry Crabb Robinson, who had kept an open mind when watching the Okey girls previously, attended the demonstration with his friend, the artist John James Masquerier. Robinson confessed himself 'disgusted' by the scenes, while Masquerier was 'made ill by what he saw'.[16] Robinson thought Elliotson made too much spectacle of the experiments and wrote: 'Unless he soon shew the application to science or medical use they will only excite disgust.' He had a point. Enjoying celebrity just as the Okeys did, Elliotson's approach was veering towards that of a professional showman, rather than a medical professional.

Yet the mesmerism show continued. A week later Elliotson staged the major demonstration of 10 May – the largest so far – when Elizabeth entertained some 300 invited guests, including the one-legged Marquess of Anglesey, with her repertoire of pantomime and ribaldry, culminating in her rendition of the musical favourite 'Jim Crow'.[17] It was at this demonstration that Elliotson revealed to his audience the moves afoot within the university to halt his experiments and gave a spirited defence of his research.

Opinions within the medical and scientific world were becoming deeply entrenched. Throughout May, most of the chief medical and scientific societies in the capital were transfixed by the subject. On 8 May, Samuel Merriman, treasurer of the Royal Medical and Chirurgical Society, proposed that the society should launch a special committee to investigate mesmerism.[18] Elliotson had served as president of the RMCS for two years, though he rarely attended since stepping down in 1835. The society's council voted emphatically against.

Within the Royal Society, however, Elliotson's supporters were actively investigating the phenomenon. Mayo had succeeded in recruiting a committee of nine leading scientists, including Elliotson and himself, all members of the RS physiological committee, as Elliotson had proudly announced at his demonstration on 10 May. This was not, as Elliotson's enemies were quick to point out, an official investigation – for the RS had no powers to undertake such an inquiry – but an ad hoc grouping of members with an interest in the field of medicine. Nevertheless, the team comprised some of the most respected scientists of the day. Faraday had been too busy to lend his aid, but alongside Mayo, Elliotson and Charles Wheatstone, the team included Peter Mark Roget, the RS permanent secretary, who would later compile the reference work for which his name is now synonymous; Robert Grant, Professor of Comparative Anatomy at UCL, who was regarded as Britain's foremost expert on his subject; and Neil Arnott, who was physician-extraordinary to Queen Victoria.

Both *The Lancet* and the *LMG* welcomed the inquiry, although the latter expressed concern that the committee's members were not all qualified doctors, since anyone unacquainted with 'the diseases of females' should beware of 'the almost marvellous things that women will do, and say, and suffer, under some forms of hysteria'.[19] The *Morning Post* was delighted mesmerism was to be submitted to 'a rigid scrutiny' by distinguished individuals who were 'not likely to fall into the sin and shame of credulity'.[20] But just in case the committee needed a lead, the newspaper added: 'Our own opinion is already formed, by frequent and attentive observation, that the extraordinary effects produced in Dr Elliotson's lecture-room are real and unsophisticated.'

Debates over whether the effects of mesmerism were real or not were also raging at the Medico-Botanical Society on 23 May when Earl Stanhope, now a committed supporter of mesmerism, took the chair.[21] One member, the society's librarian Dr John Hancock, proclaimed that mesmerism 'indisputably' provided an efficient means of pain relief to those susceptible, which could 'disarm all surgical operations of their terrors'. Another, Dr Daniel Macreight, from the Middlesex Hospital, revealed he had successfully used mesmerism to treat a patient with ulcerations of the eye as well as 'various afflictions' in children. He rejected the popular notion that mesmerism only worked on 'weakly' people – by which he meant mainly women – citing the case of an army colonel, no less, who had been put into a trance. Macreight went on to relate the story of a young woman who, in a trance, had instructed her doctor to give her a particular medicine. She had not only described the drug in question – 'a red medicine' – but told him where to find it, 'the sixth bottle on the second shelf in your medicine chest'. After taking the drug, she was soon cured. Despite his credulity, Macreight made an astute observation. Mesmerism, he said, was 'not a cure for a disease' but 'a cure for particular persons'. In other words, it worked on the minds of certain individuals rather than their bodies.

Yet George Sigmond, who had boasted of his success in mesmerising more than 100 people six months earlier, now told the society he was doubtful of mesmerism's curative powers and feared – with good reason, judging from the effects on the Okey sisters – that it might aggravate conditions such as epilepsy. Mesmerism should 'not be trifled with'. Nevertheless, he assured the meeting, he was continuing his investigations to determine which type of people were most susceptible to its influence. He speculated that mesmerism worked best on those with fair hair and blue eyes.

Discussions were even more heated a few days later at the Medical Society of London, Britain's oldest medical society, founded in 1773.[22] John Burne, a physician at Westminster Hospital, set the tone by bluntly alleging that Elizabeth Okey was an 'imposter'. Having twice witnessed the demonstrations at UCH, Burne complained that Elliotson generally announced in advance what he expected to see, which easily enabled Elizabeth to comply. This was undeniably true since Elliotson frequently commanded observers to 'watch her fall asleep' or 'mark what she does now' at which cue Elizabeth would invariably perform the expected function. Whenever Elizabeth could hear or see the professor, Burne said, her responses were perfect, yet when she could not her reactions were inconsistent. When Elliotson sat behind Elizabeth to demonstrate her ability to mimic his facial movements, 'he snapped his teeth so loudly that the noise could be distinctly heard at the distance of several feet'.

Furthermore, Burne griped, Elizabeth's eyelashes overhung her eyes so far it was impossible to tell if they were open or closed. Since 'the Magnetiser was above suspicion', Burne charged that Elizabeth and her fellow patients were acting; while critics always felt free to accuse the Okeys of deceit, it was generally inconceivable that Elliotson, a scholar and a gentleman, could be anything other than genuine.

Yet others taking part in the MSL debate were equally ardent in defending mesmerism. One physician, James Bennett, had observed that Elizabeth went through certain physiological changes in her trance, such as decreased skin temperature and a faster pulse, which were impossible to fake. He may have been on to something with this. Although the jury is still out, recent research has shown that hypnotism may produce physiological changes such as altered heartbeat, while subjects have reported experiencing changes in temperature.[23]

Such tempestuous debates, which were copiously reported in the medical press, only served to fuel further interest in mesmerism and compel more enthusiasts to throng to Elliotson's demonstrations – exactly as his colleagues had feared. Every visitor to London with a penchant for scientific marvels now had to make a detour to UCH; indeed, the *Morning Post* urged its readers to 'go, and judge for themselves' while helpfully pointing out that the doors of the hospital were 'open to every gentleman who feels an interest in the subject'.[24] This, of course, was part of the problem as far as Elliotson's beleaguered colleagues were concerned.

As well as receiving British royalty, in the first half of 1838 Elliotson paid host to a New Zealand Maori chief. The unnamed visitor was brought to ward three by Edward Gibbon Wakefield, a feckless adventurer who was promoting the colonisation of Australasia. Contradicting prevailing opinion, the chief concluded that it was Elliotson, not Elizabeth, who was the fraud; he told Wakefield 'he knew how Dr Elliotson did it: Dr Elliotson had medicine up his sleeve'.[25] The demonstrations in May also attracted Earl Grey, the former Whig prime minister who had steered through the 1832 Reform Act and the abolition of slavery. Grey, now in his seventies, joined Sydney Smith, the high-living and well-upholstered canon of St Paul's Cathedral, who was a popular writer with a ready wit.[26] Smith's repartee, however, was no match for Elizabeth, who took one look at his corpulent figure and remarked that he looked as if he had 'never been put on the low diet in *her* ward'.

Regardless of the escalating concerns within the university, the mesmerism demonstrations continued, ever growing in size. Defiantly, at the end of May Elliotson went so far as to ask the UCL council for permission to stage his next exhibition in the university's own lecture theatre – which could seat nearly 1,000 people – rather than the smaller UCH theatre in order to describe the 'important philosophical & medicinal facts of the ill appreciated and stigmatised agency commonly known by the name of animal magnetism'.[27] He needed the extra space, he explained, because his experiments had attracted 'the earnest attention & wonder of the highest scientific characters of Oxford & Cambridge, of the Royal Society, King's College &c & of the great body of medical men engaged in private practice & in the public schools' along with a 'large number of peers & members of the house of Commons'. For all his declared distaste for 'fawning and crouching', Elliotson was never above dropping a few names.

William Tooke, the university treasurer, proposed that Elliotson should be allowed to deliver one lecture on the topic in the university theatre. He was seconded by Isaac Lyon Goldsmid, the Jewish financier and university co-founder, who was already a convert to mesmerism. But after a fierce debate the council voted eight to five to refuse permission. Robinson, the diarist, who sided with the minority, was worried the vote would prompt Elliotson to resign, which would be 'a serious evil' for the university.[28]

Despite the setbacks Elliotson was undaunted. That spring the nation was enraptured by the nineteen-year-old queen who was soon to be crowned at Westminster Abbey. At the same time, the country's most respected politicians, scientists, medical practitioners and writers were entranced by the two adolescent girls from the Somers Town slums who reigned supreme on the wards at UCH. To most of the visitors, Elizabeth and Jane appeared to be acting completely under the power of Elliotson and his medical disciples. Yet as their celebrity spread, so the Okey girls, especially Elizabeth, began to assert a more dominant role. As the strange scenes at the demonstration on 10 May suggested, at times it seemed that Elizabeth – not Elliotson – was running the show. Was this simply a further manifestation of the powers of the mesmeric influence? Or was she consciously taking control of events?

The seeds of this changing relationship had been sown earlier in the year when Elizabeth had been asked to mesmerise Hannah Hunter. No longer was Elizabeth simply the passive subject of the experiments; now she was an active participant in the investigations. From that point on Elizabeth was regularly invited to mesmerise other patients, including her sister, and gradually she began to take a more decisive role. During May she began to talk of a 'negro spirit' who spoke to her during trances. Previously, in one experiment, she had lifted an 80lb weight (nearly 40kg) without obvious strain. Clarke, who witnessed this spectacle, said 'the strongest man' could not have accomplished the feat. In fact, 80lb is well below the lowest level today in Olympic women's weightlifting – 106lb (48kg) – but it was still impressive for a seventeen-year-old on the 'low diet'. In May, however, Elizabeth announced that 'her negro' had told her that lifting the weight had sprained two of her ribs and warned she would be injured if she attempted the task again.[29] The notion of a 'negro spirit' may have been inspired by the song 'Jim Crow', which she had performed with such aplomb. Whatever his origins, the spirit certainly spoke sense.

Soon afterwards, Elizabeth began making predictions about her own medical progress. The first instance took place in mid-May when she announced in a trance that she would be taken ill with a pain in her side in precisely eighty-four hours.[30] A few days later she amended the prediction to eighty-five hours. Sure enough at 4 a.m. the following day – exactly eighty-five hours from her prophecy – she was 'seized with shivering' which was immediately diagnosed by Elliotson as 'acute rheumatism' stemming from inflammation in her side. The diagnosis was typically obscure; if the attack was thought to be rheumatic fever then this was a very mild episode. Yet several other doctors who witnessed her illness were convinced it was genuine.

This strange reversal in the standard doctor–patient relationship was entirely in line with reports emanating from the Continent. Though Elliotson had remained sceptical of these accounts so far, others such as Mayo and Lardner had reported them enthusiastically. Dupotet had assured Elliotson that 'mesmeric prevision' was a typical development in highly susceptible subjects and had predicted, within Elizabeth's hearing, that he would soon see examples of clairvoyance. Dupotet had since reported in the *LMG* that Lucy Clarke, the eighteen-year-old he had first treated at UCH, was now able to prescribe for her own illnesses.[31] Lucy had first predicted that she would be completely recovered by 30 November, he said, though this eventuality had suffered something of a setback when a jar of sand had fallen on her head; she had not predicted that. Regaining control, Lucy had instructed the baron to bleed her, to excise a scab which had developed where she had been blistered and – quite rightly – to remove a seton from her neck since it was 'useless'.

Then, on 1 June, Elizabeth confided in Wood during a trance that she would undergo a dramatic change in forty-eight hours' time.[32] Rushing for a pen and paper, Wood wrote down her predictions then sealed the note with wax. Excitedly he informed Elliotson of the latest development – though not the contents of the note. Elliotson was thrilled; finally he was going to witness some of the more elusive effects of mesmerism that the baron had long promised. In the meantime, as the clock ticked down, Elliotson readied himself for a further demonstration – the biggest and most spectacular of all – in the lecture theatre of UCH on Saturday 2 June.

It was a sultry and overcast day. By afternoon dark clouds were gathering overhead as the carriages queued outside the hospital entrance. The lecture theatre filled up quickly as spectators squeezed into 'every corner'. *The Lancet* reporter George Mills lamented that 'the comfort and satisfaction' of the audience would have been much enhanced had the university authorities granted Elliotson permission to use the vast and empty theatre in the university building across the road. As it was, Edward Stanley, the Bishop of Norwich, who was approaching sixty, had to stand for the entire three-hour performance while Thomas Moore, the Irish poet, had to sit on a shelf, eventually climbing down with his jacket covered in whitewash. Among the other spectators pressed into the airless room were assorted aristocrats, MPs, clergymen, barristers, professors and medical practitioners as well as Earl Stanhope and Isaac Lyon Goldsmid, according to Mills's ten-page report published over two successive weeks in *The Lancet*.[33]

As warm-up acts Elliotson introduced two young men who responded to mesmerism with indifferent results. Quickly despatched, their seats were taken by two female patients, a twenty-three-year-old woman with epilepsy and a girl with 'hysterical lock-jaw'. The latter condition, when the jaw is locked by a muscle spasm, is usually caused by tetanus but this case plainly had a psychological root. Both had been cured by mesmerism, Elliotson declared, and they promptly demonstrated their susceptibility by falling profoundly asleep. But everyone knew the star turns were still to come. When at last Elizabeth and Jane were ushered into the theatre they were already well known to most of the audience; by now they were celebrities in their own right. And, as ever, they performed their roles to perfection.

Although many of their capers had already been witnessed at previous demonstrations, others were 'quite new and more singular', Mills noted in *The Lancet*. Both girls, Mills explained, were now subject to four distinct states. These were, firstly, their natural state when they were 'very reserved and quiet'; secondly, a delirious state when they became vivacious and familiar; thirdly, a fixed state when they could be petrified in mid-sentence by a single wave of a finger; and fourthly, a deep sleep from which they could not be roused. The sisters obligingly demonstrated all four states, though it was the comic excesses of their delirium which held the audience spellbound.

First mesmerised to sleep and then woken into delirium, Elizabeth kicked off the show by marching up to Colonel Charles Yorke, a veteran of the Battle of Waterloo, and snatching his hat. She kindly offered to 'make it tidy' – as befits a former housemaid, she was obsessed with cleanliness – then mooned over his 'beauty white eyes'. At this point she noticed the packed benches for the first time and exclaimed: 'What a many white people here are.' She started counting the guests, beginning, 'Sit away one, sit away two, sit away three' in her crazed babble before Elliotson put her to sleep. Immediately, Jane perked up, hugged her dozing sister, and declared: 'Oh, you silly thing, you shouldn't live that way.' She suddenly noticed the crowded theatre and burst out: 'Why, where the devil did you all come from?' to gales of laughter. When Wood waved his arm behind her, Jane dropped to the floor like a rag doll. Now Elizabeth was revived by Wood blowing on her eyes. She skipped around the theatre then belted out a bawdy song:

> *I went into a tailor's shop,*
> *To buy a suit of clothes,*
> *But where the money came from,*
> *God Almighty knows.*

As the audience erupted at her profanity – *The Lancet* prudishly replaced her blasphemous language with dashes – Elizabeth launched into another verse. Apprehensive of where this might lead, Elliotson fixed her to the spot by a single wave of his finger before her face. Brought to life again she blankly denied she had been asleep and exclaimed: 'Oh, Dr Elliotson, you're mad; you're quite a baby.' She now tied a knot in her handkerchief and announced she was going to 'make a parson' and had already twisted the fabric into a plausible head and cassock before Elliotson stopped her in her tracks – 'a prelate and many revered gentlemen being present', *The Lancet* reminded its readers.

Revived and entranced over and again, at one point Elizabeth regaled the guests with a comic story about a woman who had boiled a pudding in her husband's nightcap, during the narration of which members of the audience queued up to pinch her flesh without producing any reaction. After this the spectators took turns at mesmerising her. When David William Murray, the third Earl of Mansfield, pointed at Elizabeth behind her back she dropped asleep mid-sentence. 'She did not see me do that,' he announced in bewilderment, to which Elliotson, uncharacteristically attempting a joke, replied, 'No, you may cross-examine her in any way you like,' presumably in reference to the earl's great-uncle, the celebrated Lord Chief Justice.

Now Elliotson brought some cast iron weights into the theatre. In her natural state Elizabeth proved, unsurprisingly, unable to lift either a 50lb or 84lb weight. After being mesmerised, with her wrists bound to prevent injury, she was asked to try again but protested, as she had earlier, saying that 'her negro' had warned she would hurt herself if she tried to lift the heaviest weight again. Evidently the 'negro' was looking out for her welfare, even if her doctor apparently was not. Pressed once more, she succeeded in raising weights totalling 70lbs – more than 30kg – some six or seven inches from the floor. Meanwhile she kept the crowd entertained by ribald references to 'the devil' and irreverent jokes at the expense of the hospital chaplain, Mr Stebbing, to whom she had seemingly taken a dislike.

Her sister Jane, now reanimated by Elliotson after a long slumber, was scarcely less amusing. Catching sight of the spectators in the upper rows, she exclaimed: 'What a lot of heads! And faces of all sizes!' then pointing at one guest who was staring with particular intensity, she burst out: 'Look at the fool.' Observing Elliotson at one point with his back towards her, talking to someone in the audience, Jane slipped up behind him, slid her hand into his coat pocket, and remarked: 'Here, Dr Elliotson, listen at this. Train up a child in the way he should go, and when he is old he will not depart from it.' Then she slowly drew out his pocket handkerchief. It was a scene straight out of *Oliver Twist*.

For the finale, Elliotson asked Elizabeth to press her palms against his own; she drooped into a trance. Then he took her to a side door and instructed her to press her palms against the wooden panels. Instantly she fell asleep. Opening the door with a flourish, like a fairground magician unlocking a trunk, Elliotson revealed Robert Grant, the university's Professor of Comparative Anatomy, concealed in an anteroom.

With its unique mix of mysticism and magic, comedy and coquetry, Elliotson's demonstration had retained its position as the greatest show in town. Emerging from the hospital at the end of the three-hour performance, the visitors were baffled and amazed in equal measure. As Mills put it: 'The observers left the curious scene yet more puzzled than ever at "animal magnetism".'

The very next day, on Sunday 3 June, a large crowd gathered on ward three at the hour appointed by Elizabeth in the predictions Wood had secured from her two days before.[34] Earlier in the day Elizabeth had been visited by her mother and family friends when she had seemed perfectly normal – or as normal as she ever was. Now she was lying fast asleep, fully clothed, on her bed. The spectators watched the clock. At precisely 4.45 p.m. Wood woke Elizabeth by rubbing her eyebrows. Suddenly she rose up in a wild fury and raged at the observers pressed in around her like a person possessed. She fell off the bed then dragged herself along the floor with one leg bent beneath her while snatching at anyone who got in her way. When a piece of paper was thrown to her she tore it to shreds with her hands and teeth, then lunged towards Elliotson 'with the ferocity of a tiger' and growled: 'Leave me alone, you villain, do.' She tried to bite anyone who approached her and when several of the men attempted to restrain her she raved at them: 'Damn your bloody eyes, come here. Let me only get at you.' Her voice had changed; it was 'full, sepulchral, and resonant' with the 'depth and force of a powerful adult voice'. Her eyes 'glistened with fierceness' and her features were 'sharpened with intensity of feeling'. According to Mills, she was like 'an eagle, wounded in the wing, and brought to the ground, eager to tear some enemy, but imbecile from want of motive power'. It was easy to see why some had previously suspected her of 'speaking in tongues'.

For a full thirty minutes Elizabeth ranted and snarled at the alarmed crowd. She called Wood 'a bastard fool' and warned the apothecary, 'Damn you, get away'. The ward nurses insisted she had never used such language before. Poor Mills had his work cut out strewing his report for *The Lancet* with dashes. Her curses were all the more shocking since it was, of course, a Sunday; indeed there was a vicar present. When challenged or questioned, she answered with outraged contempt or meaningless absurdities and resisted all attempts to mesmerise her – even though there was a chain of ready volunteers. Finally, she grew calm and fell asleep. Now Wood produced the sealed letter but – since it had been agreed to open it the following day – four more seals were solemnly affixed to it and it was vouchsafed to the custody of the matron.

The next day, 4 June, the same party reassembled on the ward and the letter with its five unbroken seals was produced and gravely opened. By now Elizabeth had reawakened to her usual 'modest and respectful' state and was apparently so shy she would not eat her dinner while the visitors remained. The letter, of course, faithfully predicted her actions of the previous day in minute detail. Elizabeth had told Wood 'she would be very ill-tempered, cross, spiteful and mischievous, but unable to walk, and would say very bad things', that she would not recognise Wood or any other person, and if she got hold of a knife 'she will cut anybody'.

For Elliotson – and most of the observers – Elizabeth's predictions were simply further proof of the extraordinary powers of mesmerism. Only Mayo, usually among the most credulous, raised the prospect that she might deliberately be hoodwinking them. Describing the episode in the *LMG*, he acknowledged that readers might ascribe her actions to 'intentional deception'.[35] He wrote: 'It will be said she would have little difficulty in foretelling that which she could, if a clever and practised deceiver, easily act.' Mayo was convinced 'there was no attempt at deception in the matter' but he put forward two interesting alternative hypotheses to explain what had happened. Either Elizabeth had expressed her imaginings as predictions and then *'unconsciously* determined their fulfilment', or she really could foresee what would happen to her health in 'this highly excited state of the nerves'. The latter hypothesis did require, he admitted, 'a greater effort than the former to get it down'.

Were they fools? Or just fanatics? Were Elliotson and his disciples on the trail of a scientific phenomenon worthy of investigation, or the victims of one of the biggest deceptions in medical history?

Mayo may well have hit the mark. It is possible, of course, that

Elizabeth was quite deliberately duping the entire party by predicting her behaviour and then coolly acting out her prophecy. Yet it is also possible that she was unconsciously acting out the wildest extremes of her imagination. In the demonstration in the lecture theatre the previous day, she had been rewarded by laughter whenever she uttered a profanity or delivered an insult, yet she had always been pulled back by Elliotson or Wood when she overstepped the mark. In her frenzy the following day she had given full vent to all the foul language and fury she had formerly been forced to suppress. It was as if she wanted to test Elliotson's credulity to the limits. No matter what she had done or said so far, he and his devotees had encouraged her, excused her behaviour, even paraded it. Now, perhaps, she felt it had all gone too far. She wanted a way out. It was impossible after all this time simply to walk out of the hospital or ask if she could go home. And so she needed them to call a halt to the whole procedure.

Tellingly, during her raving, she repeatedly warned Elliotson and his observers to keep away, to leave her alone. 'What are you doing with me?' she asked at one point. 'Blast you, leave me alone.' Yet they would not leave her alone. For of the two possible explanations that Mayo put forward, it was the second – the most difficult to 'get it down' – that Elliotson grasped. He was unable to go back. Having staked his reputation on the power of mesmerism, Elliotson could not give up now. It was that fatal combination of stubbornness – a refusal to question his own beliefs – coupled with vanity – an inability to admit he might be wrong – which propelled him on. He was sure even more wondrous revelations would follow.

For many watching the events unfold in Gower Street, Elizabeth's crazed outburst was a step too far. Having published Mayo's accounts of the experiments at UCH since April, and Dupotet's reports before that, the *LMG* now changed tack. Quoting Elizabeth's torrent of abuse from *The Lancet*, the *LMG* expressed 'disgust' at the scenes and lambasted those 'who regard such maniacal and loathsome ravings as fit subjects for exhibition and record'.[36] Cutting short a full reprisal of events, it ended its editorial abruptly by citing Elizabeth's comment on Elliotson: 'I never saw such a d—d fool in my life.'

The weekly magazine the *Athenaeum* was even more scathing.[37] Reviewing Dupotet's latest book, the journal ridiculed the claims of 'clairvoyance' made by 'the North London illuminati' on the basis that 'it is obvious that there can be no immediate relation between the present and the future, of which the nervous system can in any imaginable state take cognizance'. Certain aspects of mesmerism might prove true, the magazine acknowledged, and if Elliotson and his supporters had confined themselves to investigating these phenomena 'in a spirit of philosophy, with modesty and doubt', they would not have encountered such hostility. But having made 'rash and hasty' generalisations from 'a few imperfect observations', it urged that 'every scientific man who regards his own character should keep aloof from them'.

Another writer, reviewing the advance of mesmerism across Europe in the *British and Foreign Medical Review*, described the latest revelations at UCH as 'equal in marvellous absurdity and incredible incredulity' to any reports from the Continent.[38] In the past, mesmerism had been 'fostered by the Germans into life, and petted by the French into a sickly existence' yet the climate of Britain had seemed 'always too cold for it'. Yet now, the journal fumed: 'In the nineteenth century, when knowledge is advancing in every direction, and when London abounds with scientific men, the *mime* called Animal Magnetism steps upon the metropolitan stage once more, waves his presuming wand, and performs with almost unbounded applause before crowded audiences.' Mockingly hailing Elizabeth the 'Prophetess of St Pancras', the magazine declared that her ravings were 'too filthy to sully our pages withal'.

Elliotson's colleagues could take no more. Having stalled Liston, Thomson and Davis throughout May, Richard Quain, the dean of the faculty, could no longer put off their demands for a hearing. All efforts at conciliation with Elliotson had failed. He had defied them by staging the exhibition of 2 June which – to add insult to injury – had been described in unsparing detail over ten pages in *The Lancet*. Quain had little alternative. He summonsed an extraordinary meeting of the medical committee 'to take into consideration certain published statements concerning Animal magnetism'.[39]

At 7.30 p.m. on 6 June six professors took their seats in the boardroom on the ground floor of UCH. Elliotson's enemies, Liston and Thomson, were ready to exact their revenge. Davis, their new recruit, was absent. Even Elliotson's usual allies, Quain, the surgeon Samuel Cooper, the physician Robert Carswell and the botanist John Lindley, felt their friendship had now been stretched far enough. All six were united in their conviction that the mesmerism mania must end. Elliotson disdained to attend the meeting in 'disgust' at the manoeuvres against him.[40] Seizing the opportunity, Thomson proposed a motion, seconded by Liston, demanding an assurance that no further public demonstrations of mesmerism would be held within the hospital. The proposal was carried unanimously.

If it seemed to Liston and Thomson that it had all been too easy, they were right. Elliotson was much too clever and far too stubborn to give in without a fight. When Cooper and Lindley called on him at his house in Conduit Street to extract his agreement, he scribbled out a letter then, having second thoughts, ripped it up and began again. This new letter had quite a different tone.

Now Elliotson vehemently defended his demonstrations and made clear his determination both to continue using mesmerism as a therapy and to teach its use to students. 'Gentlemen,' he began, 'I am so deeply impressed with the importance of the truths of Mesmerism & its utility as a remedy, that no consideration of pecuniary interest or personal arrogance could induce me to discontinue my investigations or its employment.'[41] Far from making a 'public exhibition' of mesmerism he had merely responded to 'Medical & other Scientific persons, & from Individuals whose rank & station in Society entitle them to consideration' by showing them 'the extraordinary phenomena' when asked. 'If numbers of Physicians, Surgeons & General Practitioners & persons of the highest rank & attainment have testified their anxiety to witness the facts which I have demonstrated, this only proves their conviction of the importance of my investigations.' He therefore refused to stop his exhibitions, though in mock deference to the committee he offered to submit the names of anyone applying to witness them.

However, Elliotson's enemies were equally determined not to be beaten. By now Liston and Thomson had persuaded William Sharpey, their fellow Scot who was joint Professor of Anatomy, to join them. This had not been too difficult since Sharpey would later tell a friend that although Elliotson was 'a good teacher and a *man of note*' he was 'in my opinion all along an objectionable person'.[42] Elliotson would later allege that the Irish, Welsh and four of the six Scottish professors of the medical school had conspired against him in a Celtic cabal. Considering Elliotson's letter on 13 June – Elliotson still refused to attend – the committee ruled that all 'public exhibitions' of mesmerism were 'foreign to the objects of the hospital' and must therefore stop.[43] But Liston, backed by Sharpey, pushed the committee to go further and rule that no further 'public exhibitions' of mesmerism could be sanctioned 'to any parties whatsoever'. The following day the decision was ratified by the university management committee.[44]

Elliotson was seething. First he affected nonchalance and petulantly complained that the medical committee had not sent him minutes of its meeting, but told them not to bother since 'I have not curiosity enough to induce me to take the trouble of inspecting the minute book'.[45] Ignoring the faculty's ruling, he sent the committee a list of people who had asked to see a mesmerism demonstration. He wrote 'soberly and advisedly' – although he sounded anything but – to insist that in staging further exhibitions 'I shall not be pandering to the vulgar love of the marvellous' but 'setting forth an additional view of the truths of creation, increasing our awe & our reverence for the God of the Universe'. The committee refused point blank to read his list and simply referred him to its previous decision. Finally Elliotson had no choice but to accept defeat. He had infuriated his enemies and alienated his allies. There would be no more mass demonstrations in the lecture room, no more entranced patients in the operating theatre.

The decision was roundly applauded in the *LMG*, which crowed: 'We are very glad to find that the public exhibitions at University College Hospital have been discontinued.'[46] The *LMG*'s report was repeated in *The Times*, which adopted a similar stance. In *The Lancet*, however, the gushing reports by George Mills continued unabated and Wakley still refrained from editorial comment. In fairness, he had rather more important matters on his plate.

Dividing his time between the House of Commons and his editorial desk, Wakley had been as indefatigable as ever in taking up cudgels on behalf of social and medical causes. In the first half of 1838, he had campaigned for coroners to be medically qualified and highlighted inadequate medical care in the navy.[47] He had been vigorous, too, in defending working people and their rights. In February he had presented a petition to parliament on behalf of the five leaders of the Glasgow cotton spinners' trade union who had been sentenced to five years' transportation after the murder of a strike-breaker; whether any of them had been involved in the murder would never be determined. He was likewise active in the Chartist movement which was demanding greater representation for labouring people. Yet Wakley had reserved his greatest time and energy in showing up the iniquities of the new Poor Law – the 1834 Poor Law Amendment Act – by highlighting the pernicious regimes which governed the workhouses. In the meantime, his only daughter, Elizabeth, had died at the end of May at the age of sixteen after a long and gruelling illness.[48] It was understandable, then, if Wakley did not devote his whole attention to the convolutions of mesmerism or the battle now approaching a climax between his two friends at UCH.

But if Elliotson's colleagues thought they had seen an end to mesmerism they were mistaken.

8

Humbug! Humbug! Humbug!

University College Hospital, London, 14 June 1838

A lull had descended over Bloomsbury. With parliament in recess, the aristocracy and gentry had retreated from the city stench to the fresh air of their country estates. Judges, barristers and law clerks were putting their feet up during the long summer vacation. Dickens had taken a cottage by the river at Twickenham for the summer. Traffic in Gower Street was sparse, the corridors of UCH quiet, the lecture theatre empty. But on ward three John Elliotson was as busy as ever.

Far from feeling cowed by the medical faculty's restraints on his work, Elliotson was determined to extend his research. When he had first embarked on his mesmerism experiments, he had been stoutly sceptical of the more exotic claims, yet now he knew mesmerism was not only accepted by some of the most eminent medical men in France and Germany but that many of these enthusiasts had testified to witnessing acts of clairvoyance and other strange phenomena. One physician, a member of the Royal Academy of Medicine in Paris, was even offering a prize of 3,000 francs to the first person who could prove they could read blindfolded.[1] Having witnessed Elizabeth Okey apparently predicting her own behaviour, Elliotson was convinced more extraordinary marvels must follow and his scientific integrity seemingly went out of the window. Clarke, the vigilant *Lancet* reporter who had watched the experiments from the start, observed drily that it would have been 'well for science, and well for the able lecturer himself' if he had stuck to his original plan.[2] 'But he went far beyond the line which I am certain he had then marked out for himself. No doubt, dazzled and astonished by the effects which, as appeared to himself and others, had resulted from experiments upon the O'Keys, he was encouraged to go too far.'

However, it was George Mills, rather than Clarke, who scurried up the steps of the hospital and along the quiet corridors to reach the apothecary's room on 14 June.[3] He had been summoned by a note informing him that startling new developments had occurred the previous evening. On arrival he found a small group – just Elliotson, Wood and the new apothecary, Frederick Chapman, who had taken over from Taylor in February – gathered in the room, which would have been redolent with the scents of herbs and oils. The Okey girls were brought from their ward in a delirious state. On Elliotson's orders a mug was half-filled with water from a tap and given to Elizabeth to drink. There was no change in her behaviour. Then Chapman surreptitiously dipped one finger in the water and the mug was given to her again. She raised the cup to her lips and was in the act of swallowing when she was suddenly fixed in position 'as though she had been turned to stone'. Mills was astonished – so astonished, indeed, that he insisted on the experiment being repeated. Again Elizabeth was induced to drink water from the tap, again there was no response. Then Wood and Mills each dipped a finger in the mug and upon drinking the water Elizabeth was transfixed – twice as quickly as before. Two magnetisers, Elliotson explained, doubled the effect. Neither Chapman nor Wood was able to wake Elizabeth from her trance until the little party realised that she could only be woken by both the original mesmerists – Wood and Mills – working together.

Now the experiment was repeated on Jane who responded in the same way. On waking, however, Jane appeared to be in 'great distress'. Neither Wood nor Chapman could bring her to her senses until 'it struck us that the mug from which she had drunk contained the doubly magnetised water', wrote Mills. Mills now 'lent a hand' to Wood in stroking Jane's brow and she was restored to her normal state. Baffled as he was by what he had seen, Mills was positive there had been no trickery. It was impossible, he later explained in his 'Third report of facts and experiments' for *The Lancet*, that either girl could have known in advance whether the water had been 'magnetised' since the act was done out of their sight. Furthermore, he was sure the girls were oblivious to any conversation taking place around them. To confirm this point, one of the party had asked Jane whether she had heard what the men were talking about and she had tartly retorted, 'I think you are a fool.' This response – oddly perhaps – was taken as evidence of her innocence.

Now he had convinced himself that the mesmeric influence could 'magnetise' water, Elliotson was impatient to uncover further revelations. However, since he was banned from staging demonstrations in the lecture room and operating theatre, he was forced to restrict his experiments to the wards. Even though the medical committee had expressly forbidden 'public exhibitions' of mesmerism 'to any parties whatsoever', Elliotson blithely continued to invite guests to gather round the beds and watch his experiments. Two days after the mystifying water tests, Mills was recalled to UCH for further trials on the Okey sisters as Elliotson proceeded to demonstrate that mucous surfaces were more sensitive to the mesmeric force than skin.[4]

This time the group included John Wilson, the elephant whisperer, as well as the ubiquitous Wood. Sat facing Elizabeth, Elliotson slowly extended his forefinger to touch Elizabeth's lips, then her tongue, then 'gently inserted' his finger inside her mouth, and finally touched her eyeball while an assistant gravely counted the seconds each successive trance lasted. At last, having plainly had enough of these uninvited intimacies, Elizabeth climbed on her chair and grabbed Wilson around the neck. When Elliotson remonstrated with her, she said she was 'teaching him a lesson of patience'. She was certainly trying to teach him something.

Excited by his latest successes with mesmerised water and mucous membranes, Elliotson demonstrated the results over and again to amazed visitors. But Mills, who was devoting nearly as much time to reporting the spectacles at UCH as Elliotson was to producing them, was growing increasingly uncomfortable at these intrusive experiments. Finally, when Elliotson invited one guest, Philip Crampton, surgeon-general to the forces in Ireland, to touch Elizabeth's eyeball, Mills protested. Having seen the experiment repeated three or four times – each time producing 'violent convulsions' in Elizabeth – Mills expressed 'the strongest objections'.[5] He later sent Elliotson a note requesting that 'touching of the eye ought not to be performed again'. The young journalist was evidently half in love with the seventeen-year-old girl; in the same report he described her 'beautiful statue-like form' and revealed that she had described him, albeit in a mesmeric trance, as 'a very great friend'. After two days observing the trials on Elizabeth, Crampton pronounced himself convinced by the 'perfect honesty of the somnambulist and the reality of the extraordinary events which occurred'. Yet for all his interest in the subject of the experiments, Mills was becoming less sure about the results.

Dutifully recording the repeated trials with 'magnetised' water through June, Mills had to admit the findings were frequently inconsistent. Sometimes the tests were 'strikingly successful' but at other times 'altogether contradictory'. In one test, in front of twelve visitors crowded into a lobby, the expected results all 'failed', he revealed in his 'Fourth report' for *The Lancet*.[6] Another trial, before some of Elliotson's students, 'presented additional occasions for doubt'. In this latter experiment, Elizabeth was asked to drink from six wine glasses of which the water in two had been secretly 'magnetised'. She responded as expected to five of the six but on drinking the second glass had become transfixed even though the water was not 'magnetised'. Baffled by these results, the experimenters cast about for an explanation. Elizabeth – in her mesmerised state – was quick to proffer one. She explained that the water from the second glass was still in her mouth when she drank from the third. Elliotson and his guests nodded sagely. They were completely satisfied with this account despite the fact that it was the second glass which had proved erroneous, not the third. Mills suggested the tests were being conducted with too much haste and inadequate precautions. But there was, of course, a more obvious explanation, which he now allowed himself to consider for the first time.

It was possible, Mills conjectured in *The Lancet*, that the Okey sisters were imposters, accomplished actresses, who were faking their trances and strange antics. Their failure to distinguish between pure and 'magnetised' water certainly seemed to point to deliberate deception, he observed, although it never occurred to him to question the notion that water could be 'magnetised' in the first place. Yet at other times, Mills reasoned, the girls failed to respond as expected. If they were imposters, he asked, 'why should they not on this occasion have obeyed the law upon which their whole existence as objects of interest depends?' Such inconsistencies tended rather to 'satisfy discriminating observers that the patients were not actors'.

Mills had a point – one which supports the theory that the Okeys' reactions were largely subconscious. They were neither faking their behaviour nor responding genuinely to the mesmeric force, but simply reacting subconsciously in the way most likely to meet their observers' expectations. Mills, for one, was ready to dismiss the doubts. 'The opportunities for testing the reality of the phenomena in the girls O'Key are innumerable, and they have invariably stood such tests as we could offer,' he stressed. Certainly, in their altered personalities at least, the girls were always consistent. 'That is to say, if they *be* imposters, there had never been *forgetfulness of the part to be acted*, even for a moment, on any occasion.'

In reality, of course, the idea that two adolescent girls from impoverished circumstances could fool not only an esteemed Professor of Medicine but eminent members of the scientific community seemed more implausible than the notion that they were reacting to an invisible mesmeric fluid. Moreover, the possibility that two ordinarily meek and demure girls should take improper liberties with the respectable gentlemen who came to watch them – hanging around the neck of one guest and sitting on the knee of another – without being influenced by some mystical force was also deemed unconscionable. The chief question, argued Mills, was whether the girls' trances were real or faked, for if they were imposters in this then surely all their acts were false. Yet everyone who saw them fall into a trance was certain 'at least the sleep is real'. Said Mills: 'It is strikingly real to the judgement, after every test; it is strikingly real to the eye.' And to prove his point he included in his report two sketches of the beguiling Elizabeth in her mesmeric trance.[7]

In these simple pen sketches, reproduced in *The Lancet*, Elizabeth is captured in profile with her eyes tightly shut, her flaxen hair drawn back in an elaborately plaited bun on top of her head, soft ringlets falling in front of her ears from which delicate drop earrings hang. She is wearing a decorous high-necked dress with a large lace-trimmed collar and a neat bow. She looks every inch the virtuous young lady from a decent working family, except for her extraordinary expression. In the first sketch her head is thrown back and her mouth gapes open; in the second her head droops forward and her mouth is closed. In both she appears to be profoundly asleep, as if 'turned to marble', in Elliotson's words or, as Lieutenant-Colonel Thompson put it, with all the appearance 'of a recent corpse'. The two portraits closely resemble another, rougher and less skilled sketch, drawn inside the back cover of Elliotson's casebook at some point in 1838, probably by Wood, whose name is written beside it three times. These three tantalising sketches are the only known portraits of Elizabeth Okey taken from real life. At a time when photography was in its infancy, they provided the first chance for readers to study a mesmeric trance for themselves – and see the celebrity of UCH.

Just as doubts were growing about the latest marvels being unveiled at UCH so the notoriety of the Okey girls was spreading.

In June, the *Morning Chronicle* published an anonymous poem entitled 'Animal Magnetism' which ridiculed the feats performed by Mesmer and Dupotet and added: 'To say nothing of all the wonders done/By that wizard, Dr ELLIOTSON,/When, standing as if the gods to invoke, he/Up waves his arm, and – down drops OKEY!'[8] Really an excuse to lampoon Lord Brougham, who had become politically isolated – if not a little unhinged – since turning on his former Whig allies earlier that summer, the poem also poked fun at Elliotson's Royal Society friends who were dithering in their inquiry into mesmerism. It ends:

> *In short, 'tis a case for consultation,*
> *If e'er there was one, in this thinking nation;*
> *And therefore I humbly beg to propose,*
> *That those Savans who mean, as the rumour goes,*
> *To sit on Miss OKEY's wonderful case,*
> *Should also Lord HARRY's case embrace;*
> *And inform us, in both these patients' states,*
> *Which ism it is that predominates,*
> *Whether magnetism and somnambulism,*
> *Or, simply and solely, mountebankism.*

In truth the Royal Society *savants* were taking an inordinate time to investigate mesmerism and rumours about their languorous deliberations were rife. *The Lancet* reported that the panel had watched Elliotson's experiments and 'unequivocally pronounced in favour of the reality of the coma and the somnambulism'.[9] But the now openly hostile *LMG* revealed that the members had insisted that anyone involved in the experiments at UCH – in other words Elliotson and Wood – should be excluded from the investigations to guard against 'all sources of fallacy'. At that Elliotson petulantly prohibited Elizabeth from further involvement unless either he or Wood could attend (evidently she had no say in the matter). With neither side prepared to give way the investigation had stalled. It was clear that even Elliotson's scientific allies were beginning to doubt his impartiality – not to mention his common sense. Meanwhile the *Penny Satirist* reported that the Berlin mesmeric clinic had been closed down because one of its 'fair patients' had become pregnant by its presiding doctor and professor.[10] Blind to the warning signs Elliotson ploughed relentlessly on.

Amid the swirling fug of scepticism hanging over Gower Street, events now took a sinister turn. As accusations of trickery and deceit gathered force, for the first time Elliotson himself began to harbour doubts about some of his patients – not the Okey sisters, but those displaying far more innocuous behaviour. Charlotte Bentley, a twelve-year-old girl being treated for weakness in her back and legs, had been improving under mesmerism.[11] When she fell into a trance she also withstood being pinched and other sadistic tests, though when the passes were made out of her sight she never fell asleep. Another patient, twenty-three-year-old Ann Ross, who had been exhibited in the lecture theatre on 2 June, had likewise been progressing well under mesmeric treatment. Her epileptic seizures had decreased but she was also displaying some more remarkable responses – in line with the changes seen in the Okey girls.

On 18 June Ross announced an angel had appeared to her who foretold she would be cured within three months and proposed she should have a decayed tooth removed. Promptly acting on this celestial advice, Elliotson had ordered the offending premolar be extracted in the presence of several onlookers while the girl slumbered peacefully. Since then the soothsaying angel had become increasingly vocal, predicting that Ross would have an epileptic seizure on 1 July, that her seizures would cease soon after, that she could now be mesmerised through walls and that a second tooth should be removed – as it duly was. Other patients also seemed to be asserting their own ideas about their treatment. It was becoming unclear who was in control on the wards. Were the medical staff managing the patients? Or were the patients managing the staff? It was plain that decisive action was needed to restore order. And it was not long before someone stepped forward to oblige.

On 26 June Elizabeth Okey suddenly announced that one of her fellow patients was an imposter and threatened to expose her. The following day, in a mesmeric trance, she was true to her word. Asked to unmask the imposter, she started trembling and turning from one side to the other as if unsure which direction to take. Then, walking to the table, she filled a mug with water and stirred it with a stick, as if aping Elliotson's manoeuvres with mesmerised water. Casting around the ward, she fixed on Charlotte Bentley and announced darkly: 'I want her.' Presented with the mug by Elizabeth, Charlotte sipped the water and instantly fell asleep. At Elizabeth's instigation she was woken and the action repeated. Each time Charlotte drank the water and lapsed into a trance, the spectators pinched and prodded her with their usual abandon but could evince no signs of deceit. Asked whether perhaps she was mistaken, Elizabeth promptly tipped the water over Charlotte's head. The poor girl came to her senses spluttering and burst into tears, all the while protesting that she had truly been asleep. But Elizabeth shook her head furiously and shouted: 'It won't do!'

Further trials by water ensued. Elizabeth now filled three wine glasses to the brim and made Charlotte drink from each in turn. When the girl became entranced, Elizabeth railed at her: 'Arise, or I'll limb you! Do you hear me? Get up! I say; up! or I'll surely limb you!' Despite this demonic denunciation and threats of violence, Charlotte slept on. Now in a frenzy, Elizabeth bodily lifted the girl out of her chair and shrieked: 'Get up, you wicked thing.' The terrified Charlotte begged to be allowed to go home though she still protested her innocence. Mills, himself mesmerised by Elizabeth's performance, observed: 'The eyes, countenance, and positions of the somnambulist, otherwise a diminutive and insignificant-looking personage, presented at this stage the most striking characters, inviting comparisons with those of the finest tragic actress, as she paused in fierce contemplation of the crouching object before her, which she seemed to regard as though its annihilation was within her power.' Understandably petrified, poor Charlotte appealed to Elliotson: 'Oh, Dr Elliotson, do wake her. I can't bear it. I won't do so any more. I'll go home. I'll not stop here another day.'

Charlotte was subjected to one final test. While she was apparently entranced, Elliotson loudly ordered that the 'foul end of a glyster-pipe' – a syringe used to administer enemas – be put in her mouth. At once Charlotte opened her eyes and jumped up, though even then she maintained she was not shamming. Indeed, her reaction may have been genuine – even in deep hypnosis everyone has their limits. Faking or not,

Charlotte was sharply discharged and packed off home. Asked later how she was so certain the girl had been feigning, Elizabeth coolly replied that Charlotte had gone to sleep when the water was not mesmerised as well as when it was.

Whether Elizabeth truly believed Charlotte was a fraud is unclear. She may well have been indoctrinated sufficiently to believe in such absurdities about mesmerised water as devoutly as Elliotson did. At the same time, since suggestions of fraud on the wards of UCH were being widely voiced, it was certainly convenient that the finger of suspicion should point to someone else. At a time when the vast majority of women were utterly disempowered – denied the vote, university education, entry into a profession and financial independence – the Okey sisters' rule on ward three was one way, at least, that they could assert some control. Elliotson swallowed Elizabeth's verdict on Charlotte Bentley completely – regardless of Elizabeth's own inconsistencies with 'mesmerised' water. But now that the shadow of doubt had fallen on one patient, it touched others too.

In swift succession three more patients, all of them epileptic, were discharged by Elliotson as imposters.[12] Suspicions had already centred on Ann Ross as her behaviour became increasingly perverse. Harbouring doubts about her wilder frolics, such as the prophesying angel, some of the students hatched a cunning plan to expose her. While she was supposedly entranced, they mentioned having seen some somnambulists awake when the index finger was pricked; when this was done, she immediately awoke. When they pretended Elizabeth had prophesied Ross would wake when her nose was pinched, she did just that. Finally the students said Elizabeth had predicted Ross would become delirious; sure enough the delirium came on. Watching this last scene, Elliotson was convinced she was feigning. When he challenged her to stop her nonsense, Ross freely confessed that she had felt only a slight drowsiness when mesmerised; all the rest was faked. Two more patients, Mary Anne Butler, aged eighteen, and James Isaacs, aged nineteen, were likewise accused of feigning sleep and turfed out of the hospital.

Later giving a lecture on the 'impositions of some patients', Elliotson described Ross as an 'artful patient' and claimed he 'never saw worse acting' though he failed to explain how she had sat unflinching while two of her teeth were extracted. Bentley, he had noticed, 'did not go to sleep in a natural manner', though he had to admit that she did recover from her original complaint. He suspected deceit in the other two patients, he claimed, though even then he seemed unsure whether they were really imposters – certainly Isaacs' epilepsy had improved. But because none of these patients complied with the results he had seen in the Okey girls, Elliotson concluded they must be frauds.

In fact, it is entirely possible that all four were genuine. In all likelihood Ross really was in a trance during her dental procedures at least; hypnotism is commonly used today for patients suffering from dental phobia and to combat dental pain. Charlotte Bentley also seemed impervious to pain in her trance-like state; the fact that she never responded when the mesmeriser was out of her sight makes it all the more likely she was authentic. The other two patients likewise showed every sign of being genuine. Why Elliotson was so determined to name and shame these four, yet placed so much faith in the Okeys, is hard to fathom. Other observers had certainly suspected the Okeys of acting, though just as many were persuaded of their veracity. And, for all their preposterous actions, they certainly exhibited all the classic responses attributed to hypnotism today. Like most medical mavericks, Elliotson was simply incapable of questioning his beliefs. As one contemporary would say, 'he could do nothing by halves'.[13] He had invested too much in the Okeys and their responses to his experiments to question them now.

So, despite proclaiming the four discharged patients frauds, Elliotson insisted there was no reason to suspect mesmerism itself was false. He was 'as firmly as ever convinced' of its power, he told his students, and pledged to 'continue to give to the world' and to demonstrate to small parties – since he could not, of course, exhibit his work to a larger audience – 'such facts and experiments as tended to elucidate the truth'. When he left the lecture theatre he was loudly cheered. As summer temperatures soared, Elliotson reported having witnessed a shower of frogs falling on Gower Street.[14] They were a sign, perhaps, of his growing credulity – and certainly not a good omen.

The revelation that some patients at UCH had been exposed as cheats only fuelled more certainty in some quarters that they were all frauds. Having previously argued that the test of mesmerism was whether the sleep was genuine, George Mills now had to admit that the allegation some patients had feigned sleep added 'a new page' to the need for precautions. This prompted him to ask again, in his 'Fifth report of experiments and facts' for *The Lancet*, whether the Okeys were frauds.[15] On one side, 'many able scientific men' had avowed their belief in 'the good faith of the girls'; on the other, there was no shortage of gentlemen 'who pronounce or suspect the whole to be trick'. Now thoroughly confused about where he stood himself, Mills argued that whether the Okey sisters were true or false, they were equally remarkable as 'illustrations of insanity' or as 'instances of perfection in acting and deception which defy the most vigilant scrutiny'.

Other commentators were unequivocal. The *Athenaeum* jubilantly reported that despite being paraded by Elliotson before a 'grand display' in June, Ann Ross had confessed her sleep was 'all a humbug'. Charlotte Bentley, likewise, had been unmasked when 'Elizabeth Okey (who keeps the only true original booth in the fair), fearing, we suppose, that the number of competitors would lower the profits, denounced her and threatened exposure'.[16] Writing in the *Morning Chronicle*, Dionysius Lardner was just as convinced the Okeys were genuine. Having watched innumerable trials to test Elizabeth's veracity, he pronounced that 'no one who has had an opportunity of knowing the amiable and artless character of this little girl could for a moment entertain the idea of her being an imposter (to suppose which it would also be necessary to believe her to be the most consummate actress in the world)'.[17] Consummate actress or artless little girl, Elizabeth was back in supreme position at UCH.

While the scientific laws governing mesmerised water remained frustratingly elusive, in July Elliotson launched a raft of new trials to test the mesmerising properties of a dizzying range of materials from glass and metal to paper and tea. Invited to watch these latest experiments, a dozen or more men gathered around the Okeys' beds each day with stopwatches primed to measure the girls' responses to assorted materials. At one of these bizarre sessions, Elliotson solemnly demonstrated that crumpled paper, a scrap of oilskin and a business card which fell untouched from its case had no 'magnetic' effect when Jane touched them. Yet a penknife, a pocket watch, gold coins and the same card after it had been held by its owner sent her into a trance. Carefully charting these experiments for his 'Sixth report of experiments and facts' in *The Lancet*, Mills observed breathlessly: 'A *penknife* at once acted magnetically. A piece of *oil-skin* had no influence. A watch, with the *glass*, placed on her palm affected her less quickly than when the *metal back* was grasped.'[18] Gold sovereigns produced the most profound effect, sending Jane instantly to sleep after being held in the mesmerist's hand, but having no effect when they were untouched. It was even noted that, when the trial ended, one visitor handed Jane her 'brown Holland sleeve cuff' – and she immediately stopped in her tracks.

Similar effects were produced in Elizabeth. When one cynical observer suggested Elizabeth could detect the 'mesmerised' coins because they had been warmed in the mesmerist's hand, Elliotson repeated the tests after heating the coins in warm water. According to Mills, she 'experienced stupefaction in every instance in which the money had been magnetised'. In another test, one observer secretly held two coins out of twelve, yet Elizabeth unerringly fell asleep only when she touched the chosen two.

The Reverend Henry Moseley, a skilled statistician and Professor of Natural Philosophy and Astronomy at KCL, later professed he was not convinced by any of the tests and even doubted 'the proceedings were honest'. Crampton, however, was a fervent convert to the cause. 'It is too absurd,' he declared, 'to deny that these phenomena are real.' He even went so far as to proclaim that Elliotson's trials on mesmerism were the most important discoveries being undertaken in physiology.

As these latest tests were repeated using a vast array of materials, Elliotson became convinced that some substances, especially certain metals, could conduct the mesmeric influence while others could not. So the mesmeric power could be concentrated and directed in exactly the same way as electricity. And although the idea might sound absurd to modern ears, it made sense in the context of the scientific world Elliotson inhabited and his theory of how mesmerism worked.

The first experiments on conductivity had been undertaken more than a century earlier by Stephen Gray, a Kent cloth dyer who taught himself astronomy and other natural sciences.[19] From the 1720s Gray performed a series of tests on the 'communication' of the 'electrical vertue' by hanging household objects made from different metals – including an iron poker, a silver tankard, and a copper tea kettle – from silk threads connected to a glass tube which produced static electricity when rubbed. When he found these metals conducted electricity to varying degrees, he tested other materials including bricks, tiles, fresh vegetables and – scrabbling at the back of the pantry – dried vegetables, which proved to be inferior conductors. Realising electricity operated like a 'fluid', Gray tried to transmit the force over long distances. Becoming something of a showman, he performed a party trick in which he suspended a charity schoolboy from silken ropes to show that the human body could conduct electricity too. After Gray's pioneering work, experimenters had discovered that silver, copper and gold were the most efficient electrical conductors while others, such as zinc and nickel, were less so. By the 1830s, Elliotson's friends Wheatstone and Faraday were taking research on electricity to new levels. Since Elliotson belonged to the school that believed mesmerism was an invisible physical force, it was entirely logical that he should investigate its conductivity in the same way.

Mayo, one of his chief collaborators, explained the purported logic in the *LMG*.[20] Gold, silver, platinum, water and the moisture of skin were good conductors of mesmerism, he asserted, while copper, zinc, tin and pewter were not. So the mesmeric force was largely – though not entirely – consistent with electrical conductivity. The mesmeric force could even be channelled by the mesmerist simply looking at an object, Mayo added and proclaimed: 'In this marvellous inquiry, wonder succeeds wonder.'

Whatever was really going on to produce such 'wonders', the Okeys proved remarkably consistent in their reactions to 'mesmerised' substances. No doubt they were influenced – consciously or not – by the expectations of Elliotson and others. Since Elliotson had divined that gold and silver were the best conductors, for example, it was easy enough for the girls to respond most powerfully to them. One observer shrewdly noted that Elliotson and Lardner freely discussed their theories and expected outcomes before and after the experiments in the girls' hearing 'so that it would have been extraordinary . . . if the anticipated results had not occurred'.[21]

Plainly, with hindsight, such tests were inherently flawed – though again Elliotson was simply following the prevailing research standards of the time. The Scottish naval surgeon James Lind is credited with conducting the first randomised controlled trial in 1747, when he chose twelve sailors suffering from scurvy and assigned them to take different substances including cider, seawater, lemons, oranges and a paste made up of garlic, radish and mustard seed.[22] He found the two sailors who ate the lemons and oranges recovered in six days while the others languished on – though with the usual tardy take-up of medical discoveries it took fifty more years before lemon juice was routinely issued to the navy. Though the lemons had since helped the British navy to defeat Napoleon, scientific standards remained at sea. Elliotson, like Lind and Gray, had been careful to test a variety of substances in his search for the best mesmeric conductor. But he had not, crucially, thought to vary the subjects – the Okey girls – on whom he experimented.

More significantly, Elliotson had little concept of the importance of 'blinding' both researchers and participants to avoid bias in the results. The first tests in medicine on 'blinded' patients are thought to have been performed, ironically enough, by the French Royal Commission investigating mesmerism in 1784 when some people were literally blindfolded and told they were being mesmerised even though they were not. The surgeon John Hunter had conducted a similar test around the same time, when he gave mercury to some patients and identical pills made of bread to others in tests on gonorrhoea.[23] Hunter was one of the first to understand the principle of the placebo – even tricking his wife into believing she was enjoying the health-giving benefits of Bath spa water by sticking labels onto bottles filled with water from the filthy Thames. Elliotson had, of course, blindfolded the Okeys – or hidden items from their view. But he had made no allowances for his own or his assistants' bias, which plainly influenced the outcome of the experiments. Even so, the fact that the Okeys regularly picked out which coins or glasses of water were 'mesmerised' from a line of identical items was remarkable. They were either extremely lucky or extraordinarily attuned to body language – or both.

Just as Mayo predicted, the wonders never ceased. In early July Elizabeth was suddenly able to 'see' with her hand in mesmeric trances. This seemingly inexplicable development came as little surprise to Elliotson since 'transposition of the senses', as it was known, had been widely reported by Continental mesmerists in highly responsive subjects. Accounts of mesmerised patients being able to hear, taste and smell through their fingers and toes, or read sealed letters placed on their stomachs, were ten a penny. One patient in a hospital in Bologna could apparently describe the 'form, smell, quality, and colour' of any item placed on his epigastrium – or upper abdomen.[24] A patient in Paris could purportedly read a prescription in a sealed envelope placed in her hand. Previously Elliotson had been understandably dubious about such reports, writing: 'Often have I seen Baron Dupotet speak at the epigastrium and finger ends of the ecstatic and comatose patients ... but nothing, which, till I witness such things, I must consider supernatural, has yet occurred.' Now that he had thrown caution – and scientific principle to the wind – he was delighted.

Like a proud parent showing off his offspring's talents, he demonstrated his protégée's latest gift to large groups of witnesses on 9 and 11 July. Mills described how Elizabeth used her hand 'as an *organ of vision*' not to touch objects but through 'a peculiar motion of *viewing* them with that member'.[25] With her eyes bandaged and a tea tray held under her chin, Elizabeth used her left hand to 'look for' a piece of bread and butter. Her hand quivered each time it neared the bread then 'when a clear "view" of the food seemed to be obtained, she suddenly turned round the palm, and snatched the bread'. Asked by Wood, whether she had an 'eye' in her hand, Elizabeth said she had a light there. When the test was repeated substituting a wine glass and a sovereign for the bread, Elizabeth was not interested; she clearly knew on which side her bread was buttered. Thrilled by these new developments and convinced he had finally witnessed the 'transposition of senses', Elliotson was certain the next step must be clairvoyance.

Already Elizabeth had predicted when she would fall ill, while other medical practitioners had reported patients prescribing for their own ailments. But mesmerists on the Continent had detailed cases where the subjects would routinely diagnose other patients' conditions, predict their progress and prescribe appropriate remedies. Dupotet had mesmerised a woman in Paris who had predicted a man's death – albeit after the event – by touching a lock of his hair. When tested previously, Elizabeth had failed to make any convincing pronouncements. But now that the two sisters had developed their sensitivity to a higher level, Elliotson was sure they would succeed.

On 16 July Elliotson escorted the mesmerised Jane to the bedsides of fourteen female patients on another ward. Stopping at each bed, he directed her to place a gold sovereign in each patient's hand, then take it back after a few seconds. Mills, on the spot as always, reported that Jane fell into a stupor after taking the coins from six of the patients, but showed no response with the others.[26] Charting the results as Jane moved from bed to bed, Mills reported she was immediately stupefied when taking the sovereign from one girl with secondary syphilis and another with acute rheumatism but showed no response with a patient suffering from pulmonary consumption (tuberculosis) and another with 'fever'. Mayo, who was likewise following this mystical ward round, noted that Jane went into a trance when she took the sovereign from 'a little girl in good health, but affected with ringworm' but showed no response to 'a young person, who having recently miscarried, was in a state of great bodily weakness'.[27]

What to make of these reactions? Analysing Jane's responses, Elliotson was quick to come up with a theory. He concluded that the patients who produced a stupor in Jane had only minor ailments while those who produced no effect were seriously ill. As always this appraisal was based on a liberal interpretation of Jane's responses as well as the typically imprecise nature of nineteenth-century medical diagnosis. According to Elliotson's perverse formula, the patients with consumption and fever were seriously ill – which was accurate enough – but so was a woman with catalepsy, which Elliotson believed was feigned, though the latter had gone without food for seven weeks so was probably not in the best of health. At the same time, Jane 'diagnosed' only superficial disease in a girl with secondary syphilis, another with acute rheumatism, a third with chorea and a fourth with epilepsy – all comparatively serious conditions. Obviously Elliotson was interpreting Jane's responses according to his own prognoses for the patients. Naturally the experiment was repeated a few days later using Elizabeth. Her reactions, however, were quite different. Every patient threw her into a stupor but – Elliotson now reasoned – the length of time she slept was directly proportionate to the health of each patient. There was no explanation as to why, if mesmerism was a physical force which ought to act according to fixed principles, as electricity did, the two girls should display such different reactions.

Soon afterwards, at the behest of one incredulous student, Elliotson escorted Elizabeth to a ward where neither had previously been.[28] As a further precaution, the labels denoting the diagnosis at the head of each bed were removed and every patient was covered from head to toe by bedsheets so they resembled nothing less than corpses. At the end of the trial, the bedclothes were turned down, the patients revealed and their labels checked. 'The effects were in every instance precisely proportionate to the strength of the patient in whose hand the sovereign had been placed,' Elliotson solemnly announced.

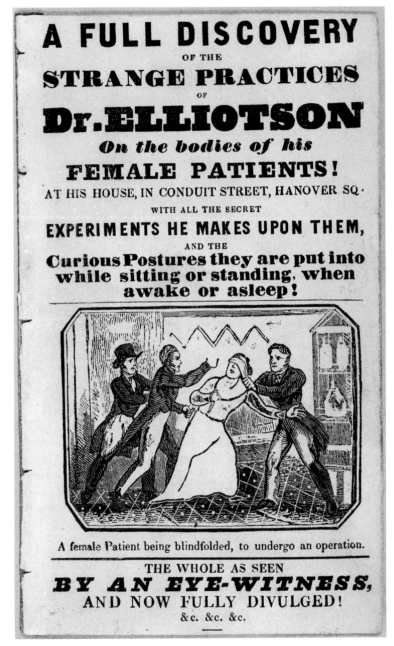

A FULL DISCOVERY

OF THE

STRANGE PRACTICES

OF

Dr. ELLIOTSON

On the bodies of his

FEMALE PATIENTS!

AT HIS HOUSE, IN CONDUIT STREET, HANOVER SQ.

WITH ALL THE SECRET

EXPERIMENTS HE MAKES UPON THEM,

AND THE

Curious Postures they are put into while sitting or standing, when awake or asleep!

A female Patient being blindfolded, to undergo an operation.

THE WHOLE AS SEEN

BY AN EYE-WITNESS,

AND NOW FULLY DIVULGED!

&c. &c. &c.

Strange but true. This sensational pamphlet promised to divulge 'all the secret experiments' that John Elliotson performed in his West End home.

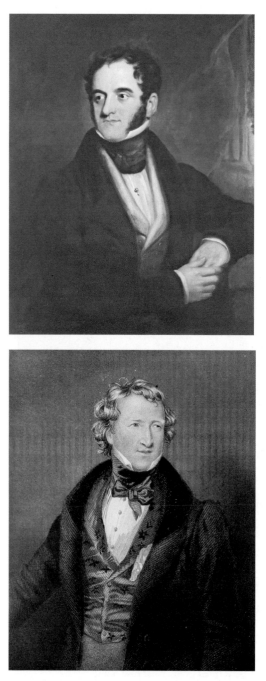

Young men in their prime. John Elliotson in a portrait by James Ramsay c. 1837 (left). Thomas Wakley is pictured in the 1830s soon after he launched *The Lancet* (bottom left).

opposite page:
Friends and foes. Baron Jules Denis Dupotet de Sennevoy (top left); Scottish surgeon Robert Liston (middle left); Charles Dickens as a young journalist and author (bottom left); William Makepeace Thackeray (top right); the only known portraits of Elizabeth Okey (bottom right).

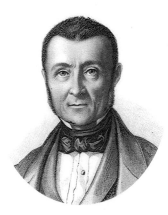
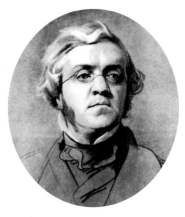
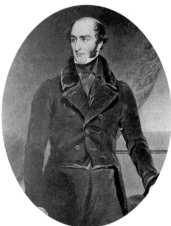
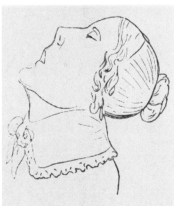
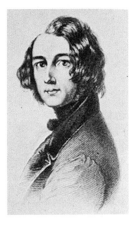
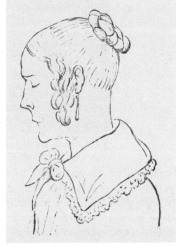

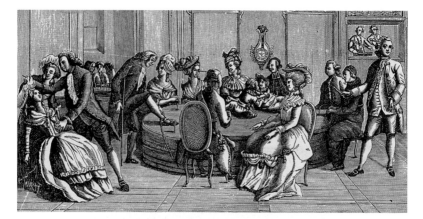

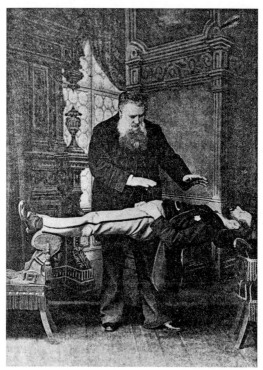

Mesmerised (clockwise from top left): Denizens of fashionable Parisian society flocked to enjoy the thrills of Franz Anton Mesmer's magnetic tub or 'baquet' in the late eighteenth century. John Elliotson is shown manipulating the mesmeric 'forces' in this 1843 cartoon in *Punch*. A frock-coated mesmerist directs the invisible magnetic rays to entrance a woman in this engraving from the 1840s. A man is suspended rigid between two chairs in a stunt which awed theatre audiences.

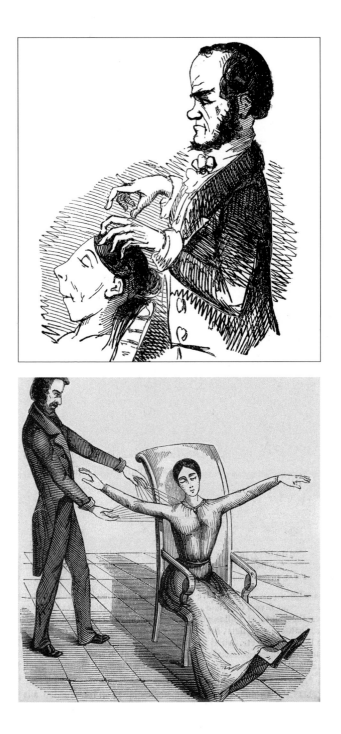

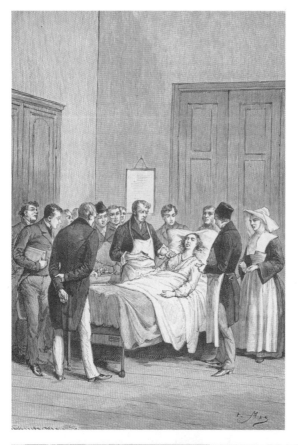

The sweetest sleep.
A Frenchwoman, Madame Plantin, had her breast amputated in the first operation performed under mesmerism in 1829 (left). A laughing gas party depicted in a colour aquatint by Thomas Rowlandson (bottom left). Robert Liston performed the first operation under ether at UCH in 1846 in this picture painted several decades later (top right). James Young Simpson and friends sample chloroform in a dinner party experiment (bottom right).

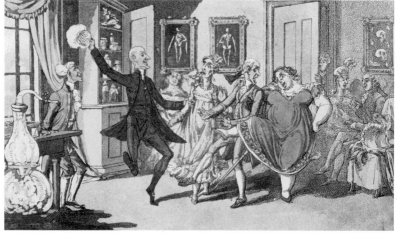

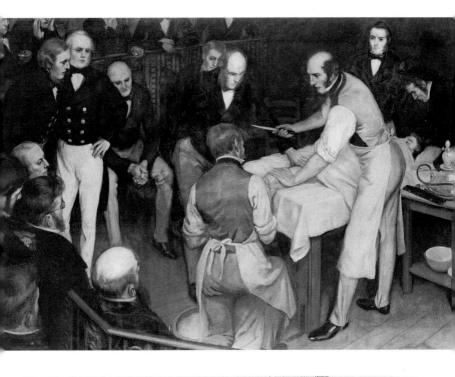

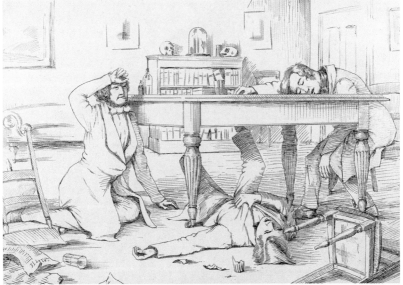

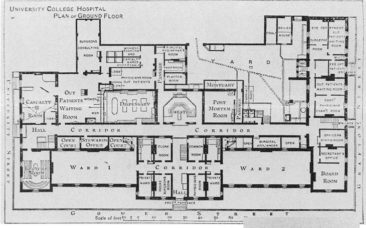

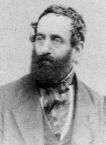

University College Hospital. The original hospital, which opened in Gower Street in 1834, is shown in this early photograph. A plan of the ground floor shows the lecture room and board room at opposite corners and the operating theatre in the centre. John Elliotson (inset) photographed in the 1860s, when he was in his seventies.

What the patients thought about their new medical consultant and her cryptic methods was left unsaid. Only once did Elizabeth appear to fail. At one of the beds her response suggested the patient was moderately ill. But when the student gleefully flung back the sheets, the patient turned out to be one of the nurses he had asked to slip into bed in an attempt to trick Elizabeth. Elliotson was not to be gainsaid, however. He pronounced the nurse 'looked very sickly' and discovered she had only lately returned to work 'very weak' after being ill. The experiment, he declared, was 'triumphant' and the cowed student felt the need to apologise the following day.

There seemed nothing left for Elliotson to do but to hand over his stethoscope and medicine chest to the Okey sisters and retire to the country. The Okeys had been elevated to the role of medical advisors; his own role had been reduced to escorting them round the wards like a hospital porter and meekly recording their pronouncements. Patients had become doctors; doctors were now passive observers. Yet the pace, if anything, now quickened. Fixated by the gathering speed of these latest revelations, Elliotson launched himself into a flurry of new activity.

In a dizzying succession of madcap trials, Elliotson tested the effects of 'mesmerised' farthings, pennies, silver shillings, gold pencils and a pencil case made from zinc and nickel on the Okey girls. He discovered that the girls could be 'fixed' in a stupor when a gold coin was put in their hands while whistling, reciting poetry or writing a letter, so that they would endlessly repeat the interrupted act. A sample of Elizabeth's writing from a letter to her father was reproduced in *The Lancet* in which she repeated the word 'my' eight times.[29] Coins were piled up to see whether the fluid travelled upwards or downwards and laid in rows to see whether the fluid could move from one end to the other. A wine glass – previously immune from the mesmeric influence – could now be magnetised when the mesmerist pointed at it, passed a hand over it or placed it near to another containing 'mesmerised' water. The rules were elastic; they could be stretched to fit each new result.

As the trials reached new heights of absurdity, a gold chain measuring several yards was procured in order to 'ascertain to what extent the magnetic or soporific fluid would travel'. The experiment simulated Wheatstone's work developing the telegraph – though with rather less useful application. Elizabeth was given one end to hold while Elliotson or Lardner held the other; after a minute or so she became stupefied. If a brass chain was twisted around the gold, the fluid 'was arrested by it' so that Elizabeth halted mid-speech. In the middle of singing Byron's 'Maid of Athens' she was 'stuck' repeating the line 'My life, I love you' like a prototype gramophone record stuck in a groove. Singing a comic air, she became stuck repeating the line 'Whether his mother would let him or no' a total of fifty times.

Observing these barmy scenes, eminent intellectuals including Wyndham Knatchbull, the Professor of Arabic at Oxford University, and John Crocker Bulteel, a former Whig MP who was the son-in-law of Earl Grey, carefully counted the girls' repetitions and timed their responses. The tests were as ludicrous as they were sadistic. Or in the words of Clarke, the student and journalist, 'so much irrelevant twaddle'.[30] As Clarke wrote: 'Experiments of this kind – and they were many – were repeated, and before audiences who for several hours together waited with the greatest patience to witness the results.' He added: 'There were so many sources of fallacy in them that it is marvellous that there could be found any persons who could place any reliance upon them.'

Finally, at the end of one long day of exhausting tests, Elizabeth was asked in her delirious state how she felt. Generally, when delirious she gabbled nonsensical rubbish or spouted vulgar street language. Now, as Elliotson's trials reached a peak of mania, Elizabeth displayed a rare instance of lucidity. 'Do you know, Dr Elliotson, I cannot talk to you, I am so ill,' she said. 'It has runned all up to my head from my hands.' Touching the various metals had burned her hands, she complained. Asked to expand, she said: 'Suppose I had a doll, and stuck a wire up it, and then pulled it, and threw its stremeties about. That's how it shoots through me.' Elliotson asked: 'Shall I bring you to yourself again?' And she replied: 'To myself? ... What do that mean? Am I ever anybody else?' It was a cry of despair. She had completely lost sight of who she was.

A hospital was meant to be a place of safety, a refuge from the outside world. Yet life on ward three of UCH had descended into madness. In this looking-glass world, in which doctors performed surreal tests and distinguished scientists noted the results, Elizabeth suddenly sounded like the lone voice of reason. She really was very ill, as was her sister. Their delirium had become almost constant and they lapsed only briefly in and out of their 'normal' selves. Most of the time they lived in an upside-down, nightmarish state that was encouraged by Elliotson and his associates. After a year on the ward, Elizabeth could hardly remember her family or home; the hospital was home, Elliotson and his assistants her family. Whether mesmerism had ever helped the girls or not, it was certainly not helping them now. Switching continually between derangement and entrancement, for the enlightenment and entertainment of others, they had lost all sight of normality. And there was nobody they could turn to, nobody they could trust. Doctors and students were intent on testing them to extremes; parents and friends were too humble to intervene; even independent observers – journalists and scientists – conspired with the lunacy. One observer expressed their plight succinctly: 'They have been cut off from a watchful parentage – placed among influential strangers – subjected to measures giving them extraordinary eclat – much caressed by persons of distinction – and is it to be wondered at that they have lost an ascendancy over themselves?'[31] Yet Elliotson was deaf to appeals, impervious to reason. He had moved so far from his position as a questioning, insightful, independent doctor and scientist that he had forgotten the basic Hippocratic Oath: do no harm.

Recording the latest taxing round of tests in his 'Seventh report of experiments and facts' for *The Lancet*, Mills praised the 'unwearied perseverance' of Elliotson and his collaborators – though he made no mention of the wearying effect of their perseverance on the subjects of the experiments. By now Mills had become as deeply embedded in Elliotson's team as Wood, Mayo and Lardner, as firmly committed to the research as they were. He frequently lent a hand with the tests and recording results. Zealously defending the investigations, Mills railed: 'As for the ridicule and imbecile denunciations of shallow observers, or of those who have not observed at all . . . it will not retard the investigation, we apprehend, one jot.' Rather giving himself away with that inclusive 'we', he thundered: 'Nothing can subdue, or long successfully combat, FACTS.'

In the twelve months since Elliotson had first introduced mesmerism to UCH, however, the nation's mood had changed. From initial fascination and good-humoured tolerance, views had become deeply ingrained and often bitterly savage. In the press, among the public and within the profession, the divisions seemed unbreachable. As the *Athenaeum* noted:

'When we first took up the subject, it was scarcely possible to join a dozen persons in any society where its professed mysteries were not a subject of serious discussion – latterly, we rarely hear them adverted to, except with a laugh.'[32] Yet *The Age* applauded the 'impartial' accounts by Lardner in its rival the *Monthly Chronicle*. The *Penny Satirist* dismissed an account of a woman who could play the piano in a trance better than normally as 'Sheer humbug!' Yet its own medical advisor praised Elliotson's investigations and argued that to deny the effects of mesmerism 'is nothing but an impudent attempt of ignorance to repress truth'. Meanwhile the weekly journal *Figaro in London*, the forerunner of *Punch*, published a cartoon of figures genuflecting before the statue of a withered old man dressed as the devil under the title 'The Worship of Humbug'. 'Whether it be to crowd the benches of a Theatre, to witness the tom-fooleries of a popular buffoon, whether it be to throng the saloons of a quack, to witness the mummery of animal magnetism,' the magazine thundered, 'it is still Humbug! Humbug! Humbug!'

Families and friends were equally split. Lady Byron, the long-suffering widow of the late poet, was a fervent disciple; her daughter, the gifted mathematician Ada, Countess of Lovelace, remained a sceptic.[33] Fanny Trollope, the prolific travel writer and novelist, was an avid supporter; her son, the future author Anthony Trollope, harboured doubts. While Dickens's interest in mesmerism was increasing, his friend Macready had already seen enough.

Even Elliotson's own students were openly feuding over the rights and wrongs of mesmerism. One student, James Blake, complained to *The Lancet* about the lack of scientific integrity in the experiments and when his letter was refused he sent it to the *LMG*.[34] Having seen the tests to 'mesmerise' water, he was adamant the Okey girls could tell the expected outcome from the expressions and comments made by Elliotson and his aides. Sometimes Elizabeth only went into a trance after Elliotson and Wood exclaimed that she was 'fixed'. When he repeated the trials himself, she frequently failed to detect which water was 'mesmerised' and which was not. He considered the tests 'one of the most shameless subterfuges ever made use of in the course of any inquiry professing to be conducted in a scientific manner'.

Another student, Edward Wooldridge, agreed that Elliotson had taken no precautions against deception and that the tests produced conflicting results.[35] Elliotson freely discussed the trials and expected outcomes in front of the Okeys, he said, and when anticipated results failed to materialise he often asked Elizabeth to confer with 'her negro' to explain the discrepancy. Wooldridge and other doubting students had repeated the tests on Elizabeth's 'seeing hand' but placed the bread and butter beyond her reach. When they whispered, 'She begins to see it', she clutched – and found nothing.

Although Wakley had restricted criticism in *The Lancet* so far – rejecting Blake's letter for example – he could not hold back the chorus of dissent any longer. He had published seven long detailed accounts of Elliotson's experiments in *The Lancet*, he had kept faith with his friend through his increasingly absurd trials and defended the professor's scientific integrity against a storm of criticism. The long-awaited inquiry by the members of the RS stumbled on without conclusion.[36] The university authorities had failed to rein in Elliotson's excesses. Even Wakley's own reporter Mills had apparently gone native. But now Wakley's patience snapped. In August, he published a letter from a London surgeon-apothecary, John Leeson, who complained that 'the grossest absurdities' were being 'palmed off as genuine science upon the learned societies of Europe'.[37] Having witnessed Elliotson's experiments on coins and water, Leeson was adamant that Elizabeth could detect the 'mesmerised' substances through the differences in temperature. Repeating the experiments in his own home, Leeson had consistently picked out the 'mesmerised' coins because they were warmer from being held in the hand. Elizabeth displayed 'the most extraordinary cunning and ability', he declared, and Elliotson was 'the victim of her impositions'. As usual, Elliotson was the blameless professional, Elizabeth the wicked imposter. In the same issue Wakley published a story revealing that a French physician had attempted to claim for his own daughter the 3,000 francs prize for someone who could read without the aid of their eyes. Supposedly the girl had read a book with her fingertips while blindfolded; when tested it was discovered she could see beneath the blindfold.[38]

Even Wakley's own staff were at loggerheads. While Mills avowed complete faith in Elliotson's tests and displayed puppy-like devotion to the Okeys, Clarke was openly scornful and proclaimed the experiments 'twaddle'.

Wakley was coming under increasing pressure from his friend Liston, and Liston's ally Sharpey, to denounce Elliotson's experiments. As a local MP he felt duty-bound to protect the students of UCL and the patients of UCH from unorthodox theories and therapies. As a UCL shareholder he shouldered a responsibility to defend the university's reputation. Students and professors were openly warring and mesmerism was being used as a weapon. Too much was at stake for Wakley to continue standing on the sidelines. His own reputation as a medical man, a journalist and an MP was under threat; the good name of *The Lancet* was being called into question. And, most significantly, Wakley believed the future of the medical profession was in jeopardy.

The battle between orthodox medicine and unconventional alternatives had reached a critical point. Although barber-surgeons, bone-setters, urine casters and itinerant herbalists had largely died out by the beginning of the nineteenth century, they had been replaced – in droves – by homoeopaths, electrical therapists and charlatans such as John St John Long. One medical practitioner had estimated in 1809 that qualified doctors were outnumbered nine to one by unqualified 'pretenders'.[39] Unlicensed chemists, grocers and tobacconists sold patent medicines such as Dr James's Fever Powder – which Elliotson had proved useless a decade earlier – and James Morison's Vegetable Universal Pills, which had made their creator a fortune, despite two of Morison's agents being found guilty of manslaughter after patients had died in the 1830s. What was more, the British public stoutly defended their freedom to shop around for health care, since unqualified practitioners and patent medicines were often cheaper than – and at least effective as – their orthodox counterparts. The laissez-faire Whig government was loath to stifle this approach.

Wakley had always taken up the battle against quacks, chasing St John Long through the courts and denouncing Morison as the 'King of Quacks'. He knew, fundamentally, that the survival of the medical profession – his readers – depended on their supremacy over their rivals. Granted, some of those qualified doctors were among the biggest enthusiasts for homoeopathy, electrical therapy and acupuncture, not to mention the detail that *The Lancet* vociferously supported phrenology. The fact that the medical orthodoxy Wakley fought to defend was at best ineffectual, frequently harmful and devoid of scientific evidence seemed to matter very little. Through his campaigns in parliament and his crusades in *The Lancet*, Wakley was determined to bring an end to the free market in medicines and free choice over medical practitioners which had characterised the Georgian era. Instead of patients enjoying unshackled liberty over who they turned to for medical advice, Wakley was adamant qualified doctors alone should be the arbiters of medical care. But he knew his efforts in parliament to establish a single regulatory body to license all doctors had a long way to go. And now mesmerism was threatening to overturn all his hard work.

In Wakley's view, Elliotson's erratic experiments were bringing the profession into disrepute. The idea that two ill-educated, half-crazed young girls were being encouraged to diagnose medical problems in place of doctors challenged every class, gender and professional convention he knew. Now forty-three, he had devoted fifteen years as editor of *The Lancet*, and three years as an MP, to his cause. He was not going to stand back and see it all destroyed. Mesmerism, in Wakley's view, was like a cancer spreading through the nation, and drastic surgery was required to cut it out. With the Royal Society panel dithering, the university council seemingly impotent, he was plainly the man to do the job.

The 'Seventh report' in *The Lancet* on Elliotson's experiments on mesmerism at UCH would be the last. Now Wakley was determined to take matters into his own hands.

9

Great Jackey

35 Bedford Square, London, 16 August 1838

The two sisters arrived at the five-storey house on the west side of Bedford Square in the heart of Bloomsbury at 3 p.m.[1] Although the square had lost some of its fashionable cachet since being developed in the 1770s, its elegant houses ranged in four terraces around an oval garden were still popular with judges, lawyers and bankers.[2] The only truly symmetrical square in London, Bedford Square retained a classical, clean-lined Georgian simplicity in the midst of the noisy Victorian metropolis. Escorted by Elliotson up the steps to the front door, the girls were admitted into the tiled hall and led up the staircase to the drawing room on the first floor.

It was not their first visit to Thomas Wakley's house – the Okey girls had been there on two occasions within the past two weeks – but it must still have been impressive to be ushered into the richly furnished drawing room of a grand townhouse rather than being shunted unceremoniously to the servants' quarters in the basement. Inside the room, whose three tall windows overlooked the plane trees in the square, six men were waiting. It was becoming a familiar scenario; the girls had been taken by Elliotson to the homes of several distinguished men – as well as to his own house – several times in the past few months. They even knew most of the men. Wakley still presented a tall, imposing figure with his piercing blue eyes and curling blond hair, though he had grown a little more corpulent in middle age. There too was their old friend Dupotet, looking as dapper as ever, the admiring young reporter from *The Lancet*, George Mills, and his rather less admiring colleague, James Fernandez Clarke. Yet for all their supposed clairvoyant talents, Elizabeth and Jane had no idea that this particular outing would prove to be a defining moment, both for them and their devoted professor.

Growing increasingly sceptical about Mills's glowing reports on the mesmerism experiments, Wakley had determined to see the phenomenon for himself. But the scenes which had enthralled Mills and enraptured so many others only convinced the independent-minded MP of the patent flaws in the trials. Wakley was adamant that they were not true scientific experiments and he did not mince his words in saying so. He did not regard them 'as tests of the reality of the phenomena displayed' but only as 'demonstrations of the supposed discoveries and . . . opinions' of Elliotson himself.[3]

Although he had not revealed his misgivings in public, privately Wakley had become convinced that the Okey sisters were calculating frauds and Elliotson their innocent dupe. His old friend, the ally of his long campaigns for medical reform and scientific progress, was plainly in thrall to the beguiling powers of these two clever girls. Since it was clear nobody else was prepared to make a stand, it seemed the task had fallen to Wakley. Pressing Elliotson to deliver the Okeys for the ultimate test, Wakley had waited impatiently.

It was already midday on 16 August when Wakley had opened a note from Elliotson offering to bring the sisters to Bedford Square at 3 p.m. that day. The short notice gave Wakley no time to assemble his own witnesses nor prepare experiments of his own design. All five men invited to observe the trials had been summoned by Elliotson. Along with Dupotet, Mills and Clarke, Elliotson had asked William Hering, the surgeon-apothecary and phrenologist who had mesmerised Charlotte Dewbury, and a Scottish physician named Dr Robert Richardson, who he probably knew from his Edinburgh days.[4] All were friends of Elliotson; all, as far as Elliotson was aware, were sympathetic to mesmerism. Nevertheless, Wakley was determined to make this a fair and final trial.

At first Elliotson took charge and requested that Elizabeth should take a chair while Jane was sent to an adjoining room. As the men watched, Elliotson produced the usual mesmeric phenomena before progressing to the more novel tests with metal and water. Plainly delighted that his friend was taking a belated personal interest in his hobby horse, Elliotson promised to show Wakley the 'quite astounding' effects he had obtained with 'mesmerised' nickel. Producing a small pellet of nickel and another, roughly the same size and weight, of lead, Elliotson explained that the effect of magnetised nickel was 'most extraordinary', while magnetised lead could be 'applied with impunity', that is, with no effect whatsoever. Chattering happily to herself, Elizabeth seemed oblivious to the proceedings as two of the men positioned a piece of cardboard in front of her face so she could see nothing behind it. She was already in a state of 'ecstatic delirium', Elliotson said. He then held the nickel pellet in his hand for several minutes to 'mesmerise' it and gave the lead piece to Wakley so he could warm it to the same temperature. Wakley seated himself in front of Elizabeth and took both metal pieces. Carefully concealing them so it was not possible to identify which was which, he rubbed first the lead and then the nickel on her hands. Elizabeth stared at the board without responding to either. The experiment was repeated; again there was no reaction. After further repetitions, Wakley applied the nickel once more and suddenly Elizabeth's body convulsed, with her back arched and her limbs rigid, her face flushed and her eyes bulging in a 'startling squint'. She was petrified in this position for the next fifteen minutes.

Elliotson was triumphant. The mesmerised nickel had worked just as he had predicted – albeit not quite as promptly as he had hoped. There was no doubt, he insisted, that Elizabeth's reaction was caused by the mesmerised nickel. Wakley scoffed, equally adamant that the experiment had proved no such thing. Any experiment was valueless, he argued, if there was no uniformity to the results. There was clearly no room for consensus. Elliotson would not back down; Wakley would not concede. Given the impasse, Wakley insisted on repeating the experiments – but this time he was determined to prove his case. And he had a clever ruse up his sleeve in order to do just that.

Again Wakley took both pieces of metal, but before beginning the tests anew he drew aside two of the men, his reporter Clarke and the surgeon Hering, and conferred with them in private. Once Elizabeth was recovered and the board back in position, Wakley performed the tests again, alternately rubbing the girl's hands with the pieces of metal concealed in his hands. For some time there was no response then just as he was about to apply the metal in his left hand, Hering urged in a loud whisper: 'Take care; don't apply the nickel too strongly.' Immediately, Elizabeth flew into a paroxysm with her body and limbs rigid, her spine arched and her face 'violently red'. At this Elliotson turned to his friend with obvious satisfaction. Delightedly he declared that 'no metal other than nickel had ever produced these effects'. Elizabeth remained fixed in position for more than half an hour as the guests shuffled their feet and stared at the floor. When finally she relaxed, Wakley insisted she leave the room since he was 'anxious to make a statement' to Elliotson in her absence. Elizabeth, however, objected to leaving. She plainly realised something was afoot. As ever Elliotson was prepared to concede control to her, so rather than forcing her to leave, he had Jane brought in to join her sister and the seven men trooped into the smaller anteroom.

Wakley could hardly contain himself. Once the men had squeezed into the room and closed the door, he looked over at Elliotson and gravely informed him he had been 'entirely deceived'. He now revealed that he had not used the nickel at all in the last trial; it was only when Hering warned in his stage whisper not to apply the nickel too strongly that Elizabeth had reacted.

Elliotson was flummoxed. He bluntly insisted the nickel must have been used; he was positive the effects could not be produced in any other way. Tempers flared; or as Clarke diplomatically put it, the discussion 'assumed an angry aspect'. While Elliotson accused Wakley of deliberate deception, Wakley was insistent that Elliotson was the one being deceived. Both stubborn men with famously quick tempers, neither would back down. At last, with a flourish worthy of a stage magician, Wakley announced there was 'a gentleman present who could confirm the accuracy of his statement'. At that moment Clarke stepped forward and produced the nickel piece from his waistcoat pocket. Wakley explained that before the experiment began, he had slipped the nickel to Clarke who had kept it in his pocket and stood for the duration of the tests in front of the window. Wakley had substituted the nickel for a farthing and had touched Elizabeth only with this and the lead.

Elliotson still refused to accept the evidence before him and urged Wakley to repeat the tests. So the men repaired to the drawing room once more and performed the tests on Elizabeth using the exact same deception; the results were precisely the same. Desperate to prove his faith in mesmerised nickel was not misplaced, Elliotson begged Wakley to try the experiments again the following day. He was confident a 'satisfactory explanation' would emerge. Fully exasperated by this point – and with good reason – Wakley retorted that he did not believe 'a single additional experiment could ever be necessary in connection with such an inquiry'. Nevertheless, for the sake of their long friendship, Wakley agreed to reconvene the next day.

The girls duly arrived at Bedford Square at 9 a.m. the following day, and this time Elliotson brought his chief disciple William Wood. Having slept on the puzzling events of the previous day, Elliotson had woken with a flash of insight. As he patiently explained to Wakley, when he applied the lead to Elizabeth's hand it must have touched the skin where the nickel had previously rubbed and reactivated the nickel effect. But Wakley was in no mood for new theories. He tartly replied that he believed Elizabeth herself could give a 'better explanation' for the results 'than any other person'. As the girls were readied for a further round of experiments, Wakley petulantly declared he could 'take no interest' in any further tests after the 'exposition' of the previous day. Nevertheless, over the next thirteen hours, from 9 a.m. to 10 p.m., Wakley presided over an exhaustive series of experiments on the Okey sisters to test and retest the nickel and lead, as well as gold sovereigns and mesmerised water.

As the second day's tests continued to produce inconsistent results, so the tension between the two men mounted. With each new result, Elliotson changed his thesis. When the nickel failed to produce a dramatic response, Elliotson urged applying it to Elizabeth's lips. When the lead produced a stronger reaction, he decided lead was just as conductive as nickel after all. And all the while he griped about the manner in which the trials were being conducted; it was 'not fair' to use the lead more often than the nickel. Wakley, understandably, was reaching the end of his tether. In a scientific test of any phenomenon, he snapped, the experimenter would be justified in using the lead 'throughout the entire day' and not employing the nickel at all. At this point, *The Lancet* recorded, 'Mr Wakley was obliged to leave the room to see a person on business' – though it seems more likely he left to stop himself swinging his renowned boxer's punch at his erstwhile friend. Elliotson too was obliged to leave; he was heading for the Continent for the start of his six-week annual tour. Nothing, not even his scientific reputation and his devotion to mesmerism, would stand in the way of his summer vacation. Besides, he remained as confident as ever that the tests were valid. This was sheer arrogance, of course. For somebody so demonstrably intelligent in youth, he had become patently obtuse in middle age. Taking Wood, and the metal pieces, with him, he left the girls at Bedford Square on the assumption that they would shortly be returned to UCH. Elizabeth was by then in 'an intense coma' with 'violent spasms'; it did not cross his mind that the 'poor little girl' would be subjected to any further trials.[5] With hindsight Elliotson would heartily regret this decision.

When Wakley returned to the room half an hour later to find Elliotson gone and the girls left behind he saw his chance. He sent Clarke out to buy more lead and nickel, then embarked on a raft of further experiments lasting five more hours. As Elliotson trundled off to the coast in merry anticipation of his summer jaunt, Wakley set out to repeat the full range of tests the professor had demonstrated at UCH in order to prove once and for all whether mesmerism was genuine or false.

In all a total of twenty-nine separate trials were conducted, using nickel, lead, gold and water. Since Elizabeth was out of sorts, the tests were commenced on Jane; she underwent twenty-two trials, and Elizabeth, once recovered, a further seven. With Elliotson and Wood out of the picture, Wakley called in a bevy of his own associates to witness the results. It was a distinguished group comprising some of the most respected medical men of the age. Along with Mills and Clarke, the party included William Farr, the brilliant statistician who would dedicate his life to improving public health, Frederick Hale Thompson, a surgeon who was co-president of the Westminster Medical Society and Dr Peter Hennis Green, an expert on childhood diseases who would shortly edit the *Provincial Medical and Surgical Journal*, the forerunner of the *British Medical Journal*.[6]

The ensuing tests proved predictably inconsistent. The 'mesmerised' water produced no effect while 'unmesmerised' water threw the girls into a seizure; the 'mesmerised' sovereigns produced no response while 'unmesmerised' coins sent the girls into paroxysms. After each set of trials, Wakley solemnly asked the assembled men to confirm their opinion that the mesmerising influence had no effect on the material tested. Each time the men unanimously concurred. After the tests on Jane were concluded, the party agreed with Wakley that 'it would be useless, and even ridiculous, to subject the alleged magnetic powers of Jane O'Key to a single additional test'. The tests on Elizabeth were equally conclusive.

By the end of the day, both girls were understandably exhausted and Elizabeth was complaining she felt sick. This was scarcely surprising since she had drunk nearly a pint of warm water, mesmerised or not. As darkness fell over the square, the girls were finally sent back to UCH to sleep off their ordeal. Once they had gone, the men unanimously affirmed a record of the experiments and jointly testified that the trials proved beyond doubt the fallacy of mesmerising metal and water. But Wakley was determined to go further. Drawing himself up to address the group, he declared that 'the effects which were said to arise from what had been denominated "animal magnetism", constituted one of the completest delusions that the human mind ever entertained'.[7]

Wakley was adamant. If the tests on 'mesmerised' water and metal had failed, then mesmerism fell in its entirety. As far as he was concerned, the experiments that had taken place at his house on 16 and 17 August proved beyond doubt that mesmerism was a total fallacy; all who believed in it were sorry dupes, and all who practised it foolish quacks. Furthermore, he was resolute that his tests proved the Okey sisters were frauds, clever actresses who had cynically tricked the honest professor along with half the nation's medical community.

Elliotson had been hoist by his own petard. By insisting that mesmerism was a physical force that could influence metal and water, he had clouded proper inquiry into its effects. And by placing his faith so entirely in the Okey girls, he had jeopardised support for mesmerism as a whole. Yet Wakley was equally remiss. In using Elliotson's ludicrous theory, and the Okey sisters, as the sole basis for testing the authenticity of mesmerism, he was blind to its real potential. He had effectively thrown out the baby with the mesmerised bathwater. The single-minded determination and pig-headed arrogance which had helped them both reach the summits of their careers were also the flaws which prevented either of them applying sound scientific principles to the entire enigma.

In reality, of course, Wakley's tests proved very little. Certainly they showed that the notion of mesmerising metal or water was a nonsense. Yet Wakley's experiments failed completely to address why the Okey girls, along with scores more patients at UCH and elsewhere, fell into deep trances, withstood extremes of pain, performed superhuman feats and showed dramatic improvements in their medical conditions.

Content simply to discredit mesmerism and the Okeys as one wholesale bundle, Wakley had turned his back on these remarkable responses and their potential benefits for medicine.

Clarke, *The Lancet* reporter who witnessed the Bedford Square tests from beginning to end, summed up the situation astutely. 'The experiments of Mr Wakley, whilst they proved some things failed to prove others; and, in fact, left the subject under discussion still more mysterious,' he wrote.[8] He argued: 'Most people doubted – indeed, denied – the reality of the prophetic power of Elizabeth O'Key, and some of the more striking phenomena exhibited by her sister Jane. But there were some experiments so fairly performed, and the results so palpable to all, that no one could fairly deny that there had been "effects," whose cause, by whatever name we might call it, was mysterious, strange, and meriting calm and deliberate inquiry.'

With hindsight there seems little doubt that the Okey sisters were genuinely affected by mesmerism, at least at first. In response to the mesmeric hand movements, they fell into trances, withstood pain and electric shocks, and underwent personality changes just as many other subjects did – and still do under hypnotism today. Then, egged on by the credulous Elliotson and his eager assistants, the Okeys extended their repertoire to satisfy the predictions of further marvels. It is likely that they subconsciously set out to 'please' their doctor and fulfil his suggestions and expectations. The wide margin of error Elliotson allowed them, and the fact that he frequently adapted his theories to fit their responses, meant whatever they did they seemed to confirm his beliefs. As the doctor's demands grew wilder, the sisters responded in kind. They were poor, vulnerable, impressionable young girls in the presence of wealthy, powerful men so it would not be surprising if they felt the need to comply.

But were they also at times consciously acting? It is impossible to be sure, yet it seems probable that, as time went on, the girls began to deliberately fake their more bizarre 'abilities', such as seeing through doors, predicting the future and diagnosing patients. Certain instances betrayed them. When Elizabeth said her 'negro' had warned her not to lift any more weights she was obviously trying to protect herself; when she announced she was no longer insensitive to pain she had clearly had enough of the sadistic trials. It was plainly in the girls' interest to retain their position as the stars of the mesmeric scene in order to continue benefiting from the shelter the hospital provided. At the same time, they were most likely enjoying their celebrity status, revelling in the media spotlight and relishing their hold over the gullible professor and all the slavering men who came to view them – just as any adolescent girls might when offered a chance of fame.

Here too Clarke offered a sage analysis. He was convinced Elizabeth 'feigned some of the phenomena' but was 'certain that others were really the product of "mesmerism"'.[9] 'Thus, I believe that the sleep, coma, and sleep-walking were the result of the passes,' he wrote, while he did not doubt that, in this trance-like state, she and Jane were insensible to pain. Yet he also believed Elizabeth's long 'jetty' eyelashes enabled her to fake sleep whenever she pleased. 'That this peculiarity gave her immense power in appearing to be asleep when she was not, I am quite convinced.' She possessed, he added, 'extraordinary cleverness and shrewdness'.

While Elliotson wandered the Swiss Alps, oblivious to events back home, Wakley lost no time in broadcasting the results of his tests. They were published in painstaking detail over seven pages in *The Lancet* on 1 September. Conscious Elliotson was still abroad and unable to defend his research, Wakley made no comment; he evidently believed the facts would speak for themselves. Yet while he was careful not to traduce his old friend Elliotson, in the same issue Wakley published excerpts from two letters written by Mayo in the *LMG*, which, Wakley assured his readers, would provide 'no small portion of amusement'.[10]

Then, on 8 September, Wakley broke his silence and published a withering attack on mesmerism and its followers in an editorial headlined: 'Life and death of animal magnetism'.[11] Given the support for mesmerism on the Continent and the firm conviction of many of its supporters, Wakley said he had felt it was his duty to report Elliotson's experiments at UCH in *The Lancet*. The authenticity of the trance, catalepsy and delirium were now widely accepted, he wrote, but these were only enacted 'through the senses', both voluntarily and involuntarily, to differing degrees in different people. His tests had proved there was no such thing as a physical magnetic force, yet Wakley was determined his discoveries would sound the death knell of mesmerism in its entirety. 'Careful investigation and a consideration of all the experiments have convinced us that the phenomena are not real, and that animal magnetism is a delusion,' he declared. Wakley roundly ridiculed Dupotet – 'the Magnetic Missionary of Britain' – along with Mayo and Lardner for their credulity, yet still he held back from criticising Elliotson; so far the bonds of friendship stayed firm. His fiercest condemnation was reserved for the Okey girls. 'O'KEY lays her hand upon a sovereign, and is fixed, or prostrated to the earth. We lay our hands upon the same sovereign and perceive no such influences . . . the experience of mankind is on one scale, the O'KEYS in the other.' Fools might predict the world would end in 1840 or that the sun would never rise again. Though not entirely impossible such things were 'infinitely improbable', wrote Wakley, and 'the same might be said with respect to the facts that O'KEY is fixed by gold, that her *negro* can foretell events, or that she can see with the back of her hand'.

A week later, in a second editorial – a masterpiece of journalistic contempt – Wakley rained down scorn on mesmerism and launched another vicious attack on the Okeys.[12] Following *The Lancet*'s exposures, the 'science' of mesmerism could no longer 'affront the common sense of the medical profession, or dare to show its face in the scientific societies', he fumed. He now laid the blame for the profession's ensnarement – and by definition, for Elliotson's delusion – entirely at the feet of the Okeys. Elizabeth was 'a genius in her line' who was 'excelled by few actresses on the stage' while Jane was 'but a tame copy of her sister'. Relating examples of Elizabeth's talent for mimicry and 'wonderful performances', Wakley proclaimed: 'Her improvisations at the mesmeric sittings, the witticisms, the sarcasms, the snatches of song, which she spouted so prodigiously, were, not unfrequently, worthy of the licensed fool of the old comedy: the audience was often amused, when the jokes derived their raciness neither from ribaldry, profanity, nor obscenity. Her very impudence was *naif*.' Elizabeth was a skilled deceiver, said Wakley, who had used her talents to entrap the poor, deluded Elliotson. 'The coaxing, flattering strain in which she addressed Dr ELLIOTSON, and her other favourites, displayed tact, consciousness of power in dealing with other minds, and a full knowledge of all the advantages of her position,' he wrote. In her delirium she took 'strange liberties with the worthy Doctor' and addressed him in 'a patronising tone'. At other times she used foul and profane language, said Wakley, helpfully supplying some of the most lurid examples. During the Bedford Square tests Elizabeth had held forth on 'affected young ladies' and challenged her audience:

"'Now what would I do with such a *fine* young lady? Why kick her a— to be sure.'"

As before, Wakley insisted that all the Okeys' reactions to the mesmerism experiments at UCH were simply a case of clever acting. And as to the argument that the 'young imposters' had no motive for such deception, he stormed that the Okeys had, in fact, motives 'as few uneducated girls could resist'. At first Elizabeth no doubt '*pitied*' the believers panting for signs and wonders which the slightest exertion of her will could produce' then she sought to 'please and astonish her dear good friends' and finally she could not resist using her talents to 'exert their utmost power over a large audience'. For the first time Wakley now published the allegations, later repeated by Clarke and others, that the Okey sisters had previously 'spoken in tongues' at Irving's evangelical services. They were plainly experienced performers, well-versed in the art of deception.

Just as Wakley heaped derision on the Okey girls so he targeted Mayo – the 'Middlesex Owl' – for ridicule again. Yet still he made no criticism of his old chum Elliotson, despite the fact that the professor was universally acknowledged as the chief proponent of mesmerism in Britain.

News of *The Lancet*'s denouncement of mesmerism and denunciation of the Okey sisters unleashed a sensation in the press. The *LMG* gleefully reported Wakley's tests and even gave its rival 'full credit for the manner in which they were conducted', while crowing that the conclusions were entirely in accordance with the opinions it had expressed for the past twelve months.[13] Magnanimously, the *LMG* declined to pronounce whether the sisters were 'shameless imposters' or 'dupes of their own imaginations' and acquitted all those who had supported mesmerism of any intention to deceive. But the journal went on to accuse Wakley of hypocrisy for attempting to 'create "a diversion" in Dr Elliotson's favour by turning the laugh against Mr Mayo', as well as for defending UCL for so long. If similar events had occurred elsewhere Wakley would surely have condemned all involved, argued the *LMG*. Instead 'the bubble has been blown to its present, or rather its recent magnitude in great measure by the fostering breath of *The Lancet*'. The journal had a point. 'Magnetism has now lived a year in England: we scarcely expected that it would survive so long,' the journal concluded. 'Once buried, may we not hope that any attempts to revive it will be . . . put aside without examination.'

The Times published the *LMG*'s vituperative reports verbatim; though it made no editorial comment, its readers could be left in no doubt of its views.[14] And newspapers up and down the country repeated the details with varying degrees of hilarity and salaciousness. Having previously praised the 'impartiality' of Lardner's accounts, the *Age* now applauded Wakley – 'cunning dog!' – for exposing the 'Mesmeric Humbug'.[15] The *Penny Satirist*'s medical advisor described Elliotson as 'the dupe of a jade' but warned against the conclusion that, because the Okeys had cheated the professor, all mesmerism was false.

Aware that Elliotson was still abroad, the intrepid reporters of the *Satirist* were eager to track down the Okeys. When they discovered the girls were staying in Dover during the professor's extended absence, they could not resist a spoof story. Headlined 'Mesmeric Sympathies' the article jested that Elizabeth had become entranced on tasting the seawater at Dover because Elliotson was bathing in the waters off Calais at the same time. The *Periscope* went further with a lascivious spoof piece about 'a young and hysterical female' who was treated for dysmenorrhoea, or painful periods, by a mesmerist who injected 'magnetized water' into her vagina and placed mesmerised nickel on her belly. The treatment was apparently successful in stopping her periods; nine months later the woman gave birth.

Meanwhile *The Lancet* was deluged with letters – 'too numerous' to print – from readers, both applauding Wakley's actions and defending mesmerism.[16] John Leeson, the surgeon-apothecary who had previously challenged the experiments at UCH, insisted *he* should take the credit for exposing the Okey girls. James Birch Sharpe, a Windsor surgeon who had taken up mesmerism with gusto, argued that whether or not the Okey sisters were imposters, mesmerism produced definite effects. Two young women he had treated were now able to mesmerise their own sisters 'with as much power as when I operate upon them', he wrote. And Dr Jones, a Southampton physician, protested that he was certain the Okeys were honest, having seen them withstand electric shocks *'without moving a muscle'* and being pinched 'to a degree which would make any person flinch'. Wakley countered by ascribing all the Okeys' behaviour to their 'remarkable powers of acting' and urged Dr Jones to 'double his precautions with his patients'. From Elliotson, however, there was silence.

*

Elliotson returned to London at the end of September and resumed his work at UCH in readiness for the autumn term. Although the Okeys remained in Dover, escaping the media circus, staff had continued to mesmerise patients during the professor's absence, according to his directions. His colleagues at UCH watched intently to see what he would do next; the profession and the press held their collective breath. Elliotson seemed chastened, even shocked by the furore his experiments had created, and was stunned by Wakley's betrayal. It was a critical moment in his career. He could have taken stock, recalibrated his support for mesmerism, pointed to the success he had had in treating certain patients but scaled down his more exotic experiments. If so, he might have acquitted himself with honour. Yet, as events had shown time and time again, Elliotson was incapable of backing down; being opposed only made him all the more determined to prove that he was right.

Mulling over the events at Bedford Square, Elliotson now heartily regretted showing Wakley the experiments and could not forgive his old ally for betraying him. He had brought the Okey girls to Wakley's home 'in an evil hour', he said.[17] He had feared all along that Wakley's aim was to discredit mesmerism in response to the volume of letters he was receiving. 'He said he was pestered with letters upon the subject; but that nineteen out of twenty were unfavourable,' Elliotson wrote. 'Nineteen persons of course purchase more *Lancets* than one, and I fancied I already saw his rejection of the evidence.' Although he had shown the editor 'a variety of the most beautiful and satisfactory experiments', Wakley had suppressed these in his report. And though Elliotson had tried to explain the discrepancies in the tests, Wakley had been 'too dull to understand' or 'had his reasons for not understanding'.

When he had left for the Continent, Elliotson had little imagined that further experiments would be made on the girls 'by a person ignorant of the subject and altogether incapable of making experiments'. He was shocked to discover on his return that Wakley had not only performed further tests but published the results – 'a most imperfect and worthless account'. And to his fury when he wrote to *The Lancet* to protest at its stance, Wakley refused even to print his letters.

The breach was complete. At first Elliotson had convinced himself that Wakley was merely misguided; he had mishandled the experiments and misinterpreted the results. Then he had allowed himself to believe the editor was acting from commercial interests – to mollify his readers.

But Wakley's continued insistence that all mesmerism was a fraud, and his refusal to let Elliotson defend himself, was the last straw. The friendship between the two medical mavericks was over, the long partnership between the two social reformers blown apart. They would never meet again and over the ensuing months and years the bitterness would only fester. Elliotson would later describe Wakley as 'a mere journalist' and a 'literary trickster'. Betraying his usual snobbery, he would call the editor an 'uneducated Somersetshire peasant' who was as ignorant about mesmerism 'as of Latin, French, or Mathematics'.[18] It was a sorry day for medicine and in the process a great opportunity was lost. Yet Elliotson clung to his belief in mesmerism as firmly as ever.

As his fellow professors and students watched with alarm, Elliotson continued to treat his patients with mesmerism and to test its effects. Soon after his return he admitted four male patients – three with epilepsy and one with 'paroxysms of imbecility' – and treated them all with mesmerism alone.[19] Then in October, to universal amazement, he readmitted Elizabeth Okey after an absence of nearly two months. Her epilepsy was now cured, he said, but she had developed a new complaint, ischuria (retention of urine) which caused her 'agonizing pain in her loins'. Jane, presumably, had returned to the family home in Somers Town. Although he did not attempt to treat Elizabeth's new ailment with mesmerism, he could not resist the temptation to continue his investigations on his prize patient. 'I frequently threw her into a mesmeric state,' he wrote, 'partly for the purpose of ascertaining facts, and partly because in it her sufferings were less.'

For all Elliotson's claim that Elizabeth was cured of epilepsy, her general state of health was clearly no better. Soon after her return to UCH her family came to visit, including Uncle Arter, her 'uncle-papa', who furnished a detailed account of the extraordinary scene for his local newspaper.[20] Elizabeth was 'in a state of idiocy' when he arrived, oblivious to her father, mother, or himself, talking 'nonsense' and using 'obscene and profane' language. 'I spoke to her (and I think the pleasure of seeing me would have thrown her off her guard, had she been acting), but she evidently did not know me, nor did her eye rest on me for an instant, nor yet on her parents, though they several times told her her uncle was come to see her.' Then Elliotson arrived and Elizabeth began talking to him 'in a most childish manner'. The doctor sent Elizabeth to sleep by rubbing her gums with a silver pencil case and laid her on the bed where she snored loudly. But when he tried to return her to her normal state neither the pencil case nor a gold ring he took from his finger would have any effect. Finally Elliotson put his gold pocket watch in her mouth while 'rubbing his forehead against hers'. At this bizarre departure from bedside etiquette she woke, sprang off the bed and wrapped her arms around her uncle then picked up an accordion and played 'several tunes in the best manner I had ever heard one played'. Even Uncle Arter, it seemed, had tendered his doubts about the veracity of his niece but after this visit he was 'satisfied that no deception was practised'.

It was business as usual. Elliotson was as deeply wedded to mesmerism as ever and the wards were busy with clerks 'pawing' patients just as before. Elliotson's colleagues were aghast. His opponents in the press were apoplectic. 'We thought that mesmerism had received its death-blow, and was defunct,' stormed the *LMG* in October, 'but we understand that since Dr Elliotson's return to town the Mesdames O'Key have made their appearance at University College Hospital, and that the learned Professor declares his faith in the *science* to be quite unimpaired.'[21] The journal exhorted Elliotson's fellow teachers to 'take immediate steps for putting an end to all such mummeries'.

For once *The Lancet* was in complete agreement with its rival. One of its reporters, either Mills or Clarke, now warned Elliotson that Wakley was determined to see mesmerism banished from the wards.[22] 'Mesmerism was now all humbug; the Okeys were depraved imposters; I was a fool; and Wakley declared that he would make the Council of University College order me to treat diseases (however successfully) with mesmerism no longer.' He was convinced Wakley was working in cahoots with Liston to bring him down. 'Mr Wakley had formed the closest, the most inseparable, intimacy with Mr Liston, and Mr Liston told him that the illustrious professors at University College were against mesmerism and me,' he wrote. It was professional jealousy – 'silly envy' he said – though there was more than a trace of jealousy too in Elliotson's description of the 'bosom' friendship between Liston and Wakley. Another observer would later say that the 'principal' mover against Elliotson was Richard Quain, the faculty dean, 'aided and abetted' by Liston intriguing with Wakley.[23] For years, said the anonymous source, *The Lancet* had 'lauded Dr Elliotson to the skies as the first practitioner of the day'. But egged on by Liston, 'Wakley turns round on his former friend, and resolves to destroy his reputation'. Working in alliance, Elliotson's former friend and his enemies were now ready for the final showdown.

In October the hospital committee, which was responsible for hospital management, demanded to know why Elizabeth Okey had now been a patient in UCH for eighteen months, excepting her two months' absence in Dover, when hospital rules stipulated a maximum stay of two months.[24] In practice this rule was routinely ignored. As Elliotson pointed out, his fellow physician Thomson had a patient who had been in hospital for fourteen months. When Elliotson explained that Elizabeth had been readmitted with a new problem, he thought the members seemed 'satisfied'. In reality they were simply biding their time.

Still alert for manifestations of new mesmeric phenomena, Elliotson was thrilled in November when Elizabeth confided to him during a spell of delirium that she had developed a new power. What fresh novelty could this be? Quite simply, she could detect when a patient was going to die. In her trance, she said, she felt a 'sense of great oppression, sickness and misery' whenever she drew near someone who was sinking. When she was delirious, she saw a figure, 'something like the representation of death', wrapped in a white robe standing beside a doomed person. The closer the patient was to dying, the taller the figure appeared. Elliotson was not quite so credulous as to take this vision of the grim reaper literally. He reasoned that just as some people were susceptible to hay fever or suffered when they were close to cats, so others might perceive certain 'emanations' from the dying which had no effect on the population at large – an allergy to impending death so to speak. 'Thus, the sensation, which she knows to arise from the influence of a person hurrying to the grave, gives her a fancy that she sees the figure, when in her delirium,' he explained. One of the nurses confirmed that Elizabeth had claimed to see such a figure hovering near certain beds and soon afterwards those patients had died. Having now parted company with all scientific logic, Elliotson could not wait to put 'this wonderful fact' to the test.

On a dark December afternoon, at about 5 p.m., Elliotson escorted Elizabeth to one of the male wards with a nurse in tow.[25] He had waited until twilight, he explained, so she would be unable to see the patients or read the charts above their beds. Silently he led her by the hand up one side of the dimly lit ward and down the other without stopping. As she passed the foot of two of the beds he felt her shudder violently.

When they left the ward she told him she had seen the figure of death, which she called 'Jack', at the end of those two beds. The nurse agreed she had felt Elizabeth shudder and at the same time heard her whisper, 'There's Jack.' Immediately Elliotson wrote down the predictions, sealed the paper and handed it to John Taylor, who had resumed his post as hospital apothecary.

The following morning the hospital was in uproar. Taylor had surmised what was in the sealed letter – quite possibly he had opened it – and had gossiped about Elizabeth's predictions to anyone who would listen. Now the patients were distraught, the medical students were running amok and the medical staff were horrified. When Clarke, *The Lancet* reporter, arrived at UCH that morning he heard that the first patient Elizabeth picked out had died overnight while the second showed signs of imminent demise. The students were 'in the wildest excitement', he said, while queues of people were clamouring to see the 'inspired girl'. Then Elliotson arrived and went directly to the lecture theatre with a posse of students in hot pursuit. He seemed 'somewhat oppressed', said Clarke, but 'not daunted' and at once launched into a lecture on the scientific principle behind Elizabeth's prophecies, explaining that people near death gave out a 'peculiar effluvia' which Okey, in her heightened state, could sense.

Within days Elliotson was summoned to the hospital committee.[26] Led by William Tooke, the university co-founder who had previously defended Elliotson's right to lecture on mesmerism, the committee first asked why Elizabeth remained in hospital after so long. Elliotson said she was 'too ill' to be discharged, although he added that she was now free of attacks of delirium except when he induced them by mesmerism.[27] At this, one committee member accused him – reasonably enough – of 'taking away this poor girl's senses'. Now Tooke turned to the real reason for the summons and demanded to know why Elliotson had taken Elizabeth to one of the male wards. Elliotson was candid: he freely admitted escorting Elizabeth to the ward and giving her prophecies to the apothecary in a sealed note. He considered it was his duty to investigate this latest development, he insisted. Henry Crabb Robinson, one of the committee members who was generally sympathetic to Elliotson, recalled, 'The Dr asserted warmly his confidence that *Okey is no imposter* and his belief that there is something real & extraordinary in the facts that have occurred.'[28]

Ordering Elliotson to wait, much to his indignation, the committee called in the nurse who had accompanied him on his twilight visit. Somewhat embellishing her earlier report, she now declared that when Elizabeth approached one patient's bed she 'gave a convulsive shudder' and exclaimed, 'Great Jackey was on the bed'.[29] When she reached another she shuddered again, though less violently, and said 'Little Jacky was seated there!' The apothecary, Taylor, confirmed that during the night the first patient had died while the second appeared to be at death's door. The committee had heard enough.

A few days later, on 22 December, the university council resolved that the hospital committee should expel Elizabeth Okey immediately and that mesmerism should be banned entirely from the hospital. Henry Crabb Robinson voted reluctantly in favour. 'I concur in substance,' he confided to his diary, 'but think the form of the first resoln. objectionable – I would rather have had Dr El: informed of the opinion that E Okey shd *not prophecy*.'[30] When the house committee approved the decision five days later, Elliotson resigned.

In truth he had no choice. No physician could maintain his professional integrity when instructed by others which patients he could treat and in what manner. His resignation letter was unequivocal. 'I have just received information that the council, *without any interview or communication with me*, has ordered my patient, Elizabeth Okey, to be instantly discharged, and forbidden me to cure my patients with mesmerism,' he wrote. 'I only am the proper person to judge when my patients are in a fit state to be discharged & what treatment is proper for their cases.'[31] He demanded that the university refund his students the fees they had paid and vowed never to enter the hospital or the university again.

He was true to his word. The following day Elliotson's resignation was accepted by the medical committee and that evening he dined quietly at home with his good friend Charles Dickens.[32]

It was a sad day for the university and the hospital, and a sorry end to a remarkable career. For seven years Elliotson had reigned supreme as the most popular teacher in the medical school. When he had joined in 1831 he had a class of ninety and by the time he left his pupils numbered nearly 200. For four years Elliotson had nurtured UCH. He had been instrumental in founding the hospital, had chosen its name and had done more than any of his colleagues to promote its welfare. More significantly, for Elliotson at least, his career and reputation were in ruins. The man hailed as the foremost physician in London, the doctor who had championed the stethoscope and quinine, had lost his position and his status in one fell swoop. At the peak of his career, at the age of forty-seven, he now faced oblivion.

As the year ended, tranquillity was restored to the wards of UCH. There would be no more patients 'pawed' over by mesmerists, no more experiments with 'mesmerised' water or metal, no more demonstrations using electric batteries or levitating cats. Staff and students resumed their old practices of bleeding, blistering and poisoning patients with customary abandon.

Elliotson's colleagues rejoiced at his departure. His fellow physician Anthony Todd Thomson exclaimed: 'Thank God we have got rid of him.'[33] Thomson boasted to students that he had not once observed Elliotson's experiments and he now made a habit of labelling every case in which he suspected a patient of feigning with the single word: 'Okeyism'. Sharpey described Elliotson's withdrawal as 'a blessed thing' since 'any body is better than he had latterly made himself'.[34] Elliotson was 'in my opinion all along an objectionable person', he wrote, though a 'good teacher and a *man of note* . . . But after the absurdities of the magnetism & the scandalous proceedings carried on by him in the Hospital he could be regarded as nothing better than a broken pitcher which could no longer *hold in* or be of any use to any body.'

The medical press was equally jubilant. The *LMG* professed itself delighted that 'the dirge of animal magnetism' had finally been sung after the 'gross absurdity' of Elliotson 'receiving from the lips of a magnetic prophetess' predictions about the likely demise of patients.[35] The *British and Foreign Medical Review* dismissed the fascination with mesmerism as 'one of those unaccountable paroxysms of credulity' during which 'weak women and weak doctors went astray' but was confident that 'scarcely any man of reputation had become a convert to it'.[36]

The Lancet, inevitably, commended the 'temperate but firm conduct' of UCL and said its actions had met with 'very hearty approval' from medical men and friends of the university.[37] Still struggling with old loyalties, Wakley said Elliotson's integrity was not 'impugned in this affair' but admitted that if the professor had stayed in his post it would have caused 'great injury' to the hospital and 'inevitable ruin' to the medical school. He was unequivocal, however, in declaring that 'such a humbug as mesmerism' could not co-exist with '*the science of medicine*' in Britain and proclaimed: 'When DR ELLIOTSON became a mesmerist, he ceased to be a "physician".' *The Times* took up the refrain, printing *The Lancet*'s report of Elizabeth's twilight excursion under the headline, 'The humbug called "mesmerism"'. The newspaper congratulated the university on its good sense in ensuring the pupils would in future be taught by a Professor of Medicine rather than 'a practitioner of humbug'.[38] If any student remained 'who believes in "Great Jackey" or "Little Jackey"', *The Times* suggested they should be despatched immediately to the county asylum at Hanwell. 'Bedlam is much too good for such a fool.'

Elliotson's students were no fools but they were certainly mad. When they heard their teacher had been forced to resign, they organised an emergency meeting.[39] Nearly 300 pupils crowded into the anatomy theatre on 4 January 1839 to debate demands to bring him back. All were agreed that Elliotson was a peerless lecturer, an inspired practitioner and a dedicated man of science, but as to whether he should return to his post, the students were split. The rowdy meeting descended into chaos as pupils attacked his demonstrations and condemned his decision to take Elizabeth Okey to the bedside of a 'dying man'. A ballot was arranged for the following day. In the event the pupils would vote by a slender majority of eleven to urge the UCL council to persuade Elliotson to return. But it was too late. For by the time the resolution reached the council meeting, its members had already voted to accept his resignation.[40] The doors of UCH, the hospital Elliotson had helped bring into existence, and UCL, the university he had done so much to support, were finally closed to him.

Wakley had helped raise Elliotson to the zenith of his career and he was instrumental in dashing him to the ground again. The doctor who was 'not surpassed by any physician in the metropolis' on his appointment at UCH had now 'ceased to be a "physician"' on his departure. What was more, in his determination to banish quackery from orthodox medical practice, Wakley had cast out one of the only therapies that had shown real potential. Concerned above all else to protect the reputation of the profession from the taint of unconventional ideas, Wakley had sacrificed his friend to the cause.

'Elliotson and mesmerism stood and fell together,' wrote the journalist Clarke. Looking back, he would later say it seemed 'marvellous' that 'a great physician, a great physiologist, a keen observer of facts, should have been so misled' and ruined by 'two illiterate and hysterical girls'. The Okeys were not illiterate, of course, but neither were they responsible for bringing down Elliotson. That distinction belonged to Wakley, but also largely to Elliotson himself, through his refusal to accept he might ever be wrong. Both as blind and stubborn as each other, Wakley had cast mesmerism to the medical fringe where it would remain for the foreseeable future, while Elliotson had thrown his lot in entirely with mesmerism without stopping to distinguish the likely medical benefits from the theatrical absurdities. Clarke mused: 'There is no chapter in the history of Medicine more astounding and bewildering than the episode of 1837–38, when for a time animal magnetism or mesmerism engrossed the attention of the Profession and the public.' As the New Year dawned, Clarke – and many others – believed that particular chapter was closed. They could not have been more wrong.

Perfect Anaesthesia

37 Conduit Street, London, 4 January 1839

Elliotson sat glumly contemplating his future at home in Conduit Street. When he walked out of UCL, he had walked out on a lucrative income from lecture fees and the substantial private business generated by his university connections. Although he had built up a considerable independent fortune, he was reliant for future income on his private practice. Yet his professional reputation had been severely tarnished. He had been traduced in the press nationally and internationally with news of his resignation published as far afield as Calcutta.[1] He had lost friends in medical and scientific circles who now thought him a dupe or a fraud. The controversy had cost him two thirds of his practice, making him £10,000 a year worse off he would later estimate.[2] He felt as if the 'whole profession' was against him 'from the royal physicians and surgeons to the humblest druggist-apothecary in a by-street'. Having numbered some of the highest-ranking people in the land among his patients, he now felt stigmatised 'as a fool, a visionary, a madman, aye, and a quack'. Isolated and bitter, both his confidence and his faith in mesmerism wavered. And then there was a knock on the door.

On the evening of Friday 4 January, two weeks after Elliotson's resignation, a surgeon named Francis Johnston called to ask Elliotson's advice.[3] A patient, a woman in her early twenties named Miss Critchley, had been seized with a severe cough after hearing a pistol fired at close quarters and this had developed into violent hiccups. Despite being bled and blistered by Johnston, her hiccups had not only continued but grown so severe she was in constant pain, vomited everything she ate and was confined to a sofa day and night. Indeed, the hiccups were so loud they could be heard in the next street. Cowed by his recent defeat, Elliotson dared not suggest mesmerism, but as he examined the woman's stomach he secretly moved his fingers in a mesmeric pass. The hiccups ceased for an hour although next morning they were as bad as ever.

Throughout January and February, the poor woman consulted one medical practitioner after another who dosed her variously with opium, morphine, camphor, creosote, ammonia and tincture of cantharides – crushed beetles – yet to the bafflement of her doctors none of these therapies worked. At last, Elliotson summoned the courage to propose mesmerism. Johnston, her own doctor, confessed he had previously 'laughed at it like others' but since every other remedy had failed he saw no objection. On 27 February Elliotson began to mesmerise the hiccupping Miss Critchley. After twenty minutes her eyes closed and the hiccups subsided. Within four weeks, after daily treatment, she was back to robust health. It was a remarkable cure. Even Lord Brougham, who had stormed out of Elliotson's demonstration a year earlier, was forced to recant. Seeing the woman mesmerised in Elliotson's drawing room, he declared himself 'convinced of the truth of mesmerism'.

For Elliotson the hiccupping triumph came not a moment too soon. 'Never was there performed a more decided, a more gratifying, a more astounding cure,' he enthused. In truth there had been – and would be – far more astounding cures but whether the hiccups had succumbed to mesmerism or had simply disappeared of their own accord, the timing was perfect. Elliotson's confidence in his medical prowess was restored, his belief in mesmerism was regained and – as news of this latest sensation spread – so his reputation began to revive. By March he was his old, ebullient self.

In a triumphal farewell letter to his former students, published in the *LMG* that month, he proclaimed his belief in mesmerism was as firm as ever.[4] 'Mesmerism is not only true, and of the highest interest in a psychological, physiological and curative point of view, but is now proceeding at a very rapid rate,' he declared. In the last few weeks alone, he said, hundreds had been converted to believing in mesmerism while a growing number of medical men were beginning to practise the therapy for themselves. The *LMG* blasted the address as 'the production of an ingenious man, very vain and very angry, whose judgment, moreover, is manifestly unsound'. But Elliotson was right: mesmerism was back in business.

Although the press continued to scoff, and the medical establishment reeled in horror, surgeons and physicians in the provinces began tentatively to dabble with mesmerism and found – to their amazement – that it frequently worked. Until this point, only a handful of practitioners had tried mesmerism, following Elliotson's lead. Undeterred by his fate they had continued to experiment and were soon joined by others who began to file reports of remarkable cures in provincial newspapers and to proclaim their success to the professional bodies. Far from being quashed by Wakley's exposures and the ensuing scandal, mesmerism was advancing once more and Elliotson was leading the charge.

Now that he had been denied a public venue, Elliotson staged demonstrations of mesmerism on the Okey sisters in his own home, helped by his ever-loyal assistant, Wood.[5] After Elizabeth was expelled from UCH on 12 January, both sisters had been taken in by Elliotson and they now lived in his housekeeper's room.[6] Their performances were as popular as ever. Although admission was by ticket only, dozens of people crammed into Elliotson's drawing room as often as five times a week.[7] At one demonstration in March, the audience numbered nearly 100 including 'noblemen, clergymen, barristers, artists, distinguished scientific and literary characters, and members of the medical profession, as well as many ladies'.[8] In addition to running through the usual repertoire with the Okey girls, Elliotson presented a young boy who had been paralysed. The lad had previously been wheeled into a demonstration on a reclining chair but after one week's treatment with mesmerism he could now walk up stairs unaided. Another demonstration was staged specifically for barristers. Watching these seemingly miraculous cures, many spectators became instant converts. 'We understand that crowds of people attend these meetings,' wrote one contemporary, 'and many who "go to scoff", return firmly persuaded of the existence of such an agent as that of animal magnetism.'[9] Presiding over these ticketed performances, Elliotson seemed akin to a theatrical impresario. One spectator even published a sensational pamphlet promising titillating details of the scenes at his house.

Styled in the manner of the 'penny dreadful' booklets which entertained working-class readers with true tales of violent crime, the pamphlet was entitled 'A full discovery of the strange practices of Dr Elliotson on the bodies of his female patients!' It promised to divulge 'all the secret experiments he makes upon them' and the 'curious postures they are put into while sitting or standing, when awake or asleep!'[10] If that was not enough to whet the appetite, the cover depicted three frock-coated men assailing a blindfolded woman wearing a low-cut dress. The illustration was captioned, 'A female Patient being blindfolded, to undergo an operation' – the operation in question being mesmerism – but looked for all the world like a violent sexual assault. The text was comparatively tame.

The anonymous writer had first visited Elliotson's 'splendid suite of rooms' in his 'elegant mansion' in Conduit Street for a private exhibition where he saw the Okey girls perform their repertoire. Intrigued by this display, he returned the following day to a public demonstration attended by thirty to forty people. This time Jane sat in a chair and lifted three iron weights totalling 86lbs. Challenged to test their strength against her, several men from the audience managed the same feat from a standing position but none could lift the weights while seated. For the finale Elliotson brought on his cockatoo which had now progressed from being sent to sleep by mesmerism to becoming a powerful mesmerist in its own right for when Elizabeth 'rubbed it with her hand, the same kind of stupor was produced in her person'. Enthralled by all he had seen, the pamphleteer proclaimed the show 'one of the most curious "sights" of London'.

Established on the London sightseeing tour and feted by Elliotson's well-connected friends, the Okey sisters had become doyennes of high society. During the next few years they would divide their time between Elliotson's house and that of an unidentified colonel's wife, while enjoying regular sojourns with the writer Fanny Trollope and her talented young sons.[11] An early convert to mesmerism, Mrs Trollope, who was one of Elliotson's patients as well as a close friend, took the Okey girls under her wing and they became much-loved figures within the family.

Thomas Trollope, elder brother of the future novelist Anthony and a prolific writer in his own right, would later describe Jane helping herself to some peas at the dinner table when she suddenly became 'fixed' by the metal spoon.[12] Another time Jane was playing the accordion – 'which she did very nicely in her magnetic state, but could not do at all in her normal state' – when Thomas, who was waving his arms in time to the music, realised he had unwittingly sent her into a trance. The Okeys would still be staying with the family in 1840 when Anthony, by then twenty-five, fell dangerously ill. Somewhat disconcertingly, the sisters kept repeating that they 'saw Jack by his side, but only up to his knee' and therefore predicted that although at death's door he would recover – as he duly did. 'Great Jackey' was also a familiar figure on the London streets – to the Okeys at least. Travelling to and from the Trollopes' house by omnibus, the girls often claimed 'they had seen "Jack" by the side of one of the passengers'. On one occasion, Thomas revealed, the sisters had noticed three children looking out of a window opposite Elliotson's house. Jane had exclaimed: 'What a pity . . . that child in the middle has Jack at him. He will die!' Within days, said Thomas, the child was indeed dead.

As the Okey girls' performances continued to dominate reports on mesmerism, so they would remain emblems of the debate. Rumours that they had confessed to cheating or been committed to a lunatic asylum were periodically rehearsed in the press.[13] The terms 'Okeyism' and 'Okeyites' became synonymous with fraud and the girls were the frequent butt of jokes. When London society was gripped in autumn 1839 by a scandal which centred on whether an unmarried former lady-in-waiting to Queen Victoria's mother, the Duchess of Kent, was pregnant, *The Lancet* suggested asking 'Okey's Negro'.[14] A few years later, in 1842, the poet Thomas Hood would dismiss rumours of his demise by jesting that 'a Miss Hoki, or Poki, even declared that she had seen the Angel of Death, whom she rather irreverently called "Great Jackey", standing beside my pillow'.[15]

Elliotson would always defend them staunchly. In the fifth and final edition of his textbook, *Human Physiology*, published in 1840, he insisted that after 'the most rigorous daily observation' of the girls over the past three years he had never once witnessed 'a shadow of inconsistency'.[16] By that point their epilepsy – had it ever existed – was completely cured and they had lost many of their old affectations. Now when they lapsed into delirium they were 'comparatively sane', talked 'very little nonsense' and were 'only rather odd'. Although for some time Elizabeth would pick up hot coals from the fireplace then stare in wonder at the blisters they produced, eventually she lost her insensibility to pain while her 'negro' also made a wise exit. At length, the girls were also reunited with their family – though this was not the happy event that might be expected.

Thomas Trollope was present at the 'very painful' scene – probably in early 1841 – when the sisters were reintroduced to their mother after a long absence.[17] 'The mother was a respectable, but poor and very un-educated woman,' he wrote, 'and of course wholly different in intelli-gence and manners from all the surroundings to which the girls had become habituated.' Having been welcomed into the smartest Victorian parlours during the previous two years, the girls could not imagine who this shabby, ill-spoken, downtrodden woman could be. At first they refused to believe Mrs Okey was their mother. Then, as the bystanders insisted it was true, the girls reacted with 'repulsion and dismay', said Trollope, 'while she, poor woman, was weeping at what appeared to her this newly developed absence of all natural affection'. Why the girls' parents, who had certainly visited them in hospital, had failed to keep in touch in the intervening years went unexplained.

Finally restored to their humble lives, the Okeys would quickly fade from the mesmerism scene. By the summer of 1841, both Jane and Eliz-abeth, now eighteen and twenty, were back in lodgings in Somers Town with their family, which now numbered nine children with another due shortly.[18] Elizabeth found work as a seamstress before marrying William Bittlestone, an engraver, in 1846. The couple settled in Islington and had four sons before Elizabeth died, aged 51, of consumption and bronchitis, in 1872. Jane also married, when she was nineteen, in 1842, and likewise had several children, settling in Hoxton. They kept in touch with the Trollopes and one of Jane's daughters later worked as a housemaid for Anthony Trollope.[19] Yet while the Okeys vanished back into the obscu-rity from which they had come, there were plenty more subjects ready to slip into their place in Elliotson's drawing-room spectacles.

Many of the individuals presented by Elliotson at his soirees had initially applied to him to be treated with mesmerism and were then persuaded to demonstrate their reactions to convince others. Miss Critchley, now thankfully free of her hiccups, appeared on several occasions from 1839 onwards. The novelist Captain Frederick Marryat, who had retired from the navy to write sea adventures, told a friend he was looking forward to meeting Elliotson and hoped 'Miss Critchley will perform again'.[20] Dickens saw her in 1841 – perhaps the time when Elliotson wrote to him: 'I am anxious that you should see human nature in a new state, and if you can come to my house tomorrow at four precisely I will shew a very curious and perfectly genuine case of mesmerism.'[21] Thomas Trollope recalled seeing a sixteen-year-old girl named Emma Melhuish, a glazier's daughter who was being treated by Elliotson for seizures, in a 'magnetic trance' in early 1839.[22]

Another patient, Rosina Barber, who was also sixteen, was first brought to Elliotson's house in August 1841 by her father after he read about the doctor's methods in his newspaper.[23] She was 'a sweet looking little daughter' with a 'blooming face and dark blue eyes', wrote Elliotson; he had an eye for a pretty face even if he was not interested in the female sex. Having suffered from epileptic seizures since she was seven along with pains in her head and chest, Rosina had been taken by her parents to numerous medical practitioners who had cupped, bled and blistered her to no avail. The girl herself was adamant mesmerism was 'a piece of perfect nonsense' yet when Elliotson began his hand movements she fell asleep in five minutes. In this trance, she moved her arms and legs at Elliotson's command and chattered spontaneously. Mesmerised four times a week, her seizures diminished and after two years she was cured. But as much as he was delighted with her medical progress, Elliotson was equally captivated by Rosina's extreme susceptibility to mesmerism. He proudly exhibited Rosina at his soirees and she became his new star.

Under mesmerism, Rosina was insensitive to pain; she was bled four times and had a tooth extracted without any hint of discomfort. Obedient to Elliotson's every movement, she rose ghostlike from her chair when he lifted his hands and slumped limply when he let his hands fall. Like the Okeys, Rosina displayed a fierce attachment to Elliotson and a repulsion towards others in her trance, so that she frowned whenever he left the room and smiled when he returned to her side. Elliotson believed she had 'occult senses' since when blindfolded she could distinguish his finger or breath from that of anyone else.

Working with Wood, Elliotson treated hundreds of patients with mesmerism without once charging a fee.[24] Many of them came from humble backgrounds and had already exhausted their hard-earned savings on conventional therapies. One patient, a thirteen-year-old girl named Mary Ann Vergo, who suffered from St Vitus's dance, was sent to Elliotson by a surgeon from Staines in August 1840.[25] Elliotson mesmerised her for half an hour a day. Within six weeks she was well enough to make a straw bonnet and after two months she was 'perfectly well'. Another patient, a nine-year-old boy from Northampton called 'Master Linnell', was brought to Elliotson when he had suddenly become ill and imbecilic after supposedly being frightened by a fire and could no longer talk, walk or stand unsupported. Within a few days of being mesmerised his movement and speech had improved and after several weeks he was completely recovered, at which point he declared himself 'very sick of sitting still to be mesmerised'.

Elliotson's house had become a kind of mesmeric clinic and teaching institute with patients being treated in his library and exhibited in his drawing room. One fellow enthusiast, calling on Elliotson, found 'your patients as usual enjoying their mesmeric nap'.[26] Whenever Elliotson was indisposed, or taking his annual holiday, Wood stepped in, and if Wood was busy, Elliotson's friend Edmond Sheppard Symes, his former pupil from St Thomas', could always be relied on to lend a hand. Symes, who was now in his early thirties and living in lodgings in Hill Street, a short stroll from Elliotson's house, mesmerised Rosina when Elliotson was called away.

Together Wood and Symes would remain Elliotson's most ardent disciples, as well as his closest companions. Writing to Dickens in early 1841, Elliotson painted a cosy domestic scene in which the trio gathered around a lamp on Friday nights to read the latest issue of the author's new periodical, *Master Humphrey's Clock*. 'Oh, how as a human being I thank you for your delightful Clock,' Elliotson gushed. 'I look forward to every friday night with impatience; for after dinner one of us reads the new number aloud. But last friday week we were beaten to the earth – Symes, who reads most beautifully, at last threw down the book & sobbed, & Wood & myself cried a deluge.'[27] Even after Symes was married – to a woman about twenty years his junior, with whom he had at least five children – he would visit Elliotson most days.[28]

Other former pupils also followed their teacher's lead. Thomas Chandler, the former UCH student who had treated a youth for rheumatism in 1838, continued to mesmerise patients with patent success.[29] Another ex-UCH student, Robert Hanham Collyer, had emigrated to America where he diversified from giving lectures on phrenology to presenting demonstrations on mesmerism. Travelling up and down the east coast of the United States and Canada, Collyer would become a colourful figure. After finding his wife in bed with the dashing Captain Marryat, Collyer would marry a second time – bigamously.[30] He would later tour the southern states with a troupe of male and female artistes who posed naked save for painted body stockings in tableaux based on famous works of art.

At the same time, other medical men, who had initially turned their backs on Elliotson, now gave his methods a try. Edward Spooner, a surgeon in Dorset, wrote to Elliotson to apologise for previously attacking mesmerism after being 'entirely misled' by Wakley's reports in *The Lancet*.[31] Now he had conducted his own experiments, he expressed 'my entire conviction of the reality of the phenomena of animal magnetism'. Support came from other influential quarters too.

In autumn 1839 a weekly medical journal, the *Medical Times*, was launched in competition with *The Lancet* and *LMG*. Whereas the older journals maintained their assault on mesmerism, the new arrival defended Elliotson and reported his investigations with serious scrutiny. One article in early 1840 argued that the potential benefits of mesmerism were worthy of scientific examination and railed against the 'noisy bullyings' of *The Lancet* whose editor had set himself up as 'self-elected censor of what shall and what shall not have the support of the medical profession'.[32] Wakley, now appointed coroner for West Middlesex on top of his parliamentary and journalistic duties, kept all mention of mesmerism out of *The Lancet* as much as possible, beyond the occasional reminder that it was he who had 'exposed' the Okeys. In truth, however, the rising tide of support for mesmerism was proving impossible, even for Wakley, to hold back.

By 1841 mesmerism was sweeping the country as scores of pamphlets, books and journals expounded its benefits and lay practitioners travelled from town to town captivating audiences with their sensational demonstrations and astounding cures. One of the most popular was a French mesmerist called Charles Lafontaine who arrived in London that spring and staged his *soirées mesmeriques* in Hanover Square before setting off on a nationwide tour.[33] A big, muscular man sporting a long black beard, Lafontaine exhibited a French youth who slavishly obeyed his commands and withstood his painful assaults. At one performance in

London in September, *The Times* reported that Lafontaine stuck pins in the boy's cheeks, hands and thighs, held sulphurous matches under his nose, and placed a lit candle close to his eyes without evincing any response. The youth was then attached to an electric battery and was 'dreadfully shaken' but seemed to suffer no pain. At another event a spectator rushed forward and thrust a scalpel into the youth's thigh – the instrument suggests the attacker was actually a surgeon – yet still the boy showed no reaction. The *LMG* assured its readers there was nothing in Lafontaine's exhibitions 'from which any member of our profession would derive either instruction or surprise' – relief from pain apparently having no medical significance. Lafontaine would return to France in 1842.

Hard on his heels came Spencer Hall, the son of a Nottinghamshire cobbler brought up in a cottage in Sherwood Forest, who was drawn to mesmerism after seeing Lafontaine perform in Sheffield in autumn 1841.[34] A clever and thoughtful man, he had begun working in the stocking industry at the age of seven but resolved to become a printer after reading Benjamin Franklin's autobiography. Hall had subsequently set up a printing firm and published his own poetry under the name 'The Sherwood Forester'. Inspired by Lafontaine, he taught himself mesmerism and began lecturing in packed theatres and halls throughout the Midlands and the north.

Hall's first public lecture in Sheffield attracted several hundred people while hundreds more were turned away; when a larger venue was booked it was filled by 3,000 and another 1,000 were disappointed. Hall not only exhibited the usual mesmeric phenomena but also treated countless people who came to his demonstrations in search of a cure. They included a seventeen-year-old girl who had been deaf for four years but after treatment could hear the quietest whisper, and a man with a limp who threw away his stick and danced a jig. Perhaps the most poignant case, however, was a youth with an appalling stammer who was propelled on stage by his employer, a shoemaker; after one session the lad could speak with perfect clarity. Hall was ahead of his time: today hypnosis is successfully used to treat speech disorders.[35]

As mesmerism gripped the national imagination, travelling practitioners sprouted like mushrooms. According to Hall's estimate, by 1845 there were 300 lay mesmerists, all competing to astonish audiences with more and more implausible tricks. While some of these lay lecturers offered mesmeric treatment, many specialised purely in theatrical spectacle. But none topped Alexis Didier, a Parisian youth from a poor background who had first been mesmerised to treat his epilepsy and had gone on to reveal startling clairvoyant powers.[36]

Brought to London by his patron, Jean Marcillet, Alexis held audiences spellbound as he played cards while blindfolded, identified items within sealed boxes and described in detail places and events he had never seen. Alexis was even invited to demonstrate his talents at one of Elliotson's soirees, where he spelled out the signature in a folded letter and described the house of one of the guests.[37] Elliotson was convinced that Alexis was truly clairvoyant despite his frequent mistakes. The youth would eventually flee back to France after an article in *The Lancet* alleged that he could see through his blindfold and was fed clues by Marcillet.

Charlatans such as Alexis did mesmerism no favours, just as stage hypnotism would later taint medical hypnotherapy. Opponents insisted that all mesmerists were fraudsters, all their subjects imposters, and that all mesmeric practice was false, dangerous and even evil. Two women persuaded their sister not to be treated by Elliotson because he was 'in league with the devil' while another who attended a demonstration at his house swore she could smell brimstone.[38] Others linked mesmerism with sexual impropriety. One doctor, writing to the *Medical Times*, painted a lurid scene in which a 'pretty girl' was sent to sleep by a mesmerist 'playing with the ringlets of her glossy hair'.[39] Another said he would kick out of the house anyone who proposed mesmerising his daughter. Some reacted with outright snobbishness. The artist and writer Elizabeth Rigby, later Lady Eastlake, dismissed mesmerism as 'an odious, disgusting and impious business'. After watching a demonstration at a friend's soiree in 1844, she blustered that it was 'advocated by women without principle, and lectured upon by men who drop their h's'.[40]

Elliotson – who could rival anyone for snobbishness – was inevitably disparaging about the craze he dubbed 'The Lecture Mania'.[41] He lamented the fact that experiments 'more suited for the quiet retirement of the philosopher's study than the bustle and turmoil of a public lecture room' were being performed to vast audiences by people 'whose previous education by no means entitles them to become expounders of the doctrine'.

While lay lecturers brought mesmerism to mass audiences, Elliotson gave it an aura of respectability. His influential connections made mesmerism popular among intellectuals, scientists, aristocrats and royalty. Through his friendship with Dickens and the Trollopes, the subject was warmly embraced by the literary world including Harriet Martineau, Edward Bulwer-Lytton and Robert Browning.[42] Other writers, including William Wordsworth, George Eliot, Elizabeth Gaskell and Charlotte Brontë, were likewise drawn to the mesmeric scene and mesmerism seeped into their poetry, plays and novels. Robert Browning and Elizabeth Barrett wrangled repeatedly over mesmerism in their letters; although Elizabeth was more sympathetic than her future husband, she thought there was 'something ghastly & repelling' in the idea of 'Dr E.'s great boney fingers seeming to "touch the stops"'.[43] Browning would later write a poem, entitled 'Mesmerism', which describes a woman being lured to her lover's house. Charlotte Brontë remained sceptical, though she confessed to undergoing a 'personal experiment'. No one, however, was more enthusiastic than Dickens.

His interest first piqued by Elliotson's demonstrations on Elizabeth Okey, Dickens attended several of Elliotson's soirees. The pair had developed a fond friendship. Dickens had sent Elliotson a copy of *Nicholas Nickleby* in 1839 'as a very feeble mark of my lasting esteem and admiration'.[44] The following year they joined a crowd of 40,000 to watch the hanging of François Courvoisier, a Swiss valet who had murdered his employer, confirming both in their opposition to the death penalty.[45] At one point Dickens sent Elliotson two dozen bottles of punch. 'You are resolved to punch out all my wits,' quipped a high-spirited Elliotson – perhaps after sampling a bottle – adding: 'Joking apart, you make me ashamed with your overflowing of the *milk* of kindness.'[46] And in August 1840 Elliotson invited Dickens to dinner to meet the Reverend Chauncy Hare Townshend, a wealthy dilettante who had been ordained but preferred to devote himself to composing poetry rather than sermons.[47]

An enthusiastic mesmerist, Townshend had published a book, *Facts in Mesmerism*, dedicated to Elliotson. Although Townshend was said to have been strikingly good-looking in his youth, now in his forties he was described as 'plain' and 'effeminate'. A self-confessed hypochondriac, he crammed his carriage with medicine bottles along with sherry, brandy, oranges, shawls and telescopes. Dickens and Townshend became friends – Dickens would dedicate *Great Expectations* to him – and they investigated mesmerism together. Dickens would always shy away from undergoing mesmerism himself – in one letter, Townshend invited Dickens to dinner but promised 'to keep my hands off you, however much they may be itching to perform mesmeric evolutions about your head' – but he became an expert mesmerist, first trying his skills on his wife, Catherine, during a visit to Pittsburgh in 1842, and later on several friends.

In time, this talent would intensify Dickens's marital woes. In 1844, while staying in Genoa, Dickens mesmerised Augusta de la Rue, the English wife of a Swiss friend, Emile, who suffered a variety of mysterious ailments.[48] After Dickens mesmerised her repeatedly she became obsessively dependent on him – much to Catherine's consternation. Returning to London, Dickens promised to mesmerise Mme de la Rue at set times and she wrote back swearing she could feel the benefits of his long-distance mesmerism. Another time, when Elliotson came to stay with him in Lausanne, Dickens mesmerised a man and 'stretched him on the dining-room floor'.[49] He told a friend that Elliotson 'holds my magnetic powers in great veneration' and later said: 'I have the perfect conviction I could magnetize a Frying Pan.'

Encouraged by Dickens, the writer and socialite Marguerite Gardiner, Countess of Blessington, became an avid enthusiast along with her lover – who happened also to be her stepson – the dandy Count D'Orsay. Both attended Elliotson's demonstrations.[50] Another aristocrat, Lady Mary Bentinck, daughter of the 4th Duke of Portland, used mesmerism to treat the poor on her estate, at one time catching typhus fever for her pains. George Spencer-Churchill, 6th Duke of Marlborough, was also an advocate; he invited Elliotson to Blenheim Palace in 1841. Even Prince Albert was said to be a supporter. Indeed one visitor to a demonstration at Elliotson's house noted that 'the fair ones of the British court' were among the guests.

As enthusiasm for mesmerism spread through all levels of society, so the clamour for the subject to be taken seriously intensified. By July 1841 even *The Times* was calling for an impartial inquiry to establish the scientific facts.[51] A Scottish surgeon with a thriving general practice in Manchester now took up that challenge.

James Braid first became interested in mesmerism after he attended a demonstration by Lafontaine in Manchester in November 1841.[52] A shrewd and practical man, Braid initially suspected a trick but a second demonstration convinced him the effects were genuine; what was more, he was sure he had divined the cause. Rushing home to conduct his own experiments, he mesmerised first his wife and then a friend by instructing them to stare at a fixed object – a sugar bowl and wine bottle respectively – held just above their line of sight (evidently he knew their respective interests). Both fell into a trance within minutes. Braid briskly dismissed the notion of an invisible mesmeric force and concluded that the sleep was 'induced by a fixed stare, absolute repose of body, fixed attention, and suppressed respiration'.

Expounding his views in five lectures in Manchester later that month, Braid was anxious to distance his theory and method from mesmerism and the prejudice it attracted. He demonstrated that the trance was most speedily produced by instructing an individual to focus on a small bright object – he favoured a silver lancet case – held between eight and fifteen inches in front of the eyes. Braid named this process hypnotism, from the Greek for 'nervous sleep', to distinguish it from mesmerism, although the outcome was exactly the same. Although he argued that hypnotism was perfectly safe, Braid believed it should only be exercised by doctors. He urged fellow practitioners to try hypnotism themselves as 'a valuable addition to our curative means' to treat numerous disorders, especially those termed 'nervous complaints', which were otherwise thought incurable.

Bringing his lectures to London in March the following year, Braid hypnotised dozens of volunteers who showed the usual insensibility to pain. At one event he attempted to mesmerise eighteen people at once; within ten minutes sixteen were in a trance. But he argued that if people were hypnotised repeatedly – as with the Okey girls – they would act as expected through imagination; in other words, suggestion. This, he said, was 'the grand source of the follies' which had 'misled ... the animal magnetisers'. Braid went on to treat numerous patients for hearing loss, chronic pain and other ailments with resounding success. His research, later published as a book entitled *Neurypnology*, attracted widespread interest among his peers. One surgeon, writing to the *Medical Times*, proclaimed that Braid 'has unpicked the lock of "Animal Magnetism"'.[53] And indeed, by reducing mesmerism to a simple explanation devoid of mystery and preposterous claims, he had. *The Lancet*, of course, did not see it that way; Wakley studiously ignored Braid's lectures and refused to publish his letters.

Rather than welcoming this long-awaited and compelling analysis of the science behind mesmerism, Elliotson – inevitably – took up cudgels with Braid. Brushing aside his research, Elliotson continued to insist that mesmerism was caused by a physical force and that hand movements were more effective than the fixed gaze. After once testing Braid's technique on a patient without success, he returned to 'the old-established modes of mesmerism' in preference to Braid's 'coarse method'.[54] Vain and dogmatic as ever, Elliotson was determined not to relinquish his crown to a Scottish upstart from Manchester. And then, in 1842, even more startling stories began to emerge of the power of mesmerism.

Ever since Mesmer had first staged his demonstrations in the 1780s, observers had noted that mesmerism produced insensibility to pain. Elliotson, of course, had repeatedly shown that the Okey girls and others were impervious to pain in a mesmeric trance. Braid, too, had demonstrated that his volunteers felt no pain in their hypnotic sleep. The hundreds of lecturers touring the country exhibited the same response to astonished audiences at packed shows every night. Yet neither the medical men nor the lay practitioners had thought to use mesmerism for its most obvious application – to render patients insensible for surgical operations.

Surgeons in Paris had performed a mastectomy using mesmerism as far back as 1829, yet this staggering feat had somehow failed to trigger an avalanche of similar operations. The fact the patient had died soon afterwards had not helped. Elliotson had seen Ann Ross have two teeth extracted at UCH without a murmur, but as she had later confessed to faking her trances he had dismissed the event. Like most physicians, Elliotson looked on surgery as a failing of medicine – a brutal last resort – rather than a vital remedy; surgery was therefore not at the forefront of his mind. Yet leading surgeons such as Liston had also obstinately ignored the potential of mesmerism, even when the demonstrations of comatose patients had taken place in their own operating theatres.

Perversely, this refusal to exploit the benefits of mesmerism for surgery was partly because surgeons were used to patients exhibiting incredible stoicism during the most brutal operations. Henry Paget, the Marquess of Anglesey, who had been so captivated by Elizabeth Okey's antics in May 1838, famously had his leg amputated after the Battle of Waterloo without uttering a sound and there were countless more examples of such endurance. But then, in 1842, the penny dropped.

Elliotson would later assert that the first operation rendered painless by mesmerism in England was the insertion of a seton into Elizabeth Okey's neck at UCH in 1838, when she displayed 'perfect anaesthesia'.[55] But this entirely gratuitous procedure was neither useful nor major surgery. The second procedure, by Elliotson's accounting, but really the first major British operation to be performed under mesmerism, was almost as little noticed and barely recorded and was carried out by a compassionate and self-effacing surgeon named William Collins Engledue.

Engledue was born in Portsea, near Portsmouth, in 1813.[56] After being apprenticed to a physician, he gained a medical degree at Edinburgh, qualified as a surgeon and obtained a licence to practise as an apothecary – all within a single year. Thus simultaneously qualified to work in all three areas of medicine, Engledue set up practice in Portsmouth where he devoted his boundless energies to treating the poor for free while gathering support for building a hospital and public baths. He became friendly with Elliotson through their shared passion for phrenology. Introduced by Elliotson to mesmerism, Engledue advocated a bizarre combination of the two theories – phreno-mesmerism – which entailed mesmerising the relevant bumps on the head. Engledue's strongly materialist views, also shared by Elliotson, led to a climactic split in the Phrenological Association in June 1842, which ultimately led to its demise.

Two months after this explosive rift, Engledue quietly performed an historic operation in Southsea on a seventeen-year-old woman, named only as 'Miss K', who had been confined to bed for eighteen months by a contraction in her knee which meant that her heel was permanently bent back to her thigh. Despite three months' treatment with mesmerism, her condition was no better. Without alerting her in advance, let alone seeking her consent, Engledue mesmerised her into a trance and then smartly severed the hamstrings behind the knee. When she awoke, the woman had no idea the operation had been performed until she noticed some blood spots on the sheet. The operation was apparently a success. Engledue, however, made no public announcement about his achievement until two years later when he published a cursory account as a letter to Elliotson. But by then the British medical profession had been stunned by a far more dramatic and controversial operation.

James Wombell, a forty-two-year-old farm labourer, was admitted to Wellow District Hospital in Nottinghamshire with a diseased left knee in June 1842.[57] After suffering agonising pain for five years, he could no longer work. The hospital surgeon, William Squire Ward, told Wombell that his leg must be amputated at the thigh. But since the poor man was terrified of surgery, Ward speculated that mesmerism might reduce the pain and so he asked a friend, the London barrister and amateur mesmerist William Topham, to try his hand. After several sessions, Wombell proved insensible to pain and the date was set for his operation. On 1 October 1842, Topham mesmerised Wombell into a trance and Ward prepared to amputate the leg.

Ward began by plunging his knife into the outside of the patient's thigh as far as the bone then slowly drew the blade around to the inside thigh. The onlookers watched with bated breath as Wombell slept on placidly. 'The stillness, at this moment, was something awful,' wrote Topham, 'the calm respiration of the sleeping man alone was heard; for all other seemed suspended.' At the second incision Wombell began to moan softly yet he continued to sleep throughout the twenty-minute operation 'in perfect stillness and repose' until he was finally woken by smelling salts. Astonished to discover his leg was gone, Wombell exclaimed: 'I bless the Lord to find it's all over!' When questioned about the experience, he said he had heard a 'kind of crunching' but had felt no pain whatsoever. The wound healed perfectly and Wombell went on to live for another thirty years.

Ward later said he had been sceptical of mesmerism until he had seen Elliotson produce a trance a few months earlier; now he hoped his fellow medical men would try for themselves 'such a boon to the surgeon'. The operation caused a sensation – but not in the way Ward had hoped.

When Topham and Ward reported details of the operation to a packed meeting of the Royal Medical and Chirurgical Society the following month, they were met with disbelief, derision and outright hostility.[58] Immediately the presentation was over, one surgeon jumped up and insisted it was common for patients to display no signs of pain during surgery while another argued that Wombell must have been trained to withstand pain. One member objected to the paper on the grounds that patients *should* suffer pain during surgery since 'they are all the better for it, and recover better'.[59] And Robert Liston cynically inquired whether the patient was now 'sufficiently advanced in his education since the operation to read with the back of his neck or his belly'.

When the meeting ended, Topham withdrew his paper, although he later published it as a pamphlet. The following month, the society voted to erase all mention of the report from its minutes; as far as the RMCS was concerned the mesmeric amputation had never happened. Elliotson promptly resigned. He had joined the society thirty years earlier as a twenty-one-year-old student, submitted many of his most important papers to it, led it for two years as president and steered it to royal patronage, even hosted its meetings in his own home. Now he turned his back on it for good.

News of the Wombell amputation was received with just as much enthusiasm in the medical press.[60] *The Lancet* reported the event under the sceptical heading 'Amputation of the thigh, during an alleged mesmeric state, professedly without the sensation of the patient' and it appealed for independent information on the surgeon, lawyer and patient; Wakley plainly hoped to discredit them. The *Provincial Medical and Surgical Journal* said the RMCS's opposition was 'most justly offered'. And the *Medico-Chirurgical Review* asked why the mesmerists had not cured the man's knee rather than amputate his leg before explaining 'the mesmerisers well knew that it was far easier to induce a peasant to feign a sleep, than to feign the cure of a disease'. Accusations of fraud would continue to hound Wombell and it would later be claimed that he had confessed himself an imposter.[61]

Yet even if the medical press was quick to dismiss this pioneering form of anaesthesia, Wombell's extraordinary operation inspired medical practitioners in Britain and beyond to test mesmerism for themselves. Surgeons, dentists and general practitioners now ventured to perform operations under mesmerism and – to counter accusations of trickery – gathered parties of witnesses to testify to what they had seen. In January 1843 in Newry, Ireland, a surgeon-apothecary named Thomas Grattan extracted two teeth under mesmerism from a woman called Sarah Moffett; several doctors signed a certificate verifying the operation.[62] In May three physicians, two surgeons and assorted lay people gathered in Edinburgh to watch Robert Nasmyth, surgeon-dentist to Queen Victoria, remove a molar from a mesmerised man named William Gill. The accounts multiplied. A month later in Leicester nearly twenty people crammed into a room in a tavern to watch a man named James Paul have a molar drawn while mesmerised and in July a thirteen-year-old girl named Eliza

Baldwin had eight molars removed at the Middlesex Hospital after being mesmerised by John Ashburner, a friend of Elliotson.

Surgeons soon became more ambitious. In January 1844, a twenty-two-year-old woman in Manchester was mesmerised to dull the pains of a long labour although she was roused for the birth.[63] Two months later in Wolverhampton forty-five-year-old John Marrien had a finger amputated in a room packed with witnesses including seven doctors, a magistrate and the editor of the local newspaper. According to one witness, 'the cutting the flaps and the dividing the bone by the nippers, was watched with breathless suspense – but there was not a muscle's quiver, nor did a sigh escape, or a finger move'. In August a twenty-two-year-old dressmaker, Mary Ann Lakin, had her leg amputated at Leicester Infirmary before several medical witnesses. Although one of the surgeons present later claimed there was 'considerable groaning, writhing, and an approach to screaming', the editor of the *Leicester Chronicle* insisted that 'the great majority of the public will have their faith in the truth and efficacy of mesmerism, as an important agent in surgical operations, strengthened'. In May 1845 a woman named Mrs Northway had an arm amputated under mesmerism in Torquay as seven medical men watched.[64] When she awoke she announced that she wished to postpone the operation to the following day.

The novelty of surgery without pain caught on elsewhere too. The first recorded operation using mesmerism in America had taken place in Providence, Rhode Island, in 1837 when a woman had four teeth extracted, a full year before Ann Ross had her teeth removed at UCH.[65] After a gap of several years, there was a flurry of mesmeric operations by American surgeons from 1843 onwards, including a leg amputation and a mastectomy. The British colonies were not to be left out. In February 1843, in Spanish Town, Jamaica, a woman had a tooth removed while mesmerised after first singing three songs. The operation was reported to the *Jamaica Standard* by Richard Tuthill, a physician with the British Army in the West Indies, and was witnessed by the island's chief police officer. Then reports began to filter back from India, where James Esdaile, a Scottish surgeon with the East India Company, was experimenting with mesmerism.

A clever and kindly surgeon, Esdaile had suffered ill health and disappointment for most of his life.[66] He had arrived in India in 1831, hoping the climate would help his asthma and bronchitis, but instead found the country 'injurious to my health and distasteful to me'. The death of his seventeen-year-old bride on the journey out, and of his second wife a few years later, did not improve his outlook and he suffered a breakdown leading to a lengthy absence. Returning to India in 1838, he was put in charge of Hooghly Hospital in a 'small obscure country station' twenty-two miles from Calcutta.

Esdaile knew nothing of mesmerism beyond having read a few newspaper 'scraps' describing Elliotson's work. But on 4 April 1845 he tried mesmerism for the first time, on a prisoner from Hooghly Jail named Mádhab Kaurá who was suffering a double hydrocele – an accumulation of fluid in the scrotum. A common problem in tropical countries due to parasitical infections, the condition can cause enormous swellings. When Esdaile began the standard treatment to drain the fluid and inject a corrosive substance, Kaurá writhed with pain. So Esdaile sat in front of him, clasped his knees between his own, and waved his hands up and down. After persevering for forty-five minutes the man's face showed 'the most perfect repose' and his pain had entirely gone. Esdaile repeated the technique several times more, then on 27 April he mesmerised a patient named Bachoo and removed a scrotal tumour, which was twice the size of a human head.

Over the next year, Esdaile would use 'Belatee Muntur' – the European charm – to perform more than 100 operations at Hooghly. In one of the most spectacular procedures he removed a scrotal tumour weighing 80lbs; it was so large the patient, a clerk, had used it as a writing desk. To conserve his energies for surgery, Esdaile trained his Hindu assistants to mesmerise the patients and invited local British doctors and dignitaries to witness his work. One observer, a Professor of Anatomy, arrived to see a row of patients being mesmerised by attendants in an open courtyard ready for Esdaile to operate on each in turn. 'At a signal from the Doctor, the first man was brought out on his bed for the removal of a large elephantoid tumour; the very size of which appeared to astonish some of the spectators,' he wrote. 'Dr Esdaile very coolly set about removing it, and he worked with a leisurely manner that convinced me he had the most certain conviction that he was giving no pain, and therefore in no hurry.'

After winning the support of British officials, in 1846 Esdaile was given charge of an 'experimental hospital' in Calcutta where he performed hundreds more operations under mesmerism. Native patients flocked to Esdaile's 'house of magic' while visitors arrived by the steamer-load to observe his work. One of the few cases Esdaile declined to treat was that of a writer, Bhugeeruth, born with both male and female sexual organs. The man – 'as this person wishes to be considered a man, I shall speak of him as such', wrote Esdaile – had travelled 281 miles to have his breasts removed. Esdaile thought it wrong to perform the operation but he would reconsider, he said, 'if the public come to think with me that he should be permitted to enjoy life in his own way'.[67]

Since Esdaile preferred to spend his time effecting cures rather than developing rival theories or new terms for mesmerism, he found a firm ally in Elliotson. In Britain Elliotson championed Esdaile's work and even sent him a bistoury – a surgical knife – to help with his amputations. Thanking him for the gift, Esdaile replied, 'I used it the other day in separating a *ninety-pounder* from its owner *without his knowledge*' and helpfully supplied a 'before' sketch of the patient with his colossal tumour.[68]

Elliotson played little active role in mesmeric surgery but he was the foremost ambassador in spreading the word about its potential. Since the medical press either derided or, worse, ignored the growing success of surgery under mesmerism, in 1843 Elliotson published a pamphlet, *Numerous cases of Surgical Operations without Pain in the Mesmeric State*, which detailed reports from around the world; it was published the same year in America. Later that year he launched a quarterly journal, the *Zoist*, to promote research on mesmerism and phrenology. Edited jointly by Elliotson and Engledue, the journal was filled with reports of successful operations as well as examples of mesmeric cures. Among the most influential of these accounts was the story of the writer Harriet Martineau.

A household name in Victorian parlours, Martineau had won popular acclaim for her travel writing, journalism and moralistic stories in the early 1830s.[69] Although she had suffered childhood illness and was almost completely deaf by the age of twenty, Martineau was no shrinking violet. She had spent two years touring America, partly on her own, and was known by friends and foes alike for her combative views and sharp tongue. But then, in 1838 at the age of thirty-six, she became seriously ill with a prolapsed uterus, probably caused by an ovarian cyst, and despite moving to Newcastle the following year to be close to her doctor, her brother-in-law Thomas Greenhow, from 1842 she was largely confined to a sofa.

Martineau had been interested in mesmerism for several years – she had dined with Elliotson in 1839 – but Greenhow deterred her from seeking a mesmeric cure. Then in June 1844 Greenhow chaired a demonstration by Spencer Hall in Newcastle and was sufficiently impressed to ask Hall to visit Martineau, who was now living in Tynemouth. After twenty minutes of being mesmerised, Martineau felt 'something very strange' but saw no obvious improvement. Since Hall was too ill to visit the following day, Martineau asked her maid to take over – with striking effect. Within one minute, she felt 'a delicious sensation of ease' which lasted all day. After three months of being mesmerised daily by her maid and a lay practitioner named Mrs Montagu Wynyard, Martineau was able to give up opiates, hear better and walk five miles a day. Within a year she was back to blooming health.

Martineau's dramatic recovery, which she related in six letters to the *Athenaeum* and published as a pamphlet, created a colossal stir, reigniting debates among the public and medical profession alike. When Greenhow published his own pamphlet suggesting her cure was due to 'the imagination and the will' rather than to mesmerism, this only heightened the furore. Martineau was not so easily dismissed, however. In a letter to a friend contradicting Greenhow's account and published in the *Zoist*, Martineau declared: 'I am in robust health, and have not had one day's illness since I avowed my cure by mesmerism.' Even the naturalist Charles Darwin was drawn into the controversy. Though sceptical about Martineau's cure he had to admit: 'With respect to mesmerism, the whole country resounds with wonderful facts or tales: the subject is most curious, whether real or false.'[70]

As accounts of mesmeric surgery and mesmeric cures accumulated, orthodox doctors felt under siege. They simply could not compete. Physicians had been tipping noxious potions down patients' throats, prescribing bloodletting, blistering and cupping for centuries without a scrap of evidence that any of it worked. Now a cheap, quick and gentle alternative not only offered success in treating numerous ailments but potentially rendered surgery free of pain and fear. For all Wakley's campaign to banish 'quackery', it was conventional medicine that was now suspect, qualified doctors who were becoming isolated. Mesmerism threatened not only their authority and status but also their livelihood. The fear and hostility reached such a pitch that in 1843 a lecture by Hall in Northampton was interrupted by an unruly mob who bayed, yelled and hissed for the entire two hours; they were not local hooligans, but qualified doctors.[71]

Many medical practitioners felt they could no longer resist the tide. A chemist in South Shields said his customers as commonly asked for mesmerism as they did for medicine and several druggists in Lancashire combined mesmerism with conventional medicine.[72] The letter writer Jane Carlyle told a friend that Martineau expected 'the whole system of medicine is going to be flung to the dogs presently, and that henceforth instead of Physicians we are to have *Magnetizers*!' And she added: 'May be so!'[73]

Even Wakley could no longer ignore the march of mesmerism. In 1845 he commissioned Charles Radclyffe Hall, a prominent physician, to undertake a comprehensive study, which ran in *The Lancet* from February to May.[74] Though Radclyffe Hall accepted mesmerism produced sleep, probably produced other effects and possibly – 'but not very probably' – induced insensibility to severe pain, he concluded it was not superior to 'more ordinary methods of influencing the mind and the body'. He did not elaborate what these ordinary methods might be, nor did he consider the effects worth pursuing further.

Many now agreed with Martineau when she complained that 'the systematic disingenuousness of some Medical Journals' towards mesmerism coupled with the attacks by the medical establishment 'looked as if they were in conflict with powerful truth, and as if they knew it'.[75] Prince Albert even went so far at a palace party as to criticise the medical profession for failing to investigate mesmerism seriously.

By 1846 Elliotson had been so far absorbed back into the establishment that he was invited to give the annual Harveian Oration – established in 1656 in honour of William Harvey – at the Royal College of Physicians.[76] Wakley was apoplectic at this honour being bestowed on his enemy and urged the fellows to protest against 'the professional pariah' and 'hero of ribald street ballads'. So furious was his tirade that the college arranged a police guard in case of disgruntled members; in the event, Elliotson's address was politely received and even applauded. Presenting himself as a martyr to science, Elliotson likened his battle to Harvey's struggle to convince his peers of the circulation of blood. He made an impassioned plea to his fellow physicians to investigate mesmerism for themselves 'for the love of truth' and 'in the name of the good of all mankind'. Elliotson delivered the lecture in Latin, according to tradition, but published it simultaneously in Latin and English to ensure as wide an audience as possible. Beside himself with rage, Wakley fumed: 'Dr ELLIOTSON must be barefaced and unabashed to an extraordinary degree to dare to draw a parallel . . . between his own mummeries and the labours of the immortal HARVEY.'

Protest as he might, Wakley sounded like an increasingly shrill and lonely voice; once in the vanguard of radical journalism and liberal reform, he now appeared to be on the side of the most conservative establishment. Instead of championing scientific inquiry, he was blocking it. *The Lancet* and other medical journals continued to publish long articles glorifying the benefits of bloodletting and blistering – along with accounts of brutal surgery – while disparaging mesmerism. Which was quackery and which was science? As Elliotson put it in the *Zoist*: 'Those who were terrified by Mr Wakley's firing and ran away, have now stopped to take breath, looked back, and found that he had no shot, produced merely noise and smoke.'[77]

Leaders of the medical establishment read accounts of mesmeric operations with growing despair. But few felt more despondent than Liston. Although he was still regarded as the best surgeon of his age, Liston was equally renowned for his hard-hearted approach to operations. How much longer would patients tolerate the terror of the knife? And then, in December 1846, Liston heard news from America that changed everything.

II

Pandora's Box

Operating theatre, University College Hospital, London, 21 December 1846

Frederick Churchill, a thirty-six-year-old butler, lay on the operating table with a handkerchief covering his face as Liston raised his amputation knife to make the first incision.[1] The theatre was even more crowded than usual as students and medical practitioners leaned forward to see. Liston ordered his pupils to check their watches then brought down his knife. He removed Churchill's leg in less than thirty seconds then tied the arteries and dressed the wound. The patient made no murmur throughout the procedure. Liston had performed the first major operation in England using ether. There was no doubting the significance of his achievement. Triumphantly he turned to his audience and exclaimed: 'This Yankee dodge, gentlemen, beats mesmerism hollow!'[2]

Timing was everything. Scientists had been aware for decades that inhaling ether, and other gases such as nitrous oxide, could induce sleep and eliminate pain.[3] In 1795 the chemist Humphry Davy had discovered that inhaling nitrous oxide produced dizziness and giggling; he named it 'laughing gas'. Five years later he reported that the gas was 'capable of destroying physical pain' and suggested it might be used 'with advantage during surgical operations'. Ether, first discovered in 1540, was found to have similar properties in the early 1800s. Yet just as many surgeons had resisted the use of mesmerism to render operations painless, so they had ignored the potential of ether and nitrous oxide. This was not through sheer callousness. Most surgeons believed that pain played an essential role in helping patients survive surgery; any means to render a patient insensible might depress their vital bodily functions. So although substances such as mandrake, henbane, opium and its derivative morphine, isolated in 1803, were known to relieve pain they were avoided in case they subdued patients to the point of no return. Shunned by surgeons, ether and nitrous oxide had become popular recreational drugs at parties – where guests indulged in 'ether frolics' – but by the 1840s, the spread of mesmerism had prompted doctors to cast around for a more 'scientific' alternative.

The spectacle of party revellers knocking into furniture with giddy oblivion could not go unheeded forever. Crawford Long, a young American doctor based in Jefferson, Georgia, was enjoying an ether party when he observed that his friends 'received falls and blows' but 'did not feel the least pain from these accidents'.[4] Eager to put this miracle to medical use, on 30 March 1842 he gave ether to a patient before removing a tumour from his neck. Afterwards the patient proclaimed he had not experienced 'the slightest degree of pain'. Long went on to perform several more operations on etherised patients but failed to publicise his landmark achievement until seven years later.

Meanwhile in Connecticut in 1844, an American dentist, Horace Wells, was intrigued by a travelling showman's demonstration of the effects of nitrous oxide. One volunteer banged his leg so hard against a wooden bench that it bled, yet he showed no sign of pain. Quickly realising the boon this could bring to his profession, Wells gamely put himself forward to have a tooth extracted under the gas; the molar was yanked out without a twinge. Yet Wells's efforts to replicate this wonder on other patients proved a dismal failure. When he gave a demonstration before doctors at Massachusetts General Hospital, Boston, the patient screamed as his tooth was pulled and the observers shouted, 'Humbug!'. Wells slid into depression and later killed himself by inhaling chloroform before slitting an artery.

A second dentist, William Morton, who was originally Wells's business partner, had more success. Having witnessed the problems with nitrous oxide, he experimented with ether. On 30 September 1846, a patient named Eben Frost asked to have a tooth extracted under mesmerism but Morton said he knew a better method. It was the first dental extraction under ether anaesthetic. Quickly realising the huge potential of his achievement, Morton was eager to share his discovery. A few days later, on 16 October 1846, Morton administered the agent he called 'Letheon' to a patient, Edward Abbott, in the operating theatre of Massachusetts General, before the senior surgeon, John Warren, removed a tumour from the slumbering patient's jaw. At that point Warren turned to the packed theatre and exclaimed: 'Gentlemen, this is no humbug.' In fact Abbott later said that the pain was like having his skin 'scratched with a hoe' but it was a step in the right direction.[5] News of this chemical alternative to mesmerism, which doctors easily identified as ether, sped across the Atlantic – or at least as fast as steam would allow. A report from Henry Jacob Bigelow, a surgeon who witnessed 'ether day', arrived in London in mid-December at the home of an American botanist, Dr Francis Boott, who quickly relayed the news to his friend Liston.

Liston was cautious. He had already seen the effects of ether in a demonstration at the RMCS in November when a volunteer – a doctor – had inhaled the vapour and smiled blithely as fellow members lined up to prick him with pins.[6] Students at UCL had often inhaled nitrous oxide and ether in their chemistry class; one pupil remembered knocking his knuckles against the desk without feeling pain. And an account of Morton's earlier success in extracting teeth under ether had been published in the *LMG* on 18 December, under the headline 'Animal Magnetism Superseded'.[7] Still Liston had hung back. He knew that any claim to be able to perform painless surgery was likely to be greeted with suspicion by his peers; perhaps ether was just another theatrical sensation and could make him the laughing stock of the profession. But when he read the account from Boston describing an operation performed under ether before a crowd of eminent medical men in an esteemed teaching hospital, Liston knew his moment had arrived. This was his chance to defeat mesmerism; this was his opportunity to vanquish Elliotson once and for all.

First Liston recruited an obliging student, William Squire, whose uncle, Peter Squire, ran a pharmacy in Oxford Street. Uncle Peter quickly knocked up an apparatus for administering ether vapour and over the next two days Liston tested its effects on the younger Squire. In the meantime, on 19 December, a dentist named James Robinson, based in Gower Street, gave ether to a patient before painlessly removing her tooth. Now that he was confident ether worked, Liston selected a suitable candidate, the butler Frederick Churchill who had been admitted in November with a damaged knee caused by a fall. If Churchill's leg had not needed amputation on admission, it certainly did now since the limb had become infected as a result of Liston cutting into the knee and inserting a grubby finger to inspect the damage. Yet Churchill was in such terror of the pain that he had refused to submit to the operation even as his condition deteriorated. With no time to lose, on 20 December Liston announced his plan to perform an amputation using ether and sent invitations to his medical friends and journalists.

At 2.25 p.m. on 21 December Frederick Churchill was brought into the operating theatre and laid on the table. William Squire administered ether vapour using his uncle's apparatus until Churchill appeared to be asleep and then Liston swiftly removed the leg. 'Not the slightest groan was heard from the patient,' the case notes recorded, 'nor was the countenance at all expressive of pain.' When Churchill awoke, five minutes later, he announced that he had changed his mind and did not want his leg to be removed after all. The students grinned at each other. Only when he sat up did the butler accept that his leg was gone. As Squire later said: 'The expressive smile of surprise and delight with which he then looked around is deeply impressed upon my memory.' Without further ado Liston performed a second operation using ether, to remove an ingrown toenail, the same afternoon.

That evening Liston wrote jubilantly to his friend James Miller in Edinburgh: 'Hurrah! Rejoice! Mesmerism, and its professors, have met with a heavy blow, and great discouragement.'[8] Within six months, Liston predicted, 'no operation will be performed without this famous preparation'. In fact, though Liston would never get to hear of it, another Scottish surgeon, William Scott, who had also received the news from Boston, had probably pipped him to the post. Scott later claimed to have amputated a patient's leg using ether at Dumfries and Galloway Royal Infirmary on 19 December – beating Liston by two days – but he would only assert his precedence twenty-six years later.[9]

As news of Liston's operation swept through Britain and across the Continent, ether was welcomed with open arms as the long-awaited substitute for mesmerism. Broadcasting the Boston operation and Liston's subsequent success across four pages in *The Lancet*, Wakley enthused: 'We suppose we shall now hear no more of mesmerism and its absurdities as preparatives for surgical operations.'[10] Driving home his point, he added: 'The destruction of one limb of this mesmeric quackery will be one not inconsiderable merit of this most valuable discovery.' The *LMG*, which had scooped its rival in reporting the Boston news, acclaimed this 'new mode of cheating pain'. Up and down the country surgeons and dentists now fell over themselves to test ether before crowds of awed colleagues. During the next few weeks, ether was used to perform operations and dental extractions in hospitals across London, including Guy's, St Thomas', St George's, the Westminster, the London, King's College and St Bartholomew's.[11] Outside the capital, ether was just as speedily taken up in Edinburgh, Bristol, Liverpool, Birmingham, Newcastle, Derby, Wolverhampton and Maidstone. By the end of January 1847 – just six weeks after Liston's pioneering surgery – more than fifty etherised operations and nearly 100 dental extractions had been reported in *The Lancet*. Ether was even used a few weeks later by veterinary surgeons to perform operations on a sheep and a horse at the Royal Veterinary College in London.

Intoxicating accounts of these pioneering procedures filled the columns of the medical press. A labourer whose ankle had been shattered when a sugar cask fell on his leg agreed to an amputation only when assured he would feel no pain. A man who had earlier refused to undergo an operation on his foreskin because he was convinced – no doubt correctly – that it would be agonising was astonished when he came round to find his operation was over. Surgeons at St Bartholomew's even used ether for a Caesarean delivery on a woman with a deformed pelvis who was unable to give birth normally (although she died thirty-six hours later, her baby survived).

Operations on children, previously dreaded by surgeons almost as much as by parents, were now performed on infants sleeping as peacefully as cherubs. At Guy's a fourteen-year-old boy had a bladder stone excised 'without the slightest manifestation of pain'. Another boy had a piece of bone removed from his leg at St George's and 'did not shed a tear'. Two nine-year-old boys had squints corrected at Liverpool without major discomfort. The surgeon who performed the latter two procedures declared that ether provided 'a most powerful means of alleviating human suffering' especially in children 'whose struggles during the performance of an operation are generally the greatest difficulty a surgeon has to contend with'.

Whether young or old, rich or poor, patients were equally effusive about being delivered from pain. Exhilarated by the novelty of slicing flesh and sawing bone on peacefully dozing patients, surgeons embraced operations under ether as a safer, more effective, more reliable alternative to mesmeric surgery. In fact it was none of these things.

As those same surgeons and dentists soon discovered, ether was not the trouble-free miracle it had first seemed. It was difficult to administer and variable in its effects; it smelled vile and caused serious side effects. Some patients reacted violently, becoming excited or aggressive instead of stupefied, while others remained completely unaffected. One London dentist reported that a brawny Irishman became so belligerent under ether that he had to flee his surgery, while a second patient, a hospital porter, stayed wide awake despite inhaling large amounts of the gas.[12] Another dentist said one of his patients, a solicitor, awoke from ether and invited him to dance the polka. One woman opened her eyes in the middle of having her leg amputated and happily observed: 'You are sawing,' but later assured surgeons she had felt nothing. Yet a miner who broke his leg falling down a shaft had his leg amputated with the usual degree of agony when ether failed to take effect. In addition, ether irritated the airways, causing coughing and sometimes vomiting. William Squire, Liston's student volunteer, was one of the first to suffer this effect. Travelling home on the roof of a coach during a snowstorm after a week of overenthusiastic experiments on himself at UCH, he had coughed so much he had to sit inside.[13] Several operations had to be abandoned because the patients were coughing so violently.

Doubts soon set in. One of the first to experience problems was Liston. In the first week of January he attempted to etherise one patient for ten minutes and another for twenty minutes without effect; their operations then went ahead 'with the usual amount of pain'.[14] Within weeks of his pioneering operation he was on the verge of abandoning ether alto-gether. By March even the *LMG* was raising concerns.[15] The responses of patients varied so enormously that it was impossible to determine the dose in advance, it complained. Surgeons were turning operations into public spectacles, it said, yet were not being honest about reporting the failings. *The Lancet* voiced similar worries. Within three months of ether making its appearance, the number of operations performed in London hospitals had doubled, said Wakley, yet surgeons were withholding vital information about the outcomes. Wakley's eldest son, twenty-five-year-old Thomas Wakley junior, who had trained under Liston and now practised as a surgeon at the Royal Free Hospital, appealed for details.

One young doctor did his utmost to assuage concerns and render ether safe to use.[16] John Snow, the son of a Yorkshire labourer, who would later make his name by identifying the source of cholera, had closely studied the respiratory system and also had a keen interest in chemistry. He quickly realised that the main challenge was to deliver the correct dose of ether at the right strength and so immediately set about designing an inhaler that would administer the gas more safely and effectively. After first volunteering to administer ether to dental out-patients at St George's, Snow was soon employed to anaesthetise patients for major surgery there and at UCH. Diligently refining his technique and apparatus, Snow would corner the market in administering ether in London hospitals and advised on its use nationwide.

Yet despite Snow's valiant efforts the ether euphoria soon began to evaporate. In March, a twenty-one-year-old woman named Ann Parkinson, from Spittlegate in Lincolnshire, was given ether to have a tumour removed from her leg and never regained consciousness.[17] An inquest blamed ether for her death but exonerated her surgeon, William Robbs, from a possible charge of manslaughter.

Concerns about ether's safety now dominated the newspapers and enthusiasm for the gas was fading fast. One correspondent in *The Lancet* remarked that from the 'outburst attending its first annunciation' it seemed 'another blessing had . . . escaped Pandora's box'.[18] But now the 'high hopes' had vanished, the storm of excitement had been 'lulled to a calm' and it was time to examine the facts and 'see if the whole matter is but as a bubble burst'. The *Medical Times*, which had always been sympathetic to mesmerism, asked whether the use of ether should be abandoned entirely. And although ether was lauded as a 'scientific' solution, surgeons had no more clue as to how it engendered unconsciousness than they had about mesmerism. Another alternative was needed – and quickly.

Before the year was out, James Young Simpson, Professor of Obstetrics at Edinburgh, provided the answer.[19]

*

Simpson had never signed up to the theory of pain as a vital stimulant. As a medical student in Edinburgh, watching Liston perform a mastectomy, he had been so distressed by the patient's screams that he had almost abandoned medicine for a career in law. Instead he had vowed to devote himself to finding an antidote to pain. As a young house-surgeon in 1836 Simpson had asked: 'Cannot something be done to render the patient unconscious while under acute pain, without interfering with the free and healthy play of natural functions?' As part of this quest for painless surgery, Simpson had investigated mesmerism. In 1842 he attended a demonstration at Elliotson's house and told his brother that having previously 'laughed at it all' now he had 'seen enough to stagger me'.[20] But although he had adopted mesmerism for a while he soon gave it up.

When the use of ether crossed the Atlantic, Simpson had welcomed this new development with gusto. Within weeks of Liston's triumph, Simpson gave ether to a woman in labour and from March he used it routinely in midwifery. In one case he reported a woman had slept so soundly through childbirth that when presented with the newborn baby she refused to believe it was hers. Simpson would vehemently oppose religious fanatics who argued that eliminating pain in childbirth was 'reprehensible and heretical' because it had been ordained in the Bible that women give birth 'in sorrow'. But he was quick to realise that ether brought its own problems and set to work looking for a solution.

Experimenting around the dinner table on a nightly basis, Simpson and his friends sampled innumerable vapours before trying a clear liquid with a 'fragrant, fruit-like odour' on 4 November 1847. Within minutes the imbibers were prattling merrily and soon afterwards they were discovered unconscious 'under the mahogany'. Simpson had found his elixir: chloroform. More potent than ether and easier to administer – half a teaspoonful on a handkerchief rendered most patients unconscious – chloroform was also distinctly more palatable.

A few days later Simpson gave chloroform to a woman in childbirth, and on 10 November he administered the gas to three patients undergoing major operations at Edinburgh Royal Infirmary. The first, a boy about five years old who spoke only Gaelic, had the radius bone in his forearm removed during a 'sound snoring sleep' and woke to declare – via a student interpreter – that he had felt no pain. An elated Simpson reported his success that same evening to the Edinburgh

Medico-Chirurgical Society and a week later he published his findings in a pamphlet, which sold out within days.

Chloroform was quickly adopted as the anaesthetic drug of choice. The *Caledonian Mercury* announced Simpson's discovery under the headline 'New anaesthetic agent – Ether superseded'. In London Liston lost no time in testing his former pupil's discovery and pronounced chloroform 'a vast advance upon ether' adding magnanimously: 'Simpson deserves all laudation.'[21] Yet here too, excitement soon gave way to despondency.

The first death attributed to chloroform occurred within three months, on 28 January 1848. A fifteen-year-old girl named Hannah Greener from Winlaton, near Newcastle, had already had an ingrown toenail removed under ether a few months earlier.[22] When she needed a second toenail excised, her surgeon, Thomas Meggison, proposed chloroform. Meggison held a cloth soaked in the chemical over her nose and she fell asleep in thirty seconds but minutes later she expired, despite attempts to revive her with brandy and the inevitable bloodletting. An inquest blamed her death on chloroform inhalation. Desperate to subdue further public panic over anaesthesia, Simpson argued that the brandy was to blame, while Snow insisted that the mode of application was at fault and immediately set to work devising safety guidelines.

As the medical press did its level best to promote the 'scientific' benefits of chloroform over 'quackish' mesmerism, so Wakley became entangled in the controversy over its lethal effects. In July 1848 the *London Daily News* reported an inquest on a twenty-three-year-old man, Walter Badger, who had died in the dentist's chair under chloroform.[23] The dentist administering the gas was James Robinson, who had first trialled ether; the coroner was Wakley. The verdict, however, was unclear. The newspaper reported that death was due to chloroform acting on a diseased heart and enlarged liver but Robinson immediately responded to insist that chloroform had not been implicated. The newspaper now threw the blame on Wakley for failing to provide sufficient notice for journalists to attend the inquest in person. This, it alleged, was so that Wakley could be the first to publish the results in *The Lancet*.

Deaths from chloroform began to fill the newspaper columns. In Boston surgeons returned to ether as a less dangerous alternative, but in

Britain chloroform prevailed. Having let the pain-relieving vapour out of the bottle, it was impossible to replace the stopper. Charles Dickens, for all his skills in mesmerism, arranged for his wife Catherine to have chloroform during a difficult labour in 1849.[24] The Marquess of Anglesey, who had so stoically endured his amputation in 1815, turned to chloroform in 1850 to ease the lingering pain in his stump. And chloroform won the royal seal of approval in 1853 when Snow administered it to Queen Victoria for the birth of her eighth child, Prince Leopold. A year later, when Britain became embroiled in the Crimean War, chloroform brought blessed relief to innumerable soldiers wounded on the battlefield – though some diehard surgeons still stuck rigidly to the 'pain is best' principle.

As the medical press continued to champion chemical anaesthesia and Snow worked doggedly to reduce its risks, more than fifty more deaths would be attributed to chloroform by 1858. Five years later, an inquiry by the RMCS would implicate chloroform in a total of 163 deaths and come to the conclusion – long argued by Snow – that an excess of chloroform paralysed the heart muscle as well as causing long-term liver damage. Yet despite all the dangers, chloroform continued to permeate hospitals and sickrooms throughout the land. Chemical anaesthesia was here to stay.

In time chloroform would be superseded by safer, more potent, more accurate agents including nerve blocks and epidural anaesthesia along with safer methods of administration – although sudden deaths and side effects would remain a problem up to the present day. But chemical anaesthesia had given doctors something that mesmerism never could: control. With patients rendered mute and immobile, surgeons could perform increasingly long, complex and invasive operations. Having discovered that pain was not the boon they thought it was, surgeons found they rather liked this silent, tranquil and – in time – sterile environment. Moreover, since qualified doctors were the only people who generally had access to chloroform and knew how to administer it safely, they alone could dispense its benefits. As one medical practitioner put it in *The Lancet*: 'As yet, this gift from heaven to all is held by us of the medical profession in sole and exclusive trust.'[25]

Chemical anaesthesia had shifted the balance of the therapeutic relationship. Doctors reigned supreme in the operating theatre; patients would be forever silent and subservient. But mesmerism was not yet ready to roll over and die.

As doctors wrangled over the relative hazards of ether and chloroform, and patients sometimes confessed themselves more afraid of dying from anaesthesia than from the surgery itself, mesmerism continued to thrive. Mesmeric treatment and surgery were still banished from most public hospitals and remained largely ignored by the medical press. Indeed, Frederick Knight Hunt, editor of the *Medical Times*, the only medical journal which had been at all sympathetic towards Elliotson, was hounded out of his post and forced to sell the title in 1841 because of threats of libel action over his support for mesmerism.[26] Yet a significant number of dentists and surgeons in the provinces and overseas continued to practise it in their private consulting rooms and patients' homes. Others who initially adopted chemical anaesthesia returned to mesmerism when they realised the risks.

One surgeon, John Parker, based in Exeter, carried out more than 100 operations using mesmerism as well as twenty procedures on the eye and numerous dental and minor operations before 1851.[27] In York, a surgeon named Henry Thompson abandoned ether after a few months because of the dangers of fatality and reverted to mesmerism.[28] Another surgeon, William Tubbs, who worked in the Cambridgeshire fens, was about to mesmerise a woman for a leg amputation when her sister objected; he gave her chloroform instead but mesmerised her every time he dressed the wound.[29] Beyond British shores other doctors also kept faith with mesmerism. In Cherbourg, France, surgeons performed numerous operations using mesmerism. Three patients who underwent surgery there in June 1847 were watched by a crowd of nearly seventy onlookers including barristers, clergymen and army officers.[30] Likewise in Boston, Dr Francis Dana stayed true to mesmerism on the grounds that it was more effective than ether and had been more widely tested.[31] But nobody contributed more to mesmeric surgery than James Esdaile.

Having quietly continued to perform operations under mesmerism with the help of his Hindu attendants in Calcutta, Esdaile had garnered support from medical colleagues, government officials and Bengali nobility as well as the Indian press.[32] In 1848, Esdaile's 'experimental hospital' in Calcutta even won the approval of Lord Dalhousie, the new

Governor-General of India, and Esdaile introduced mesmeric surgery into five more hospitals in the district. That same year, Dalhousie promoted Esdaile to the coveted post of presidency surgeon – and two years later to marine surgeon – in recognition of his services to humanity 'by mitigating largely its sufferings'.

Always open to innovation, Esdaile had been one of the first surgeons to try ether as soon as news of Liston's triumph reached Calcutta in February 1847. He tested the vapour on two patients but immediately encountered problems. One man became 'very drunk' but still felt pinpricks while the other fell into such a sound sleep he was impossible to rouse for several hours. The effects of ether were 'very uncertain, being often transient, or so intense as to be alarming', Esdaile concluded, while the smell was 'disgusting'. Mesmerism, by contrast, was 'perfectly safe, manageable, and curative'. By 1851 he had performed 261 major operations, including the removal of 200 scrotal tumours, plus many more dental extractions and procedures under mesmerism. His mortality rate for the tumour operations was a remarkable five per cent, and even those deaths were largely attributed to concurrent diseases. Esdaile was proud to boast that *'painless Surgery* was as common in my hospitals, long before ether or chloroform were heard of, as it has become in the hospitals of England since the discovery of the anaesthetic virtues of these drugs'. Yet in India, just as elsewhere, chemical anaesthesia soon gained a stranglehold.

As officials realised that chloroform was quicker and easier to use than mesmerism, support for Esdaile withered and his mesmeric hospital closed. Medical colleagues who had previously acclaimed his success now recanted their testimonies and embraced chloroform.[33] Esdaile was appalled his fellow doctors favoured chemical anaesthesia over mesmerism and was saddened when he heard of the first deaths in India from chloroform – a five-year-old girl having a facial tumour excised, and a man having a scrotal tumour removed in 1849.[34]

Back in Britain influential support for Esdaile's achievements likewise evaporated. His fellow Scot, James Simpson, had initially urged Esdaile to send details of his scrotal tumour operations and promised to see them published in an Edinburgh medical journal that Simpson co-edited. But after despatching his account Esdaile heard no more. Challenged by Esdaile, Simpson blustered that his fellow editors had decided the article was not 'sufficiently practical' although he assured

Esdaile his low mortality rate was 'one of the most remarkable things in the history of Surgery'. Even the mild-mannered Snow thought Esdaile had been duped by 'dishonest and designing patients'. Other critics said Esdaile's success only applied to native patients – 'one would suppose they were monkeys,' he fumed – despite the fact this still meant relief for 120 million 'fellow men'.

At least Esdaile could always count on support from one quarter: John Elliotson. Since Esdaile's achievements in India had been studiously ignored by the press in Britain, Elliotson published detailed case studies in the *Zoist*. 'Dr Esdaile's merits are transcendent,' he enthused. 'I regard him as one of the most glorious men of our profession.'[35]

Not surprisingly, both Elliotson and Esdaile were scathing about the hypocrisy of the medical press as it championed operations under ether and chloroform while stifling reports of mesmeric surgery. After his account of scrotal tumour operations was rejected by Simpson and his cronies, Esdaile published it privately and challenged readers to decide whether it had been turned down because it really was 'impractical' or 'simply because the Editors have resolved that Mesmerism in any shape shall not be true, and are determined that you shall have no opportunity, in their pages, of judging for yourselves'.[36] The notion of a free medical press in Britain was 'a mockery and a delusion', he said, when medical men were not allowed to be heard 'if what they advance is contrary to the prejudices and foregone conclusions of the Editors'.

Elliotson was equally damning. For years the medical press had dismissed accounts of painless surgery under mesmerism as fraudulent and had even argued that 'agony in operations' was 'an excellent thing'.[37] If any patient groaned or moved during mesmeric operations this was seized on as proof of their fraud. Yet with the arrival of ether and chloroform, the medical journals had suddenly welcomed the notion of painless surgery and freely accepted patients' testimonies when they said they felt no pain no matter how much they had moaned or writhed. As always Elliotson reserved his bitterest ire for Wakley and *The Lancet*. After ignoring painless operations under mesmerism for five years, he said, Wakley had offered up 'thanksgivings' to God for putting it 'in the power of man to operate without pain on his fellow-creatures'.

As the death toll from chloroform continued to mount, Elliotson accused the medical profession and medical press of suppressing reports of fatal operations. Deaths under chloroform were being 'hushed up' and inquests 'avoided', he claimed. Determined to expose the truth, he catalogued deaths associated with chloroform in the *Zoist*. 'It is now time for mesmerists to speak without reserve,' he declared. 'Ether and chloroform, when inhaled, are capricious poisons, very *uncertain* in their good effects, and *occasionally injurious and even fatal* in spite of every precaution.'

It was plain, however, that no matter how much Elliotson stamped his feet, mesmerism was not going to be allowed back into public hospitals or medical schools any time soon. So he applied himself instead to establishing a hospital that would be entirely dedicated to the practice and teaching of mesmerism. And he found the perfect place to site it.

12

The Sweetest Sleep

Bedford Street, London, January 1850

Ragged and wretched, sick and starving, the poor of north London flocked to the new hospital just as they had crowded at the steps of UCH sixteen years earlier. The London Mesmeric Infirmary opened its doors in January 1850, after four years of fund-raising, at 9 Bedford Street, a five-minute stroll from UCH and – in an almost deliberate affront – just around the corner from Thomas Wakley's house in Bedford Square.[1] Though Wakley, of course, would never visit – and probably crossed the road to avoid passing its doors – the hospital was an immediate and resounding success.

Elliotson had been the driving force in founding, running and keeping the LMI afloat and as always he drew a wide array of powerful friends to his cause. Its founding supporters included Richard Whately, the Archbishop of Dublin, who had first witnessed Elliotson's demonstrations at UCH; Lord Stanhope, who was now a skilled mesmerist in his own right; Isaac Lyon Goldsmid, the co-founder of UCL; and the writer and Liberal MP Richard Monckton Milnes. The Whig politician Henry Moreton, Earl of Ducie, agreed to be president and, after returning from India in 1851, James Esdaile would become vice-president. Elliotson took the post of treasurer and threw his energies into raising funds with his customary zeal. Wisely giving a wide berth to the supernatural claims that still dogged mesmerism, the LMI was dedicated solely to medical treatment and teaching. It was funded by voluntary donations and – in common with all hospitals at the time – treated only the poor who were charged what they could afford up to one guinea. There were no in-patient beds and so there were few major operations, but patients walked long distances to and from the hospital for daily treatment.

At first the LMI employed only one full-time mesmerist, William Fisher, who was supervised by William Tubbs, the Cambridgeshire surgeon, but within weeks it was deluged by so many requests for aid that Tubbs quickly trained up a second mesmerist, Charles Mayhew. Within a few years, as demand increased, the team would be joined by a matron, a resident secretary and several more mesmerists, including two women, Mrs Acott and Mrs Lickfold, who practised on an equal basis with the men more than twenty years before the medical profession suffered women to join its ranks. In time Fisher's wife would also become a mesmerist.

Although Elliotson would remain involved in the LMI all his life, he never served there as a mesmerist. In truth he was never a particularly skilful mesmerist, probably because he was so intent on manipulating the 'invisible force'. Hospital affairs were run by a medical and general council assisted by a committee of ladies, one of whom visited every day, partly to dispel 'the suspicions of low and vulgar minds' that lingered around mesmerism like a cheap perfume. As well as treating poor patients for low fees, the infirmary offered training in mesmerism for free and regardless of gender.

Most of the patients who flocked to the LMI from 1850 onwards were desperately poor and many were desperately ill. Some were 'almost shoeless, scantily clad, and half starved', said one annual report.[2] One benefactor provided woollen slippers for patients to wear while their sodden shoes dried before the waiting-room fire. Many had already expended what little savings they had on orthodox doctors and vast quantities of worthless medicines. Yet many of these wretched patients donated to the hospital their hard-earned farthings and halfpennies, or presented hand-made gifts to staff, in gratitude for their care. One patient gave the secretary's young son a painted horse, another an ebony toy. And despite the cynicism of conventional medical practitioners and the medical press, many who attended the LMI apparently walked away cured when all other efforts had failed.

*

Within its first year the LMI treated ninety-one patients but had to turn away many more due to lack of resources. Demand increased year on year. In the twelve months up to June 1855, the hospital treated 247 patients of whom sixty-nine were declared cured and forty-nine improved. A further nine were said to be 'nearly cured' while forty-one were still under treatment. The largest proportion, seventy-one patients, had given up their treatment after one or two appointments, apparently disappointed at not being cured instantly. The hospital kept diligent casebooks, just as Elliotson had done at UCH, and they described some remarkable results.

One boy, diagnosed with St Vitus's dance, who dribbled and gabbled, had been liberally dosed with purges, potions and pills by his medical practitioner to no avail. After two months of mesmerism, however, he was perfectly recovered. A sixteen-year-old girl with neuralgia and asthma who suffered severe pain when walking upstairs had been treated by a conventional practitioner for two years without relief. After being mesmerised for two months by Mrs Acott she was able to run to and from the hospital. Many similar successes filled the annual reports. Even the pageboy who opened the doors of the LMI to patients each day had been cured by mesmerism of a diseased shoulder.

Among the most dramatic recoveries was that of a Mrs Granger, the forty-six-year-old wife of a brick-maker, who lived in the optimistically named Teetotal Row, near Uxbridge.[3] Having suffered violent pains and swelling in her abdomen for six years, she had been diagnosed with an ovarian tumour causing 'dropsy' – fluid retention or oedema. She may have had a rare, benign condition called massive ovarian oedema. Mrs Granger had spent six months in UCH and had had her abdomen 'tapped' – punctured to draw off fluid – at UCH and elsewhere a colossal fifty-five times with as much as ninety-six pints being drained at once. By 1851 she measured five feet around the waist and her surgeon had predicted she had not much longer to live. In desperation her sister had suggested mesmerism. Since Mrs Granger could not afford the travel costs to and from the LMI, William Fisher went by rail to visit her after his usual day's work. He visited her every day for nine months despite being jeered at by villagers who called him 'the devil's imp'. When the toll began to tell on the commuting mesmerist, Elliotson and his friends clubbed together to pay Mrs Granger's train fare. Within twelve months, her dropsy had gone and she declared herself in perfect health. She even attended the LMI's annual meeting a few years later to demonstrate her well-being.

Another poignant case concerned a three-year-old boy, George Townsend, who had wounded his knee when falling from his crib at the age of fifteen months.[4] His mother took him to a surgeon, who leeched and blistered the leg for six weeks without relief. Unable to walk and weakened by pain, the boy kept repeating the pitiful words, 'Bad knee, bad knee.' When he was taken to the Middlesex Hospital, surgeons recommended amputation as the only course. Then a relative suggested the LMI. After George's third visit, the pain was so improved that now he only cried if he was not taken to the hospital at the usual time. Three months later, the swelling had reduced, the pain was gone and George was playing as happily as any small boy.

As word of the LMI's success spread, so it was deluged by patients from all walks of life. At the annual meeting in 1856 the hospital's resident mesmerist Thomas Capern paraded several soldiers who had been injured during the Crimean War but who declared themselves cured.[5] A true evangelist, Capern was in the habit of stopping people in the street who were limping or walking with crutches, and luring them back to the LMI or into local pubs and shops for treatment. One man was on his way to see doctors at St Mary's Hospital, Paddington, when Capern spotted him and promptly offered to treat him; he later returned his crutches to the surgeons at St Mary's and jubilantly informed them of his cure.

With hindsight it is impossible to determine precisely how mesmerism effected such striking results. Discounting the seventy-one people who had abandoned their treatment in 1854, the LMI cured more than one in three of its patients. Adding those who were 'nearly cured' or 'improved' suggests that more than half enjoyed some relief from their ailments – a laudable success rate for any therapy. With the limited understanding of the day, some patients had no doubt been misdiagnosed and had less serious conditions than supposed, while some problems might have resolved naturally or gone into remission. Many patients must have felt better simply by virtue of stopping the sadistic therapies and toxic medicines that orthodox medicine tortured them with; the LMI strictly banned all other treatments. In many cases, mesmerism may have worked as a powerful placebo.

Research on the placebo effect has shown that dummy pills, fake therapies and even sham surgery can produce significant improvements in patients.[6] One landmark study has found that one in three patients recovered from their ailments simply by taking placebo medicines – a figure that closely reflects the LMI's success rate. Placebos are not all equally effective. Studies have shown that four dummy pills work better than two in clearing gastric ulcers while saltwater injections are more effective than sugar pills in combating pain. Likewise 'morphine' dummy tablets work better than 'paracetamol' ones, even though both placebos are fundamentally the same. Most research suggests placebos work through suggestion and expectation; people get better because their practitioner suggests they will and because advertising and media reports tell us that certain drugs and therapies will make us well. But this improvement in health is not simply due to imagination or willpower. Brain scans have revealed that placebo therapies produce physiological changes in the body, such as the release of pain-relieving chemicals in the brain, in much the same way that chemical drugs do.

Certain studies have shown that empathetic practitioners are better at triggering the placebo response and some researchers attribute the success of complementary remedies to the attentive, unhurried approach of such therapists. In particular, the placebo effect is known to be most successful in treating illnesses with a psychosomatic root. Placebos cannot kill viruses or cure cancer but they can be remarkably successful in alleviating depression, anxiety, insomnia, nausea, asthma, gastroenterological problems and other conditions with a psychological element. Precisely how the placebo response brings about physical changes in the body is still under investigation. And whether hypnotism works simply through the placebo effect – by manipulating suggestion and expectation – or because there is an additional factor at play is still hotly debated.

Elliotson and his staff at the LMI clearly extended a compassionate approach towards their patients – that much can be seen from the woollen slippers and the voluntary donations. They also believed emphatically in their therapy and devoted long hours to treating individuals. Many conditions treated at the LMI were plainly psychological. One man attended because he was unable to swallow but after ten minutes of mesmerism he could swallow his own saliva and on returning home he wolfed down a rasher of bacon.[7] A six-year-old boy had become deluded into thinking a monkey was sitting on his bed but recovered completely after two months' treatment. The LMI treated a wide range of other ailments, including neuralgia, asthma, digestive problems and paralysis, as well as insanity and depression. Many were chronic conditions associated with pain. Mesmerists rarely treated acute problems – although there were cases of wounds being said to heal more quickly and even claims of cancers being cured.

Yet many of the LMI's patients had been treated by conventional practitioners, who believed just as fervently in their useless therapies, with no apparent placebo effect. And the reported cures of some of the most intractable problems, such as Mrs Granger with her dropsy and little George Townsend with his 'bad knee', still defy explanation. Was there some additional factor that made mesmerism work? While many of the cures claimed by the LMI took weeks or months to take effect and remain shrouded in mystery, the marvels of mesmeric surgery were both immediate and obvious. One of the infirmary's most spectacular successes was a dramatic operation performed in 1854.

Jane Flowerday, a thirty-year-old woman from Upwell in Cambridgeshire with four young children, had been aware of a lump in her right breast for two years but had put off consulting her doctor, William Tubbs, until March 1854.[8] At that point Tubbs diagnosed breast cancer and warned Mrs Flowerday she would die without an operation to amputate the breast. Despite being a keen mesmerist, Tubbs regularly used chloroform to perform surgery because of the stigma attached to mesmerism. But since Mrs Flowerday was subject to fainting fits and a cough, he feared she might not survive an operation with chloroform. So Mrs Flowerday agreed to place her faith in mesmerism.

Mrs Flowerday and her husband, a gardener, travelled from their village to the LMI on 25 April. The following day Mrs Flowerday was shown into a treatment room and sat in a reclining chair. The surgical instruments had been screened from view to soothe her nerves, although the presence of eighteen medical men and mesmerists crowding around her could not have done much to put her mind at ease. Standing behind her chair, Tubbs stared steadily into Mrs Flowerday's uplifted eyes and within nine minutes she was in a deep trance. Assisted by a fellow Cambridgeshire surgeon, Smith Burman, Tubbs commenced the operation. One of the observers, a dentist named Theodosius Purland, later described the procedure in suitably melodramatic language.

Watched in 'breathless silence' by the hushed onlookers, including Elliotson and Symes, Tubbs made the first incision. All eyes focused on the patient's face yet 'not a muscle moved – not a sigh!' Mrs Flowerday maintained 'the same placid smile' as Tubbs slowly dissected the breast then probed with his fingers for any remaining tumour and finally cut away the last remnants 'as coolly as if trying his weapon upon a dead body'. As the patient continued to sleep, the wound was stitched and dressed. When she was woken, Mrs Flowerday confirmed she had felt no pain then walked up two flights of stairs to her bedroom 'as if nothing had occurred!'

A week later *The Times*, in a rare reference to mesmerism, reported the operation in full.[9] Stressing that Mrs Flowerday was 'a most respectable married woman' – not some skittish servant girl or Hindu native – the newspaper said she had sat throughout the operation 'perfectly still, silent, and relaxed, like any one in the sweetest sleep'.

Although Mrs Flowerday's remarkable operation was widely reported, in general the achievements of the LMI were rarely noticed by the media except as the target of ridicule. Typically, *The Lancet* had heralded the plans to open the infirmary with a comical ditty, entitled 'The Mesmeric Hospital'.[10] It punned:

> *Dr E—will, of course, be the leading physician –*
> *A man of acknowledged and vast erudition,*
> *Well versed in the art; and the cream of the joke is,*
> *He has booked, for the nurses, the two little Okeys!*

Yet as news of the LMI's success spread by word of mouth, its support increased, funds rolled in and demand grew. Wealthy members of the nobility, including the Earl of Carlisle, the Earl of Dunraven, the Countess of Buckingham and the Marchioness of Downshire, gave continuing support to the hospital.[11] Its subscribers also numbered MPs, army officers, clergymen, surgeons and writers as well as numerous well-wishers who had benefited from mesmerism. Dickens donated 4 guineas, Martineau sent 10 guineas and Elliotson's publisher, Hippolyte Baillière, gave 5 guineas after his daughter was treated with mesmerism. By 1852, the annual meeting proved so popular it had to be moved to a ballroom where nearly 700 people squeezed in. The following year – when more than 1,200 people packed the meeting – the hospital itself moved to larger premises, a mansion in Fitzroy Square. But opposition from local residents, who accused the hospital of 'evil spiritual works', forced a third move, to a modest house in Weymouth Street, on the western edge of Bloomsbury. Meanwhile mesmeric infirmaries were founded in Bristol, Exeter, Dublin and Edinburgh.

Mesmerism enjoyed its zenith in the 1850s, providing Victorian Britain with entertainment in town halls, conversation over the dinner table and solace in the sickroom. Mesmeric surgery offered a safe and effective alternative to ether or chloroform, while mesmeric treatment brought relief to thousands who preferred its gentle, holistic approach over the brutality of conventional remedies. For a time mesmerism and orthodox medicine vied for supremacy. And with little wonder, since mesmerism could demonstrate clear evidence of its effectiveness while most conventional treatments still showed none.

Yet despite their all too patent failings, traditional practices gradually regained the ascendancy. Medical schools continued to teach the outdated theories; examining authorities failed students who did not parrot the ancient methods; colleges insisted their members slavishly follow the flawed and failed practices; and the medical press reinforced the age-old doctrines. At least in the operating theatre surgeons could now deliver patients from pain using chloroform – providing they survived. Yet bloodletting would continue as a dominant therapy until the end of the nineteenth century while leeches maintained their sucker hold for nearly as long. The battery of useless therapies and medicines staunchly defended by the profession would only finally fall away in the early 1900s when laboratories in Germany and France introduced effective new pharmaceuticals and British chemists developed antibiotics which vanquished a raft of deadly infectious diseases. In the meantime mesmerism was battered and bruised but it remained unbeaten – until a new and even more powerful vogue captured the public imagination.

In 1848, two sisters, Kate and Margaret Fox, aged eleven and thirteen, from a poor farming family in rural New York, became the centre of a sensation.[12] Whenever they were together in the house, loud raps or knocks were heard. Their mother decided that the noises came from spirits and the house was soon crowded with friends and neighbours seeking answers to questions which were rapped out by the obliging ghosts. The girls' brother introduced the idea of reciting the alphabet so the spirits could spell out messages by rapping when the appropriate letter was reached. Shrewdly spotting a money-spinner, their older sister promoted the girls as 'mediums' and whisked them off to New York City where they held audiences enraptured. Spiritualism became a craze which swept America, spawning hundreds of imitators. Much later, the Fox sisters would confess that they had made the rapping noises by clicking their toes and other bones. But the spiritualism mania had become unstoppable and thousands were taken in by accomplished mediums who developed a range of tricks including spinning and raising tables, dimming lights and producing ghostly hands.

It was not long before spiritualism drifted across the Atlantic. In early 1853, Maria Hayden, a medium from Boston, arrived in London and enthralled audiences with her spectacular séances. Spiritualism took Europe by storm and table-turning parties, with or without mediums, became a favourite Victorian pastime. Often these mystifying diversions attracted the very same people who had been captivated by mesmerism, including Bulwer-Lytton, Elizabeth Barrett Browning and the Trollopes. At one session in 1855 Bulwer-Lytton leapt to his feet in astonishment when he felt his hand being grasped under the table.[13] At another séance, Thomas Trollope was amazed to see the heavy mahogany table 'raised bodily from the ground' and hovering four or five inches from the floor.

Arguments raged over how the phenomena were produced. While advocates insisted that supernatural forces were at work, sceptics sought a scientific explanation. Michael Faraday devised experiments to demonstrate that participants were unconsciously moving the tables through involuntary muscle movements. Even mesmerists were drawn into the controversy. The physician John Ashburner, a long-time mesmerist and close friend of Elliotson's, had no doubt that departed souls were tilting the tables, while James Braid proposed that – as with his theory of hypnotism – the movements were entirely due to collective suggestion.[14]

John Elliotson became one of the most vocal opponents of spiritualism. Having stoutly defended the Okey sisters all his life, he was not going to be taken in by the Foxes. He scorned the idea of spirit messages as an 'ignorant and preposterous absurdity' and proposed that invisible mesmeric forces were causing the tables to tip and spin.[15] Scoffing at the way spiritualism was spreading, he wrote: 'Everyone now says their table turned be it Buckingham Palace or a room which serves for kitchen and parlour.' He broke off his long friendship with Ashburner and repudiated Townshend, who was likewise a convert. Despite his scepticism, Elliotson joined friends at several parties devoted to table-spinning but never observed any movement – either by spirits or mesmerism – except once when 'the table turned very slowly a short distance'. Whatever explanations were posited or discounted, by the end of the decade spiritualism in its various guises would more or less oust mesmerism in the popular imagination. But mesmerism had no intention of being completely spirited away.

Staying faithful to mesmerism through its fluctuating fortunes, by the 1850s Elliotson had largely recovered his popularity as a medical practitioner and had almost been absorbed back into the medical establishment. Now secure in his position as literary London's favourite physician, Elliotson continued to treat the Dickens and Macready families as well as attending Forster and Thackeray. Dickens called in Elliotson to treat his wife, Catherine, in 1844 and his sister-in-law, Georgina, in 1862, though whether he later asked his old friend to attend his mistress, Nelly Ternan, went unrecorded.[16] Elliotson tended Macready's nineteen-year-old daughter, Nina, when she fell ill in 1850, but despite his best attentions – in conjunction with the former Guy's physician Richard Bright – she died soon after. 'They spoke to me, and from their language I collected that the case was desperate,' a devastated Macready wrote.[17]

Thackeray was convinced he owed his life to Elliotson after he fell seriously ill with a fever in September 1849, in the middle of writing his serialised novel *Pendennis*.[18] Cholera was suspected, although Elliotson diagnosed 'intermittent fever' – malaria – and rather than proposing mesmerism, he dosed him with his old standard: quinine. As Thackeray worsened and feared that death was 'near at hand', Elliotson visited him devotedly while refusing to take a fee. After four weeks, the writer was pronounced out of danger and by November he felt strong enough to throw 'the physic-bottles out of the window'. When *Pendennis* was published in book form a year later, Thackeray dedicated it fondly to Elliotson with the inscription: 'My dear Doctor, Thirteen months ago, when it seemed likely that this story had come to a close, a kind friend brought you to my bedside, whence, in all probability I never should have risen but for your constant watchfulness and skill.' In *Pendennis*, Thackeray immortalised Elliotson as the compassionate 'Dr Goodenough', who 'came like an angel' into the sickroom. At one point the 'kind-hearted physician' tends the child of an impoverished porter; another time he treats the family of a writer and 'laughed at the idea of taking a fee from a literary man, or the widow of a brother practitioner'.

Elliotson's literary friends well knew that Thackeray's portrait was no fiction. He rarely charged writers, actors or artists, and never expected a fee from the working poor. Ever since he had befriended the swindler Moscati in 1833, Elliotson had also supported appeals to the Royal Literary Fund from destitute writers and their families. In one instance, in 1855, he and Dickens jointly appealed through *The Times* for donations to help the children's writer Maria Goodluck, who was struggling to support herself and her ailing sister.[19] Dickens sent another impoverished writer, a carpenter named John Overs who had turned his hand to poetry, to Elliotson when he fell ill and told Macready he 'has gone into his case as if he were Prince Albert'. Instructing Overs to stay off work, Elliotson gave him £5 to help him survive.[20] Dickens was so touched by Elliotson's generosity, he declared, 'I could almost bear the Tories for five years out of pleasure in knowing such things.' When Overs published his poetry in 1844, he dedicated the volume to Elliotson. A few months later when Overs died and was buried in a pauper's grave, Dickens helped raise money for his widow and six children while Elliotson advised her on investing it.

Elliotson provided inspiration for other writers too. Bulwer-Lytton, who had reported Elliotson's experiments so enthusiastically in 1838, paid tribute to Elliotson in his novel *A Strange Story*, serialised in 1861. Countering scepticism about mesmeric clairvoyance from the young hero, an elderly physician commends 'those who, like our bold contemporary, Elliotson, have braved scoff and sacrificed dross in seeking to extract what is practical in uses, what can be tested by experiment, from those exceptional phenomena on which magic sought to found a philosophy'.[21] Wilkie Collins, who had become a close friend of Dickens in the 1850s, had Elliotson to thank for one of his most famous novelistic twists. He used a case from Elliotson's *Human Physiology* – about an Irish porter who forgot when sober what he had done when drunk but when drunk remembered his former actions – as a crucial plot device in *The Moonstone* in 1868.[22] The porter, in Elliotson's anecdote, lost a parcel when he was drunk but the next time he became intoxicated remembered where he had left it. In *The Moonstone*, when the unwitting thief is induced to take opium a second time he retraces his steps to reveal the fate of the lost diamond. But Dickens, characteristically, had most fun with depicting mesmerism.

In 1848 Dickens revived an eighteenth-century play entitled *Animal Magnetism*, written at the height of public fascination with Mesmer, and staged several amateur productions with himself in the role of the mesmerist.[23] Nine years later he collaborated with Collins on writing a play, *The Frozen Deep*, which was inspired by the efforts of mesmeric clairvoyants to trace the lost Arctic explorer John Franklin in the 1840s.[24] The play was staged in January 1857, with Dickens in the starring role, and was reprised at a special performance for Queen Victoria that summer. It was at a later showing in Manchester that Dickens became besotted with Nelly Ternan.

Elliotson was feted by American writers too. When Nathaniel Hawthorne visited London in 1856 he was eager to meet the famous British mesmerist. Hawthorne's 1851 novel, *The House of the Seven Gables*, had entwined tales of witchcraft and ghosts with the sinister story of a man who used hypnotism to drive a young woman to her death. Hawthorne described Elliotson in suitably gothic style as a 'dark, sombre, taciturn, powerful-looking man, with coal-black hair, and a beard as black, fringing around his face'.[25]

At the same time, Elliotson was fully reinstated in fashionable London society, resuming his place as a guest at soirees and conversaziones in the city's plushest drawing rooms, and tending the nobility and gentry in their well-appointed sickrooms. According to the *Morning Post*, his practice was now even larger than before his resignation from UCL.[26] For all his banishment from teaching, *Human Physiology* remained the standard textbook in medical schools. And despite some sniffs from the medical establishment he frequently attended consultations in conjunction with prominent medical figures.

Elliotson's passion for mesmerism was now treated with fond affection as often as with sneering derision. In 1856 Elliotson gave evidence in a trial over the death of a sixty-eight-year-old mentally ill man, Daniel Dolley, in Wandsworth Asylum. Elliotson blamed the man's death on the medical superintendent who had forced him to stand under a cold shower for twenty-eight minutes; having tried the shower himself, Elliotson testified he could only withstand eight minutes.[27] The defendant's lawyer raised a laugh when he quipped: 'It was not so agreeable as Mesmerism.' Elliotson smartly put him down by responding: 'I should like you to try the difference.'

Even if his wit was as quick as ever and his physical stamina remained undiminished, Elliotson was slowing down. By 1856, at the age of sixty-five, he had effectively retired from medical practice and the same year he published the final issue of the *Zoist*. After thirteen years of 'amassing facts so they are no longer questioned except by the most ignorant', he had achieved his object, he proclaimed in the last edition.[28] The LMI continued for the time being without his active input. Now a grand old man of medicine as much as mesmerism, Elliotson even attended the annual dinner of UCL medical school in 1863, twenty-five years after his resignation, along with his erstwhile enemy William Sharpey. His old foe, Liston, had died from an aneurysm in December 1847. Since the event was held in a concert hall near Regent Street, he did not have to break his vow never to set foot in the university again. Reporting the evening, *The Lancet* wistfully remarked: 'The most remarkable circumstance of the meeting was the presence again of Dr Elliotson among his old pupils and colleagues.'[29] Sadly, even though he was now rehabilitated in the pages of *The Lancet*, Elliotson was never reconciled with his old friend Wakley.

Having worked a sixteen-hour day for most of his life, in 1851 Wakley had collapsed.[30] He was found unconscious at midnight outside the doors of *The Lancet*, after a day spent presiding over seven inquests and attending Parliament. Reluctantly he reduced his workload. The following year he gave up his parliamentary seat and began to hand over the reins of *The Lancet* to his eldest and youngest sons, Thomas and James, though he continued his role as a coroner; his middle son, Henry, now a barrister, deputised for him at inquests.

The younger generation introduced a gentler, less combative style of journalism to *The Lancet* and the magazine would continue as a family business into the twentieth century. In 1857 Wakley was bereft when his wife, Elizabeth, died after a long illness. Three years later, the telltale signs of consumption appeared and Wakley sailed for Madeira in the hope that warmer climes would help. Though he rallied briefly, on 11

May 1862 he slipped while disembarking from a boat and five days later he died, aged sixty-six. His body was shipped home for burial in Kensal Green Cemetery.

From relatively humble beginnings, Wakley had made an unprecedented contribution to Victorian public life. He had tirelessly championed medical reform, culminating in the Medical Act of 1858, which regulated the medical profession for the first time. He had helped bring about major social change and brought rigorous scrutiny to inquests. He had transformed medical journalism and campaigned doggedly against quackery. Even though the targets of his mission were sometimes misplaced – as with mesmerism – he unfailingly fought for a robust approach to research that would eventually bear fruit. *The Lancet* has continued to be one of the most important scientific journals in the world, to this day maintaining the fierce spirit of independence and integrity that Wakley had engendered when he watched the first edition emerge from the press in that tiny office in The Strand in 1823.

Despite their climactic break over the Okey sisters in 1838, Wakley and Elliotson had travelled along parallel lines for the remainder of their lives. In *The Lancet* and in parliament, Wakley had exposed the scandals of the workhouses, fought for workers' rights, condemned army flogging and battled against food adulteration. In the *Zoist*, interspersed with his articles on mesmerism, Elliotson had railed against capital punishment, damned treatment of the mentally ill and called for a national education system. Yet Elliotson later denied that he and Wakley had ever been friends and dismissed their relationship as merely a 'speaking acquaintance'.[31] Taking issue with the *Medical Times* for describing them as 'chums', he said he had 'never tasted food or drink with him under the same roof all my life' because 'my taste did not and could not allow of any further acquaintance with him'. Condemning Wakley's denouncement of the Okey girls, Elliotson declared 'the character of the Okeys stands far above yours'.

Elliotson's health was now failing too, as were his powers of judgement. While staying in Dieppe in 1863, Elliotson, now seventy-two, met the celebrated medium Daniel Dunglas Home.[32] Born in Scotland, Home had spent his early life in the United States, where he had embraced spiritualism and become one of its most adept performers. Travelling Europe from the 1850s onwards, the charismatic Home was feted by intellectuals and royalty who were rapt by his displays of clairvoyance and messages relayed from the spirit world. Observers testified that Home could levitate to the ceiling, float in and out of first-floor windows and elongate his body by as much as eleven inches. Dickens, who described Home as having long, yellow hair and 'large, glittering, and sharp teeth', was adamant the Scot was an imposter and Elliotson had long shared the same opinion. At the chance meeting in Dieppe, Home challenged Elliotson to attend a séance that same evening. Elliotson was instantly converted. Smitten by Home and his flamboyant brand of spiritualism, in 1867 Elliotson helped found a society, the Spiritual Athenaeum, to promote spiritualism and provide a base, in Sloane Street, for séances. Elliotson not only embraced spiritualism but, having been a religious sceptic if not an outright atheist all his adult life, he now became devoutly Christian. It was rather late in the day for such a conversion.

Two years earlier Elliotson had lost most of his wealth in a reckless speculation. He gave up his house in Conduit Street and moved into the home of his life-long friend Symes and his family in Hill Street, Mayfair.[33] Now a widower, his wife having died ten years earlier, sixty-year-old Symes had three sons and two daughters aged ten to nineteen. Three photographs of Elliotson taken at about this time show a grizzled face still framed by a dense black beard.[34] Though his curling black hair had receded, his dark brown eyes were as penetrating as ever. The pictures were probably taken for the LMI; in 1864 he apologised to a friend for being unable to supply him with one but directed him to the hospital. His faculties were fading fast. It is likely he suffered from a stroke or dementia in the late 1860s. According to *The Times*, his last years were 'more or less a blank' when he was 'carefully watched over' by Symes. In April 1868 *The Times* even published a premature obituary which Symes hastily contradicted in *The Lancet*, saying: 'I have no idea how such a report could have arisen, as he is no worse than he has been for months past.'[35] According to the *Morning Post*, correcting its own report of Elliotson's death, the doctor 'continues to be very feeble, both physically and mentally'.

Elliotson survived three more months before he died at Symes's house on 29 July 1868 at the age of seventy-seven. Having never proved personally susceptible to mesmerism in life, he now slipped into the 'sweetest sleep'. He left no will; he had nothing left to leave. He was buried in

Kensal Green Cemetery, not far from his one-time friend and long-time enemy Wakley. There were no descendants. His younger brother, Thomas, had predeceased him in Malta, aged only fifty, in 1850; his un-married sisters, Emma and Eliza, had lived together in Clapham until Emma's death in 1865. When Eliza, the last member of the family, died in 1885, the instructions in her will were solemnly performed: the keys to the family vault were thrown through the hole in the door.[36]

John Elliotson had been born into the Georgian world at the end of the eighteenth century and he died a celebrated figure of Victorian society in the second half of the nineteenth. One of the brightest medical minds of his generation, he had introduced the stethoscope into general use, popularised quinine and divined the cause of hay fever. One of the great-est medical teachers of his time, he had transformed medical education, produced the standard medical textbook of the era and had helped found University College Hospital. At the height of his career he was one of the most popular and highest-earning doctors of the Victorian age. Yet he forfeited his professional reputation and academic career in the cause of mesmerism. As Bulwer-Lytton put it: 'No man has sacrificed more for the cause of mesmerism than Dr Elliotson.'[37] *The Times*, in its prema-ture obituary, described him as 'one of the most distinguished scientific men of the age' while the *Morning Post* said he was 'held in the greatest esteem for the daring and successful character of his innovations' but was 'persecuted' by his brethren for his 'bold utterance of the truth'.[38] And *The Lancet*, which had devoted its columns to reviling him for thirty years, now said he was 'unrivalled' as a clinical teacher and 'gifted with singular powers of observation' yet maintained to the last that he had been tricked into espousing mesmerism by the 'consummate actor' Elizabeth Okey and her sister Jane. Most remarkably, *The Lancet* added that if Elliotson made enemies 'he had the happy power of conciliating and making friends', even though he had never been reconciled with the journal's late editor.

Elliotson never expressed a single regret over the path he had chosen. Looking back on his decision in later life, he acknowledged that his refusal to reject mesmerism had almost ruined his professional career, diminished his wealth and wrecked many friendships. Yet his faith in the idea had brought him deeper friendships and introduced him to sincere and pure-minded people among the poor patients he treated. 'I would cheerfully bear double what I have borne from my profession and others,' he wrote, 'rather than lose the elevated happiness which I thus owe daily to mesmerism.'[39]

Having lost its foremost champion, mesmerism faded from the British consciousness. A year after Elliotson's death, the London Mesmeric Infirmary closed its doors. But mesmerism was only sleeping. Before long it would reawaken under a new guise – as hypnotism and hypnotherapy.

Influenced by James Braid's work, physicians in Paris began to explore the mind using hypnotism.[40] Their leader was Jean-Martin Charcot, chief physician at the Salpêtrière asylum for women, who used hypnosis extensively to experiment on female patients in the 1880s. Staging dramatic exhibitions attended by large crowds, Charcot sought to demonstrate that the hypnotic state was a form of hysteria almost exclusive to women. Opponents asserted that he was being duped by some of his patients, echoing the charges aimed at Elliotson. By contrast, physicians in Nancy led by Hippolyte Bernheim adopted a gentler approach. They investigated the therapeutic and anaesthetic effects of hypnosis, mainly on male patients, and argued – correctly – that the hypnotic state could be invoked in most people. Both centres attracted visitors from across Europe, including Sigmund Freud, who adopted hypnosis as a tool in his early work.

In Britain the medical press reported Charcot's exotic demonstrations with due fascination while several British doctors were drawn to the Nancy school. With hypnotism finally being investigated seriously by the scientific community, the first International Congress of Hypnotism was held in Paris in 1889. As hypnotism gained impetus, an investigation by the British Medical Association in 1893 concluded that hypnosis was effective in relieving pain and alleviating numerous ailments but argued that its practice should be restricted to doctors.[41]

After this brief heyday, hypnotism languished during the first half of the twentieth century as mainstream medicine advanced in leaps and bounds. Interest in hypnotism resurfaced in the 1950s, however, both in the laboratory and the consulting room. During World War II a handful of dentists and surgeons in the British army had become intrigued by the spectacle of stage hypnotists entertaining the troops.[42] They learned the technique for themselves and after the war some introduced hypnotism into civilian practice. As interest grew, in 1955 the BMA launched another inquiry into hypnotism, which concluded that hypnosis was a useful anaesthetic for surgery, dentistry and childbirth and should be incorporated into medical training – an idea that was stoutly ignored. The following year doctors joined with dentists to form the Medical Society for the Study of Hypnosis which would later merge with other groups to become today's British Society of Clinical and Academic Hypnosis. In 1978, the Royal Society of Medicine, successor to the Royal Medical and Chirurgical Society once led by John Elliotson, set up a section on medical and dental hypnosis that thrives to this day.

Meanwhile research led by America from the 1950s onwards focused on trying to explain the hypnotic process.[43] Investigators divided into two distinct camps: one side argued that hypnotism induces a special and unique 'state' in which subjects perform involuntary acts beyond their normal waking powers, while others – the 'non-statists' – maintained that subjects were simply responding to expectations and retained conscious control, at some level, over their behaviour. Although the two camps have converged in recent years, differing explanations persist. Since the 1980s, brain-imaging scans have shown that unique brain activity occurs under hypnosis, yet the debate about the existence or non-existence of a 'trance' continues. Researchers at Stanford University in the US developed tests to gauge individual responses to hypnosis, now known as the Stanford Scales of Hypnotic Susceptibility. These, and subsequent versions, suggest that at least ninety per cent of us are susceptible to hypnosis, with one in five people being highly susceptible.

Despite this resurgence of interest, hypnosis remained on the fringes of medicine throughout the twentieth century as the growing evidence of its therapeutic benefits was overshadowed by the absurdity of stage hypnotists provoking people to eat onions or remove their clothes. In 1952 a Hypnotism Act was introduced in the UK to regulate public exhibitions after an American hypnotist performing in Britain was sued by a woman claiming she had suffered mental derangement after attending a show. Even now hypnotism is disdained by many in the medical profession through its association with stage hypnosis.

Today, understanding of precisely how hypnosis acts on the human mind remains tantalisingly elusive while its potential for medicine is still largely untapped. Thousands of hypnotherapists currently offer treatment in the UK for a range of problems, and a few are even contracted by the NHS. In 2005 University College London Hospital, which includes the former UCH, became the first NHS trust to develop a hypnotherapy service.[44] The therapeutic benefits of clinical hypnosis are now broadly accepted within mainstream psychology. Yet hypnotherapy remains unregulated so that practitioners may be highly skilled and experienced – many are qualified doctors or psychotherapists – or completely untrained, and potentially dangerous.

Since the 1980s a growing number of studies have found that hypnosis is effective in treating a wide range of medical conditions including obesity, smoking cessation, anxiety, post-traumatic stress, asthma and irritable bowel syndrome.[45] At the same time, studies have shown hypnosis is highly effective in relieving pain from headaches, labour, burns and cancer as well as during dental treatment and surgery. One large review found that clinical hypnosis provides substantial pain relief for as many as seventy-five per cent of people. Yet despite the growing evidence, hypnotherapy remains widely undervalued by the medical profession.

At the same time, the idea of undergoing surgery with only hypnosis to control the pain remains as controversial as ever. Interest in using hypnosis as a form of anaesthetic was revived in the 1950s but research is still hampered by problems in conducting the experiments. It is impossible to perform 'blind' trials since both hypnotist and patient are inevitably aware of the intervention and it is ethically problematic to recruit patients to undergo surgery using only hypnosis. Recent studies, however, have shown that hypnosis significantly reduces pain levels in volunteers, while brain imaging scans have revealed that hypnosis produces alterations in parts of the brain involved in pain perception.[46] Research is now centred on using hypnosis in combination with chemical anaesthesia – an approach known as 'hypnoanaesthesia'.

Several trials have demonstrated that hypnotising patients prior to them being anaesthetised for surgery leads to reduced anxiety and nausea, less pain, shorter hospital stays and better surgical recovery with fewer complications.[47] Particularly promising results have emerged from using hypnosis combined with conscious sedation. In Belgium surgeons have performed more than 9,000 procedures using hypnosis in conjunction with local anaesthesia and a mild sedative. Their results show that patients undergoing hypnosis suffer less pain, nausea, fatigue and anxiety, need fewer drugs, suffer milder complications and return to work up to two weeks earlier.[48] Some anaesthetists are now arguing that combined hypnosis and anaesthesia should become routine. Others have gone even further.

In the past decade a small but significant number of people have undergone major operations without general anaesthetic after being hypnotised or using self-hypnosis. A thirty-six-year-old man from Kent had a hernia repaired in 2006 after being hypnotised. Two years later a sixty-seven-year-old woman in Peterborough underwent keyhole surgery on her knee using self-hypnosis. One man from Surrey has undergone six operations, including an ankle joint replacement, after being hypnotised. And in Paris in 2014 a singer had a tumour removed from a throat gland while under hypnosis; she sang throughout her operation.

Despite the advances, the power of the human mind to heal the body and conquer pain is scarcely better understood than it was when Franz Mesmer first toured Europe more than two centuries ago. Medical reactions today are almost as sceptical as when John Elliotson exhibited the marvels of mesmerism to astonished audiences at UCH. And the idea of undergoing surgery with only hypnotism to dull the pain remains for most of us as terrifying and shocking as it was when James Wombell had his leg amputated in 1842.

For all the progress, mainstream medicine and hypnosis remain almost as far apart as ever – a direct legacy of the two men who adopted such entrenched positions in the early Victorian era. John Elliotson and Thomas Wakley were both brilliant, clever, compassionate men who wanted to push forward the boundaries of medicine. Together they promoted vital scientific advances; shoulder to shoulder they worked to reform the antiquated medical institutions and overhaul medical education. Yet because they were both implacably single-minded, stubborn and vain, they collided over one crucial debate: mesmerism. Both of them were right. Elliotson was correct in his belief that mesmerism – hypnotism – could alleviate distressing medical conditions and banish pain. Wakley was justified in demanding scientific proof and rejecting the ludicrous claims over mesmerised water and clairvoyance. Elliotson was too proud to listen to reasoned objections, too credulous not to realise when he was being duped. Bewitched by the Okey sisters he ignored sound scientific methods and abandoned all semblance of scientific integrity. Wakley sealed his former friend's fate, but he too was remiss – in blindly insisting that all mesmerism was false in the face of clear evidence of its success. Motivated by his mission to safeguard the medical profession at all costs, Wakley ensured mesmerism was banished to the medical fringe. If nothing else their story should remind us all of the value of open debate over closed minds, of the need for a sound scientific approach over superstition and credulity. All in all, the journalist James Fernandez Clarke was right when he said there has been 'no chapter in the history of Medicine more astounding and bewildering'. For the marvels of mesmerism remain as alluring as ever.

ACKNOWLEDGEMENTS

As with all my books, writing *The Mesmerist* has only been possible through the generous help and support of many individuals and organisations. In particular I wish to pay tribute again to the librarians and archivists who zealously safeguard our national history against a background of steadily encroaching cutbacks. I am especially grateful to the Wellcome Trust for a Medical Humanities Research grant [no 108790/Z/15/Z] to help with research expenses. One of the pleasures of writing this book has been the excuse to spend many months immersed in the Wellcome Library – always a favourite place to be – and I would like to thank all staff there for their courteous and friendly help as ever. Likewise I have enjoyed many enlightening months at the British Library and would like to thank all staff there, especially in the Rare Books and Music Room, for their unstinting help.

My thanks are due to numerous archives and libraries for permission to view and quote from documents. I am grateful to UCL Library Services, Special Collections, especially to Mandy Wise for her tireless efforts in organising material for my viewing. My thanks too to the Royal Society of Medicine library and archives, especially to Robert Greenwood for his help and enlivening conversations. I am grateful to staff at King's College London and London Metropolitan Archives for help in viewing their respective St Thomas' Hospital archives. The quotations from Henry Crabb Robinson's diary are given by kind permission of the Trustees of Dr Williams's Library, London, and my thanks are due to director David Wykes for his patient help. My thanks to the National Library of Scotland for permission to quote from the Combe correspondence and especially to Tom Holland. I am grateful to Wisbech and Fenland Museum for permission to quote from the Townshend Manuscript Collection. I wish to thank staff at the archives of the Royal College of Physicians, especially archive manager Pamela Forde.

I am grateful to Eleanor Gawne, librarian at the Architectural Association School of Architecture, for allowing me to view Thomas Wakley's former house in Bedford Square, now part of the association's headquarters. I would also like to thank staff at the Dana Research Centre and Library of the Science Museum, London; the Cadbury Research Library, Special Collections, of the University of Birmingham; Edinburgh University Library Special Collections; the Medical Society of London archives; The National Archives (TNA); Westminster City Archives; Southwark Local History Library and Archive; and Hertfordshire Archives Centre. Reference to the Purland Album, in the Theodosius Purland Collection of Materials on Mesmerism, is made courtesy of the National Library of Medicine, Maryland, in the US. Additionally I wish to thank staff of the New York Public Library, Astor, Lenox and Tilden Foundations, for permission to quote from the Carl H. Pforzheimer Collection of Shelley and his Circle; and the Huntington Library, San Marino, California, for permission to quote from the Huntington Manuscripts.

Many individual people have generously helped me in researching the story of John Elliotson and the Okey sisters. First and foremost I wish to thank the various members of the Royal Society of Medicine's Hypnosis and Psychosomatic Medicine Section who gave me their advice and support. In particular I want to thank former president Dr Rumi Peynovska who not only provided generous help but gave me my first experience of hypnosis – to remarkable effect – and president-elect Dr Raj Sharma, head of the hypnosis and cognitive therapy unit at UCLH NHS Foundation Trust, for his enthusiasm and advice. I am grateful to Dr Sofia Eriksson, consultant neurologist in the Department of Clinical and Experimental Epilepsy of the National Hospital for Neurology and Neurosurgery at UCLH, for her advice on epilepsy. My thanks to hypnotherapist Chris Gillies for his discussions on hypnosis. Dr Nicholas Cambridge gave his timely advice, as ever, on myriad medical matters as well as insights on experiments on electricity and Charles Dickens. Evan Stone QC also kindly gave advice on Elliotson's relationship with Dickens. Jacky Worthington proved invaluable as usual for her genealogical detective work in helping me track down the ancestry of the Okey family. John Ford answered my obscure queries about pharmacy with his characteristic speed and enthusiasm. Lucy Inglis gave me useful advice on opium – for research purposes of course. My thanks too to

Danny Rees, Simon Chaplin and Sandra Hempel for general support and encouragement.

As always I have felt blessed to enjoy the guidance and friendship of my twin pillars of support in publishing – my agent Patrick Walsh of PEW Literary Agency and my editor Kirsty Dunseath at Weidenfeld and Nicolson. Patrick gave his unstinting time and impeccable advice as ever in helping me to develop and shape my ideas. Kirsty provided her spot-on guidance as usual to help me prune, polish and improve my book in the kindest possible way while enabling me to keep it quintessentially my own work. My thanks also to Jennifer Kerslake for her help in picture research and editing. Finally I want to thank family and friends who have patiently encouraged or endured my mesmerism mania and most especially Peter, Sam and Susie for their unfailing support.

PICTURE ACKNOWLEDGEMENTS

1. Title page of 'A full discovery of the strange practices of Dr Elliotson on the bodies of his female patients!' London, 1842. (Wellcome Library, London)
2. John Elliotson by James Ramsay, c. 1837 (Royal College of Physicians); Thomas Wakley by W. H. Egleton after K. Meadows (Wellcome Library, London)
3. Baron Jules Dupotet by unknown artist from Dupotet, *La magie dévoilée* (Paris, 1852); Robert Liston by Charles Turner, 1840 (Wellcome Library, London); Charles Dickens by Margaret Gillies, exhibited 1844 (Charles Dickens Museum); William Makepeace Thackeray by Samuel Laurence, c. 1864 (Bridgeman Images); Elizabeth Okey by unknown artist (*The Lancet*, 1838)
4. Mesmer's Tub. Wood engraving by Henri Thiriat, 19th century (Wellcome Library, London); The cataleptic state by D. Younger, 1887 (Wellcome Library, London)
5. John Elliotson mesmerising a woman (*Punch*, 1843); A Mesmerist using Animal Magnetism on a female patient. Wood engraving by unknown artist, c. 1845. (Wellcome Library, London)
6. Operation on Madame Plantin from Louis Figuier, *Les Mystères de la Science* (Paris, c. 1880); Doctor and Mrs Syntax, with a party of friends, experimenting with laughing gas. Coloured aquatint by William Combe after Thomas Rowlandson. (Wellcome Library, London)
7. Robert Liston operating. Oil by Ernest Board c. 1912 (Wellcome Library, London); Sir James Young Simpson and friends drink liquid chloroform in an experiment. Pen and ink, c. 1840s. (Wellcome Library, London)

8. Old University College Hospital, photograph 1911 (Wellcome Library, London); Ground plan of UCH (UCL Archives); John Elliotson, photograph c. 1860s (Science Museum/Science and Society Picture Library)

NOTES

ABBREVIATIONS

GC – George Combe
CD – Charles Dickens
JE – John Elliotson
KCL – King's College London
RL – Robert Liston
LMA – London Metropolitan Archives
LMG – London Medical Gazette
NLM – National Library of Medicine, Maryland, US
NLS – National Library of Scotland
NYPL – New York Public Library
ODNB – Oxford Dictionary of National Biography
RCP – Royal College of Physicians
RSM – Royal Society of Medicine (formerly Medical and Chirurgical Society, then Royal Medical and Chirurgical Society)
UCH – University College Hospital
UCL – University College London
WL – Wellcome Library, London

CHAPTER 1: YOU'RE A FOOL, DR ELLISSON. HA! HA!

[1] Details of the demonstration on 10 May 1838 are from *The Lancet*, 26 May 1838, pp. 282–8 and *Morning Post*, 11 May 1838, unless otherwise stated. Elizabeth's appearance is described in *The Lancet*, 9 Sep 1837 and 26 May 1838, pp. 836–40 and 282–8. No women are mentioned in any of the reports and it is fair to assume the audience was entirely or almost entirely male. When the scientist Mary Somerville watched a different demonstration this was worthy of special mention: *LMG*, 26 May 1838, p. 392. The weather is reported in *Athenaeum*, 1838, p. 410. Although some writers have suggested this demonstration took place in the operating theatre, the *Morning Post* refers to the hospital 'lecture-room'.

[2] A building report describes the anatomy theatre as having seats for 250 people but adds that it often accommodates 350 students sitting on the steps or standing: UCL Council Minutes, vol. 3 (1835–43), 17 Jun 1837, UCL archives.

[3] *Athenaeum*, 21 Jul 1838, p. 515.

[4] Both visited on 29 Mar 1838: *Morning Post*, 3 Apr 1838; *The Lancet*, 26 May 1838, p. 320.

[5] Dickens and Cruikshank visited the wards on 4 Jan 1838 according to JE's case-books, UCL, UCH/MR/1/9. Dickens attended a later public demonstration, on 2 June, and may also have been at the 10 May exhibition.

[6] Biographical details about Elliotson are from 'Memoir of Dr Elliotson', *The Lancet*, 8 Jun 1833, pp. 341–4; obituary *The Lancet*, 8 Aug 1868, pp. 203–4; obituary (premature) *The Times*, 14 Apr 1868.

[7] On his appointment to University of London: *The Lancet*, 14 May 1831, pp. 209–10.

[8] *The Lancet*, 26 May 1838, pp. 282–8.

[9] Herbert Mayo, Professor of Physiology and Pathological Anatomy at King's College, suggested this term: *LMG*, 21 Apr 1838.

[10] Elizabeth Okey was born 9 Dec 1820 and baptised 16 Jan 1821 at St Pancras Church, London.

[11] *Freeman's Journal* (Dublin), 21 Apr 1838; *Belfast News-Letter*, 24 Apr 1838.

[12] For a full and fascinating analysis of the theatrical nature of Elizabeth Okey's performances see Lehman. Winter also discusses Elizabeth's acts in the context of Victorian theatre: Winter, pp. 81–93.

[13] Anglesey, 'Paget, Henry William, first marquess of Anglesey (1768–1854)', *ODNB*, online edn, accessed 15 May 2015.

[14] See for example http://news.bbc.co.uk/1/hi/magazine/8135928.stm, accessed 2 Aug 2016.

[15] *Monthly Chronicle*, vol. 2 (1838), p. 19.

[16] Phyllis Hartnoll (ed.), *Oxford Companion to the Theatre* (London, 3rd ed, 1967), p. 799.

[17] *Morning Post*, 27 Sep 1836.

[18] *Morning Post*, 11 May 1838.

[19] *The Lancet*, 26 May 1838, pp. 282–8.

CHAPTER 2: THE SIGN OF THE GOLDEN KEY

[1] Guy's and St Thomas' Pupils and Dressers register 1755–1823, KCL archives G/FP1/1, p. 172; General entry Guy's 1805–13, KCL archives G/FP2/1.

[2] St Saviour baptisms, marriages and burials 1538–1812. He was baptised on 20 Nov 1791 in St Saviour's Church, now Southwark Cathedral.

[3] John's grandfather, Thomas Elliotson, had a shop at the same address from at least 1777 according to trade directories and fire insurance registers. The shops are detailed in *Johnstone's London Commercial Guide* (London, 1817), pp. 55–8. The sign of the golden key is mentioned in John Timbs, *Curiosities of London* (London, 1868), p. 742.

[4] South, p. 1. Background on chemists and druggists is from Irvine Loudon, 'The vile race of quacks with which this country is infested,' in Bynum and Porter (1987), pp. 106–28; Leslie Matthews, *History of Pharmacy in Britain* (London,

1962); and Jane Eastoe, *Victorian Pharmacy: Rediscovering Forgotten Remedies and Recipes* (London, 2010).

5 Classified advertisements in the *Telegraph*, 31 Dec 1796 and *Morning Post*, 19 Sep 1800, mentioning Elliotson's business.

6 M. Dorothy George, *London Life in the Eighteenth Century* (Harmondsworth, 1976), p. 399.

7 The dates of the surviving siblings are: Thomas, born 17 May 1800; Emma, born 3 Aug 1802; and Eliza born 21 Dec 1808: St Saviour baptisms, marriages and burials 1538–1812.

8 Background on Southwark is from Richard Tames, *Southwark Past* (Andover, 2001); R. M. Wingent, *Historical Notes on the Borough and the Borough Hospitals* (London, 1913); Peter Ackroyd, *London: The Biography* (London, 2000), pp. 689–97; Leonard Reilly, *Southwark: An Illustrated History* (London, 1998).

9 Clarke (1874), p. 179.

10 Anon (1839), vol. 1, pp. 273–85. Although the entry is headed 'Dr Thomas Elliotson' the details make clear it is John. Munk's Roll, RCP, pp. 258–62.

11 University of Edinburgh matriculation albums [1762–1826], Edinburgh University Library Special Collections. Elliotson enrolled in 1805 and returned in 1808 and 1809. Information on Edinburgh University and its medical school is from Lisa Rosner, *Medical Education in the Age of Improvement: Edinburgh Students and Apprentices, 1760–1826* (Edinburgh, 1991); Alastair Hugh Bailey Masson, 'The Edinburgh medical school', in *History of Medicine*, 4, no. 4 (1972–3), pp. 3–7; and John D. Comrie, *History of Scottish Medicine to 1860* (London, 1927).

12 Evidence of JE, *Report from the Select Committee on Medical Education* (London, 1834), part 1, pp. 104–117.

13 Historical information on Guy's and St Thomas' is from Ford; Eilidh Margaret McInnes, *St Thomas' Hospital* (London, 1963); Charles Graves, *The Story of St Thomas's*, 1106–1947 (London, 1947).

14 George Eliot, *Middlemarch* (Harmondsworth, 1965), p. 119. The novel was first published in 1871 but set in 1829.

15 South, p. 27. Background on medical education at Guy's and St Thomas' is from South; Ford; and Hale-White.

16 Newman, pp. 27–8; Nicolson.

17 'Dr Elliotson's clinical lectures' in *LMG*, 9 Oct 1830, pp. 33–7.

18 South, p. 27.

19 South, p. 36; Hampton Weekes to Richard Weekes, 8 Oct 1801, in Ford, p. 49.

20 South, p. 74. Biographical information on Cooper is from Blake Cooper; Druin Burch, *Digging up the Dead* (London, 2007); and South. Information on Cline is from South, pp. 34 and 48. Information on Lucas is from Hale-White, pp. 17–8; South, p. 52.

21 South, pp. 58–60; Blake Cooper, pp. 309–12.

22 South, pp. 28–30.

23 Information on body-snatching is from South, pp. 90–101; Clarke (1874), pp. 104–6.

[24] JE, 'On the Medicinal Properties of Creosote', *Medico-Chirurgical Transactions*, 19 (1835), p. 217.

[25] Anon (1839), vol. 1, pp. 273–85.

[26] Anon (1839), vol. 1, pp. 273–85.

[27] JE signed up for a second year on 23 Jun 1807: General entry Guy's 1805–13, KCL archives G/FP2/1. He returned to Edinburgh in 1808 and obtained his MD in 1810: University of Edinburgh matriculation albums [1762–1826], Edinburgh University Library Special Collections; Anon, *List of the graduates in medicine in the University of Edinburgh, from MDCCV to MDCCCLXVI* (1867), p. 42. James Gray, *History of the Royal Medical Society 1737–1937* (1952), p. 318.

[28] JE was admitted a licentiate in 1810 and became a fellow in 1822: Munk's Roll, RCP.

[29] JE was admitted a fellow-commoner to Jesus College on 10 Oct 1810: Cambridge alumni database http://venn.lib.cam.ac.uk/acad/2016/search-2016.html, accessed 22 May 2014. He attained his bachelor of medicine in 1816 and doctorate in 1821: Munk's Roll, RCP.

[30] JE to George Combe, 11 April 1822, MS 7208 and 1 Nov 1824, MS 7213: Combe correspondence, NLS.

[31] *Report from the Select Committee on Medical Education* (London, 1834), part 1, pp. 104–117.

[32] JE (1835–40), p. 402.

[33] Newman, pp. 47-8; Susan C. Lawrence, 'Medical education' in Bynum and Porter (1993), vol. 2, pp. 1151–79; Nicolson.

[34] JE told the select committee he had visited medical schools in Germany and Italy: *Report from the Select Committee on Medical Education* (London, 1834), part 1, pp. 104–17. He referred to visiting Switzerland, Spain and France in his lectures at St Thomas': Notes of Lectures on the Theory and Practice of Medicine by John Elliotson MD FRS given at St Thomas' Hospital, KCL archives TH/PP23, vol. 9, p. 197 and vol. 12, p. 113.

[35] The first edition (1815) contains 260 pages including 20 pages of Elliotson's notes. The second, in 1817, contains 150 pages of notes. It was described as a 'typographical curiosity' in the *Morning Chronicle*, 3 Feb 1817. The third, 1820, added 200 pages of notes. The fourth, 1824, added 350 pages of notes which therefore exceeded the original text. The fifth (1835–40) was published as *Human Physiology*. The quotations are from the 2nd edition, pp. 401–2, 417–8 and 403–5.

[36] JE to Combe, 11 Jan 1823, MS 7210 and 11 Dec 1822, MS 7208, Combe correspondence, NLS.

[37] Preface to the 2nd edition of his Blumenbach translation dated Dec 1816: JE (1817). JE to Mr Battley (druggist), 20 May 1822 and JE to William Nunn (surgeon), 29 May 1829, RCP archives ALS/E17 and 19.

[38] *The Lancet*, 8 Jun 1833, pp. 341–4. JE's father had a house in Clapham High Street. JE said he lived there during the summer in a letter to Combe, 11 Apr 1822, MS 7207, Combe correspondence, NLS.

[39] His friends included Thomas Barrett-Lennard, radical MP for Ipswich, and

William Rookes Crompton (later William Rookes Crompton Stansfield), heir to an estate in Yorkshire, both Cambridge contemporaries. They are mentioned in letters to Combe, Combe correspondence, NLS. His lectures on forensic medicine were dedicated to Barrett-Lennard.

[40] JE was proposed on 21 Jan 1812 by Curry, Alexander Marcet, Dr Laird (all at Guy's) and Dr Bree, who was MCS vice-president at the time: Minutes of the MCS 1805–17, MCS/B1, p. 386, RSM archives. Background on the history of the Royal Medical and Chirurgical Society (Royal Society of Medicine) is from Hunting.

[41] Lawrence, pp. 57–8.

[42] JE was beaten by Robert Williams by 22 votes to 49 in a ballot on 4 Sep 1816. He beat William King by 63 votes to 30 on 10 Oct 1817. General Court of Governors minute book, St Thomas' Hospital, 1784–1849, LMA H01/ST, pp. 214 and 224. *The Lancet* reported that JE won the post 'through the interest of his friends' and his father's influence with the governors: *The Lancet*, 8 Jun 1833, pp. 341–4.

[43] Prout, *Chemistry, Meteorology and the Functions of Digestion* (London, 1834), p. 100. W. H. Brock, 'The Life and Work of William Prout' in *Medical History*, 9, no. 2 (1965), pp. 101–26. Iodine deficiency is still the commonest cause of goitre worldwide although the widespread use of iodised salt means the condition is relatively rare in the developed world.

[44] Grand Committee minute book, St Thomas' Hospital, 1811–27, LMA H01/ST, 7 Jun 1820; JE's request was discussed on 10 Oct 1821. The argument is described in *The Lancet*, 8 Jun 1833, pp. 341–4.

[45] JE to Combe, 11 Jan 1823, MS 7210, Combe correspondence, NLS.

[46] Background on Edward Grainger is from South, pp. 106–112.

[47] JE (1821). The remainder of the course was not published.

[48] Sandra Hempel, *The Inheritor's Powder: A Cautionary Tale of Poison, Betrayal and Greed* (London, 2013), pp. 130–4.

[49] JE to Combe, 10 Oct 1822, MS 7208, Combe correspondence, NLS; Notes of Lectures on the Theory and Practice of Medicine by John Elliotson MD FRS given at St Thomas' Hospital, KCL archives TH/PP23, vol. 17, p. 182.

[50] JE's evidence to the Select Committee, *Report from the Select Committee on Medical Education* (London, 1834), part 1, pp. 104–17. Details of JE's appointment are from General Court of Governors minute book, St Thomas' Hospital, 1784–1849, LMA H01/ST, 22 Jan 1823.

[51] *The Lancet*, 8 Jun 1833, pp. 341–4; David Davis to UCL Council (recommending JE for his post at UCL), 9 May 1831, UCL correspondence 2105; anonymous comment in letter from Eliza Wallace (mesmerist) in Purland Album, vol. 4, NLM.

[52] The *DNB* says he adopted trousers in 1826: Stephen and Lee, vol. 17, p. 264–6. JE (1835–40), p. 703.

[53] Lawrence, pp. 13–5; Nicolson; Stanley Joel Reiser, 'The science of diagnosis: diagnostic technique,' in Bynum and Porter (1993), vol. 2, pp. 826–51 and 'Aspects of role of the stethoscope in the introduction of auscultation to Great Britain and the United States' in *Proceedings of the XXIII International Congress of the History*

of Medicine (London, 1972), pp. 832–40; P J Bishop, 'Reception of the stethoscope and Laennec's book' in *Thorax*, 36 (1981) pp. 487–92.

54 Hunting, p. 80.

55 *The Lancet* obituary said he was 'one of the first, if not the first, in this country to advocate the use of the stethoscope': *The Lancet*, 8 Aug 1868, pp. 203–4. By 1889 the *DNB* described him as 'the first' to use it: Stephen and Lee, vol. 17, p. 264–66. JE himself said simply that when Laennec published his work 'I procured a stethoscope and investigated his statements': JE (1835–40), p. 398.

56 JE, Notes of Lectures, KCL archives TH/PP23, vol. 11, pp. 119 and 221; JE (1830), pp. 16 and 12.

57 JE to William Nunn, 12 May 1829: RCP archives ALS/E19.

58 JE (1835–40), pp. 398–9; *The Lancet*, 8 Aug 1868, pp. 203–4.

59 JE (1835–40), p. 402. Background on phrenology in Britain is from Cooter (1984; 1989).

60 Combe to JE, 8 Apr 1825, MS 7215, Combe correspondence, NLS.

61 A study of London taxi drivers published in 2000 showed that the hippocampus – believed to govern navigational skill – was larger than in a control group. http:// www.ncbi.nlm.nih.gov/pubmed/17024677, accessed March 2014.

62 *Transactions of the Phrenological Society 1820–23* (Edinburgh, 1824). Thomas joined 22 Nov 1821 and JE 22 Nov 1822. The correspondence between JE and Combe is held in the NLS. Although the first letter dates from 1822 it refers to an earlier letter in 1821. The correspondence came to an end in 1829 apart from a few further formal exchanges in 1836 and 1838. The Combe correspondence is discussed in Miller; Ridgway (part 1); and Cooter (1984).

63 JE to GC, 10 Mar and 13 Jun 1823, MS 7210, Combe correspondence, NLS. Deville's name was also spelled De Ville or DeVille.

64 JE to GC, Dec [?] 1823, MS 7210, Combe correspondence, NLS.

65 JE to GC, 17 Jan and 14 Feb 1824, MS 7213, Combe correspondence, NLS.

66 JE to GC, 10 and 19 Mar 1823, MS 7210, Combe correspondence, NLS.

67 JE, Notes of Lectures, KCL archives TH/PP23, vol. 17, p. 1.

68 JE to GC, 27 Oct 1823, MS 7210, Combe correspondence, NLS.

69 Cooter (1984) provides an astute analysis of Elliotson's contradictory character, which he attributes to his social insecurity and diminutive height: pp. 52–3.

70 GC to JE, 5 Apr 1824, MS 7213, Combe correspondence, NLS.

71 JE to GC 1 Apr 1824 MS 7213; 27 Oct 1823; and 11 Jan 1823 MS 7210, Combe correspondence, NLS.

72 JE to GC, 4 Dec 1826, MS 7217, Combe correspondence, NLS.

73 GC to JE, 4 Nov 1824, MS 7213; 9 Jun 1828, MS 7221; and 25 Jul 1829, MS 7223: Combe correspondence, NLS.

CHAPTER 3: THE TALK OF THE TOWN

1 Biographical information on Wakley is from Sprigge; Brook; Hostettler and Clarke (1874). No letters or family papers survive – they are believed to have been

destroyed by Sprigge – but Wakley's life is amply illuminated in the pages of *The Lancet* and other contemporary media.

[2] Sprigge, pp. 37–69 and *Morning Chronicle*, 28 Aug 1820.

[3] In 1826 Wakley successfully sued James Johnson, editor of the *Medico-Chirurgical Review*, for libel after Johnson called him a 'firebrand' who was 'extinguishing debts by means of fire-engines': Hostettler, p. 33. As late as 1844, a fellow MP accused him of 'incendiarism': Brook, p. 130.

[4] Wakley's granddaughter confirmed the pronunciation in the 1940s: Brook, p. 10. Wakley was born 11 Jul 1795 in Membury, Devon.

[5] Hostettler, p. 75. Wakley was speaking at a meeting to support the Reform Bill on 4 Nov 1831.

[6] Wakley enrolled on 14 Dec 1815: Surgeons' Pupils of Guy's and St Thomas' Hospitals 1812–25, KCL archives G/FP4/1.

[7] Sprigge, p. 70.

[8] *The Lancet*, 5 Oct 1823, p. 2.

[9] Sprigge, p. 86–7; Clarke (1874), pp. 16–8.

[10] *The Lancet*, 23 Feb 1828, pp. 786–9.

[11] *The Lancet*, 5 Jun 1824, pp. 315–6.

[12] *The Lancet*, 29 Mar 1828, pp. 959–60.

[13] *The Lancet*, 11 Jan 1824, pp. 55–62. This is the first mention of JE in *The Lancet*.

[14] John Forbes and Robert Willis quoted in Hostettler, p. 88.

[15] Miller, p. 185.

[16] Brook, p. 130. Wakley was speaking in the House of Commons in 1844.

[17] Wakley's campaign against the RCS is detailed in Brook, pp. 80–90; and Sprigge, pp. 180–90.

[18] Letter JE to the editor, *The Lancet*, 24 Jun 1826, pp. 409–12.

[19] JE's evidence, *Report from the Select Committee on Medical Education* (London, 1834), part 1, pp. 104–17.

[20] JE to Combe, 2 Mar 1824, MS 7213, Combe correspondence, NLS.

[21] JE, 'Illustrations of the Medical Properties of Quinina', *Medico-Chirurgical Transactions*, 12 (1823), part 2, pp. 543–64.

[22] JE, 'On the Medical Properties of the Subcarbonate of Iron'; 'On the Use of the Sulphate of Copper in Chronic Diarrhoea'; and 'On the Medicinal Properties of Creosote' in *Medico-Chirurgical Transactions*, 13 (1827), part 1, pp. 232–53 and part 2, pp. 451–68; and 19 (1835), pp. 217–37.

[23] JE, 'On the Glanders in the Human Subject', *Medico-Chirurgical Transactions*, 16 (1831), part 1, pp. 171–218.

[24] JE, clinical lecture, delivered 31 Mar 1831, *LMG*, 8 (1831), pp. 411–3; Kathryn J. Waite, 'Blackley and the development of hay fever as a disease of civilization in the nineteenth century', *Medical History*, 39 (1995), pp. 186–96. Bostock's paper was published in 1819; he published a second in 1828.

[25] JE, 'On the Medical Properties of the Subcarbonate of Iron' in *Medico-Chirurgical Transactions*, 13 (1827), part 1, pp. 232–53.

[26] *The Lancet*, 6 May 1826, p. 190; 7 Jan 1826, pp. 519–20.

27 JE to GC, 2 Mar 1824, MS 7213, Combe correspondence, NLS.

28 Brook, p. 144.

29 Sprigge, p. 360; Brook, 147–8.

30 Sprigge, p. 441.

31 *The Lancet*, 16 Apr and 18 Mar 1825, pp. 41 and 349.

32 Cooter (1989), p. 334; JE to GC, 7 Feb 1824, MS 7213, Combe correspondence, NLS.

33 JE, 'On the Use of the Sulphate of Copper in Chronic Diarrhoea', *Medico-Chirurgical Transactions*, 13 (1828), part 2, pp. 451–68. Acupuncture is still recommended as a therapy for low back pain by the UK government health watchdog NICE although the evidence for effectiveness is slight: NICE guidelines, Low back pain (2009) https://www.nice.org.uk/guidance/cg88/chapter/guidance, accessed May 2014.

34 *The Lancet*, 7 Jan 1826, pp. 524–5.

35 Kate Williams, *Becoming Queen* (London, 2009), pp. 146–7.

36 Keats died on 23 Feb 1821. Details of his death are from Hale-White (Oxford, 1938), p. 63.

37 *The Lancet*, 5 Jul 1828, pp. 443–4.

38 JE to GC, 8 Feb 1826, MS 7217 and 5 May 1823, MS 7210, Combe correspondence, NLS.

39 Abel Campbell to Astley Cooper, 26 Jan 1825, St Thomas' Letter Book, LMA, ST/A86/4.

40 JE to St Thomas' board, 26 Jan and 27 Apr 1825, and minutes 29 Jun 1825, Grand Committee minutes 1811–27, LMA H01/ST. The first request was refused but several other physicians weighed in with the same demand and the board resolved it would no longer 'interfere' in the appointment of lecturers.

41 *The Lancet,* 20 Aug 1825, pp. 206–9. JE to GC, 9 Oct 1825, MS 7215, Combe correspondence, NLS.

42 The lectures were announced in *The Lancet*, 1 Oct 1825, p. 22. One pupil filled 17 volumes with notes. JE, Notes of Lectures, KCL archives TH/PP23.

43 'Abstract of a clinical lecture by Dr Elliotson', *The Lancet*, 24 Oct 1829, p. 141.

44 Clarke (1874), pp. 300–2. Clarke was describing JE's clinical lectures at UCL but they were first introduced at St Thomas'.

45 *The Lancet*, 17 Apr 1830, p. 86.

46 Clarke (1874), p. 180.

47 JE, 'Introductory Lecture at London University', *LMG*, 19 (1831), p. 23.

48 Anon (1839), vol. 1, pp. 273–85.

49 He was proposed by Prout, Faraday and Halford, among others: Royal Society archives, EC/1829/16.

50 Background on London University and its medical school is from Rosemary Ashton, *Victorian Bloomsbury* (New Haven, 2012); Merrington.

51 Clarke (1874), p. 318.

52 The title was later changed to Professor of the Principles and Practice of Medicine. JE to council, n. d. [1831] college correspondence, 1996; David Davis to

council, 9 May 1831, college correspondence, 2105; and JE to council, 16 Jun 1831, college correspondence, 2464, UCL archives; *The Lancet*, 14 May 1831, p. 210.

53 JE to council, 16 Jun 1831, college correspondence, 2464, UCL archives.

54 JE, 'Introductory Lecture at London University', *The Lancet*, 8 Oct 1831, pp. 64–70. The lecture was also published in the *LMG*, 9 (1831), pp. 23–30 and *Morning Chronicle*, 3 Oct 1832.

55 Clarke (1874), p. 36. Medical student numbers rose from 248 in 1831–32 to 351 in 1833–34: JE to council, May 1834, college correspondence, 3223, UCL archives.

56 John Hogg, *London As It Is* (London, 1838). Hogg lived at the dispensary for six years and later became an assistant at North London Hospital. His exposition of the capital's public health problems was significantly ahead of its time.

57 JE, 'Introductory Lecture at London University', *LMG*, 9 (1831–32), pp. 23–30.

58 UCH annual reports 1835 and 1838, UCL archives.

59 JE to council, 10 Jul 1834, college correspondence, 3243; JE to council, n. d. [1835], college correspondence, 3437, UCL archives. In the event the council raised a loan for £2,500 to cover building and fittings.

60 Plan of the ground floor of the original UCH: Merrington.

61 JE's letter of resignation was received 19 Aug 1834: St Thomas' General Court of Governors minute book, St Thomas' Hospital, 1784–1849, LMA H01/ST, p. 312.

62 JE wrote twice to the council after first meeting with a refusal. JE to council, n. d. [1835] and 17 Jan 1837, UCL archives.

63 The prizes were funded by the philanthropist Robert Fellowes, who said he owed his life to 'the great medical judgement, promptitude and sagacity of Dr Elliotson': UCL council minutes, vol. 3 (1835–43), 28 Jan 1837, UCL archives.

64 Clarke (1874), p. 180.

65 JE first gives his address as Conduit Street in Apr 1832: JE to Thomas Coates, Apr 1832, college correspondence, 2517, UCL archives. Westminster rates books refer to the coach house and stables: rates books 1634–1900, Westminster archives. The servants are listed in the Census 1841 when there were six staff; it is reasonable to suppose they were in place in the 1830s when he was at the height of his success. Other information on the house is revealed in anon (1842) and Moscati. The soiree is described in the *Morning Post*, 7 Feb 1834.

66 *Morning Post*, 31 Dec 1833; *Standard* 20 Apr 1838.

67 *The Lancet*, 8 Jun 1833, pp. 341–4.

68 Council minutes of the RMCS, A2, 1817–37; General minutes 1824–34, B5, and 1834–40, B6, RSM archives.

69 *Morning Post*, 3 Mar 1835; Queen Victoria's Journals, 28 Aug 1835, p. 282: http://www.queenvictoriasjournals.org, accessed 11 May 2014.

70 'John Elliotson' by James Ramsay, c. 1830–40. Elliotson's brother, Thomas, was also painted by Ramsay and his portrait exhibited at the Royal Academy in 1837. Both portraits are owned by the RCP. The portrait of Thomas was presented by his sisters, Emma and Eliza; the portrait of John was presented by Emma.

71 JE, 'Introductory Lecture at London University', *LMG*, 9 (1831), pp. 23–30.

72 *LMG*, 17 Nov 1832, pp. 213–23.

[73] *Morning Post*, 12 Feb 1835; RLF correspondence: BL Loan 96 RLF 1/756 (1833-39); Moscati.

[74] Wakley's political career is best described in Hostettler.

[75] Obituary, *The Lancet*, 8 Aug 1868, pp. 203–4.

CHAPTER 4: A NEW POWER IS REVEALED TO THE WORLD

[1] Clarke (1874), p. 161; Richard Harte, *Hypnotism and the Doctors* (New York, 1903). vol. 2, pp. 44–6. The first advertisement in *The Times* appeared on 23 Jun 1837. Dupotet describes his visit in Dupotet (1840), pp. 186–256. He styled himself Du Potet but was generally known in Britain as Dupotet.

[2] Dupotet (1840), pp. 186–7.

[3] Paul F. Cranefield, 'Mayo, Herbert (1796–1852)', *ODNB*, online edn, accessed 20 Mar 2014; Report of senate committee re. applications and testimonies for professor of anatomy and physiology, Oct 1836: UCL college correspondence, UCL archives, AM/3/1.

[4] Mackay, pp. 319–25; Colquhoun (1833), pp. 46–73; Gauld, pp. 1–17; Waterfield, pp. 64–90. Elliotson also refers to Mesmer in *Human Physiology*: JE (1835–40), pp. 662–3.

[5] Elliotson gives a good description of the history of such rites: JE (1835–40), pp. 664–7.

[6] Mackay, p. 325.

[7] The inquiry focused its investigations on the work of one of Mesmer's disciples, D'Eslon, rather than Mesmer himself, but the principles were the same.

[8] Waterfield, pp. 105–8 and 121.

[9] Colquhoun; Dupotet also describes his demonstrations in Dupotet (1838), pp. 40–6.

[10] Dupotet (1838), pp. 48–50; *Monthly Chronicle*, 1 (1838) pp. 305–6.

[11] JE (1835–40), p. 663. Elliotson recalled a Miss Preston in Bloomsbury Square who had lately died and a man in Kennington who had practised about 20 years earlier.

[12] Dupotet (1838), p. 117; Percy Bysshe Shelley, 'The Magnetic Lady to Her Patient', 1822.

[13] Colquhoun; Alan Gauld, 'Colquhoun, John Campbell (1785–1854)', *ODNB*, online edn, accessed 14 Sep 2015.

[14] JE (1835–40), p. 663; *Monthly Chronicle*, 1 (1838), pp. 301–2; the views of Cuvier and Laplace are given in JE (1835–40), pp. 678–9.

[15] JE (1835–40), pp. 680–1; Melyvn C. Usselman, 'Chenevix, Richard (1774–1830)', *ODNB*, online edn, accessed 20 Mar 2014; Gauld, pp. 198–9; Fred Kaplan, '"The Mesmeric Mania": The Early Victorians and Animal Magnetism', *Journal of the History of Ideas*, 35 (1974), pp. 691–702.

[16] *LMPJ*, 62 (1829), pp. 114–25; 210–20; 315–24. JE's addendum is in the latter.

[17] JE, the *Zoist*, 1 (1843–44), pp. 77–9.

[18] *LMPJ*, 61 (1829), pp. 219–30; *The Lancet*, 13 Jun 1829, pp. 341–4.

[19] *The Lancet*, 24 Jun 1837, pp. 469–71.

[20] George Tradescant Lay to JE, 21 Jun 1837, UCL correspondence 4362.

[21] John Elliotson sr died 30 May 1836; his wife, Elizabeth, was buried on 7 Jul 1837. Elliotson sr left all his wealth and estates at Southwark and Clapham to his son Thomas and his household goods to his wife. There was no mention in the will of John: Will of John Elliotson, proved 22 Jul 1836.

[22] JE's casebooks: Male Case Book 1836–37, UCH/MR/1/7, UCL archives. Orton eventually requested not to be mesmerised any further and 'to trust to medicines for his cure'. Orton and the other three patients first mesmerised by Dupotet are described in JE (1835–40), pp. 682–3 although Orton is not named there.

[23] Clarke (1874), p. 161.

[24] JE describes the three female patients in JE (1835–40), pp. 682–3. One of the epileptic girls was Elizabeth Okey but it is not clear from the casebooks who the second was. The hysterical girl was probably Charlotte Shea, aged 18, admitted on 4 Jul 1837 and first mesmerised 9 Jul. Their treatment is also described in JE's lecture published in *The Lancet* 9 Sep 1837, pp. 866–73. I have used the terms 'sleep' or 'trance' throughout the text although technically the hypnotic effect is not the same as sleep and some practitioners today deny the existence of a trance altogether.

[25] See Elaine Showalter, 'Hysteria, Feminism, and Gender' in Sander L. Gilman et al (eds), *Hysteria beyond Freud* (Berkeley, 1993), pp. 286–344, and Roy Porter, 'The Body and the Mind, the Doctor and the Patient', in same, pp. 225–85, for a discussion of hysteria in Victorian times.

[26] JE, 'Abstract of a clinical lecture by Dr Elliotson', *The Lancet*, 9 Sep 1837, pp. 866–73.

[27] Studies suggest women are marginally more responsive to hypnosis: Heap (2012), p. 6.

[28] Female Case Book no 2, 1837, UCH/MR/1/9, UCL archives.

[29] JE (1835–40), pp. 662–71. Elliotson was writing in Sep 1837, shortly after his first experiments with Dupotet.

[30] JE (1835–40), p. 683. Lucy Clarke's reactions are described on pp. 683–4 although she is not named there. Her response and treatment are also reported by Dupotet in *LMG*, 11 May 1838, pp. 334–5.

[31] JE (1835–40), p. 688. Elliotson said he had watched the baron's demonstrations for two months and was therefore writing in early Sep 1837.

[32] Female Case Book no 2, 1837, UCH/MR/1/9, UCL archives. The entry begins on p. 142. There are 15 pages devoted to her case running at intervals in the book while most patients warrant a single paragraph. JE also describes her history and early responses in JE (1835–40), pp. 628–30, 682 and 684; and in his first lecture on the subject in *The Lancet*, 9 Sep 1837, pp. 866–73.

[33] The anonymous letter is dated 28 Aug: *The Lancet*, 9 Sep 1837, pp. 836–40; Clarke (1874), p. 163.

[34] Jane was admitted on 14 Feb 1837 and discharged again on 6 Jun: Female Case Book no 2, 1837, UCH/MR/1/9, UCL archives.

35 Elizabeth Okey, born 9 Dec 1820, bapt. 16 Jan 1821: parish records St Andrew's Holborn. Her father's occupation is then given as 'chaser' and their address as Euston Crescent. Jane Okey, born 20 Jan 1823, bapt. 16 Feb 1823: parish records Old Church St Pancras. The family had by then moved to Crescent Street, one street away. Their siblings' baptism records give various addresses in the same area. George Talbot Okey married Jane Mundell, 2 Nov 1818: parish records St Martin's in the Fields, London. George's apprenticeship indenture to William Frisbee is dated 4 Dec 1811. Background on Somers Town and the surrounding areas is from Clarke (1992); Jerry White, *London in the Nineteenth Century* (London, 2007); J. R. Howard Roberts and Walter H. Godfrey (eds), *Survey of London* (London, 1949), vol. 21, p. 119; Walford, *Old and New London* (6 vols, London, 1879–85), vol. 5, pp. 340–52. The sisters have been assumed to be poor Irish immigrants by successive writers on mesmerism including Hughes, Pintar and Lynn, Waterfield and Winter.

36 Tomalin (2011), p. 27. Dickens lived at 29 Johnson Street (now Cranleigh Street) from 1824–27.

37 Quoted in Clarke (1992), pp. 257–8.

38 Letter to the *Hampshire Telegraph and Sussex Chronicle*, 3 Dec 1838.

39 The baptisms of Sarah, Edward, Henry and James were all registered on the same day – 20 Jul 1837 – at the Dissenters' Library, originally established by Dr Daniel Williams: National Archives, Protestant Dissenters' Register, RG5/150. At that time the family was living in Denton's Buildings.

40 Clarke (1874), p. 163.

41 Munk's Roll, RCP, vol. IV, p. 64; *The Lancet*, 15 Sep 1860, pp. 276–7. Thompson lectured on medicine at Grosvenor Place School of Medicine and Anatomy adjoining St George's Hospital at Hyde Park Corner and would later work at the Brompton Hospital.

42 Background on the history of epilepsy is from Owsei Temkin, *The Falling Sickness* (Baltimore, 1994). The Hippocratic texts are thought to have emanated from a group of physicians following the doctrines originally taught by Hippocrates.

43 JE, Notes of Lectures, KCL archives TH/PP23, lecture 29, vol. 8, pp. 63–143; the quote is from p. 117.

44 Female Case Book no 2, 1837, UCH/MR/1/9, UCL archives. My thanks to John Ford for advice on the medication and dosage.

45 This change is described in JE (1835–40), pp. 628–30 and in his first lecture on the subject in *The Lancet*, 9 Sep 1837, pp. 866–73.

46 *Monthly Chronicle*, 2 (1838), p. 19.

47 Letter to the Editor, signed 'T', *The Lancet*, 9 Sep 1837, pp. 836–40. He is identified by Antonio Melechi, *Servants of the Supernatural: The Night Side of the Victorian Mind* (London, 2008), p. 8; Michael J. Turner, 'Thompson, Thomas Perronet (1783–1869)', *ODNB*, online edn, accessed 7 Oct 2015.

48 The problems are described in UCL council minutes, vol. 3 (1835–43), 17 Jun 1837, UCL archives. His lecture was published in *The Lancet*, 9 Sep 1837, pp. 866–73 when it was said to have taken place 'last week'.

[49] JE (1835–40), pp. 628–30 and 660–93; later he added another 32 pages providing 69 pages in all: pp. 1163–94.

[50] *The Lancet*, 4 and 11 May 1833, pp. 175–83 and 205–18.

[51] Hostettler, pp. 98–101 and 117; Sprigge, p. 320.

[52] Dupotet, letter to editor, *The Lancet*, 16 Sep 1837, pp. 905–6.

[53] JE, the *Zoist*, 1 (1843–44), p. 89; Dupotet (1840), p. 201.

CHAPTER 5: DAGGERS DRAWN

[1] *The Lancet*, 14 Oct 1837, pp. 99–101. The description of Dupotet's experiments are from here unless otherwise stated.

[2] JE, the *Zoist*, 1 (1843–44), p. 89.

[3] *The Lancet*, 14 Oct 1837, pp. 99–101. The anonymous letter was dated 25 Sep.

[4] *LMG*, 16 Sep 1837, pp. 913–8.

[5] *The Times*, 20 Sep 1837; *Patriot*, reprinted in the *Liverpool Mercury*, 24 Nov 1837; *Satirist*, 10 Dec 1837; *Blackwood's Edinburgh Magazine*, cited in the *Belfast News-Letter*, 8 Sep 1837.

[6] According to *The Lancet* the demonstrations were stopped by the medical committee; JE confirmed this. In fact the medical committee did not meet from the end of August to the beginning of October so the move was probably informal.

[7] Clarke (1874), p. 308.

[8] D'A. Power, 'Liston, Robert (1794–1847)', rev. Jean Loudon, *ODNB*, online edn, accessed 2 Dec 2014; Percy Flemming, 'Robert Liston, the first Professor of Clinical Surgery at UCH', *UCH Magazine*, 2 (1926), no. 4, pp. 176–85.

[9] Richardson, p. 327, n.103; Anon (1839), vol. 1, pp. 356–60.

[10] Anon (1839), vol. 1, pp. 356–60.

[11] Brook, p. 145.

[12] Richard Gordon, *Great Medical Disasters* (New York, 1983), pp. 19–21. Gordon makes the comment about 300 per cent mortality.

[13] Cock (1911a). Cock interviewed a 77-year-old man who had his leg amputated by Liston at the age of 13 and witnessed the surgeon dragging his victim out of the lavatory.

[14] *The Lancet*, 6 Feb 1836, p. 754.

[15] Clarke (1874), p. 322.

[16] JE to Richard Quain, 21 Dec 1835: Medical Faculty Correspondence, UCL archives.

[17] Clarke (1874), p. 308.

[18] RL to James Miller, 7 May 1835, WL MS 6095; UCL council minutes, vol. 3 (1835–43), 23 Oct 1837, UCL archives. Although some of the originals of Liston's letters are preserved at the WL as MS 6084 and 6085, I have generally used the transcripts made by Liston's brother, David Liston, in MS 6095.

[19] UCH medical committee, 13 Oct 1835, UCHoff/1/1, UCL archives; RL to James Miller, 24 Oct 1835, WL MS 6095.

[20] UCL council minutes, vol. 3 (1835–43), 8 and 11 Aug 1836, UCL archives.

21 RL to James Miller, 1 Jan 1836; 16 Jan and 29 Feb 1837, WL MS 6095.

22 Clarke (1874), pp. 308–11.

23 Clarke (1874), pp. 81 and 142. Clarke was born in 1813.

24 Clarke (1874), pp. 309 and 313.

25 *The Lancet*, 11 Apr 1835, pp. 40–3; 17 Oct 1835, pp. 123–5; 11 Mar 1837, p. 877; 17 Dec 1835, p. 47.

26 *The Lancet*, 26 Dec 1835, pp. 519–20; 25 Nov 1837, pp. 317–21.

27 RL to James Miller, 24 Oct 1835, WL MS 6095.

28 *The Lancet*, 19 Dec 1835, pp. 447–8; Jan 9 1836, pp. 592–3.

29 RL to James Miller, 1 Jan 1836, WL MS 6095.

30 *The Lancet*, 23 Jan 1836, pp. 668–80 and 6 Feb 1836, pp. 753–5.

31 RL to James Miller, 11 Jan 1836, WL MS 6095.

32 UCH medical committee, 16 Feb 1837, UCHoff/1/1; UCL council minutes, vol. 3 (1835–43), 17 Jun 1837; UCH medical committee, 19 May 1837, UCHoff/1/1, UCL archives.

33 RL to James Miller, 7 Mar 1837, WL MS 6095.

34 UCH medical committee, 1 and 29 Aug, 1 Sep 1837, UCHoff/1/1, UCL archives. The article in *The Lancet* was published on 19 Aug 1837, pp. 779–80.

35 JE (1835–40), p. 688; JE, the *Zoist*, 1 (1843–4), p. 89.

36 *The Mirror of Literature, Amusement, and Instruction* (1838), vol. XXX, pp. 185–6.

37 Dupotet (1840), pp. 255 and 212.

38 JE, the *Zoist*, 1 (1843–44), p. 90.

39 JE (1835–40), pp. 692–3.

40 *The Lancet*, 21 Oct 1837, pp. 122–4.

41 UCH medical committee, 25 Nov 1837, UCHoff/1/1, UCL archives.

42 RL to James Miller, 14 Nov 1837, WL MS 6095.

43 Waterfield, pp. 110–2; Dupotet (1838), pp. 17–8.

44 JE (1835–40), pp. 679, 685.

45 Female Case Book no 2, 1837, UCH/MR/1/9, UCL archives. Elizabeth was mesmerised on 27 occasions in October, 12 in November and 17 in December.

46 Wood, letter to the editor, *The Lancet*, 28 Oct 1837, pp. 163–5.

47 *The Lancet*, 25 Nov 1837, pp. 295–8.

48 *Morning Post*, 12 Jul 1837 and various regional newspapers.

49 Dupotet (1840), p. 257. He was the 4th Earl Stanhope.

50 *The Lancet*, 9 Dec 1837, pp. 387–9.

51 *The Lancet*, 6 Jan 1838, pp. 522–4.

CHAPTER 6: I AM A BELIEVER

1 Female Case Book no 2, 4 Jan 1837, UCH/MR/1/9, UCL archives. A note at the end of the entry but in a different hand and ink states: 'Messrs Cruikshanks and Dickens were present.' Kaplan gives the date of Dickens's visit as 14 Jan 1838 but the UCH casebooks clearly record it on 4 Jan. The error stems from an article in the *UCH Magazine* which erroneously gives the date as 14 Jan: T. R. E. 'John

Elliotson, M. D. Camb., F. R. S.', *University College Hospital Magazine*, 1 (1911), pp. 272–84; Kaplan (1975), pp. 3 and 27.

² Biographical information on Dickens is from Forster; Tomalin; Peter Rowland (ed.) *Charles Dickens: My Early Times* (London, 1988).

³ The first mention of Elliotson in Dickens's letters is 24 Nov 1838 and in his diary on 28 Dec 1838: CD to George Cruikshank, in House and Storey, vol. 1, pp. 461 and 637.

⁴ Clarke (1874), p. 156.

⁵ JE to CD, Thursday evening [Feb 1841], vol. 1, p. 210 n.1; CD to Dr Robert Collyer, 27 Jan 1842, vol. 3, pp. 22–3; CD to John Overs, 24 Aug 1841, vol. 2, pp. 369–71; CD to Augustus Tracey, 11 May 1841, vol. 2, p. 281, all in House and Storey.

⁶ Dr Thomas Buzzard to anon, 7 Jul 1880, referring to an anecdote related by the lawyer William Ballantine: RCP archives, ALS/B362A8.

⁷ CD, 'Full report of the first meeting of the Mudfog Association for the Advancement of Everything', *Bentley's Miscellany*, 2 (1837), pp. 397–413, particularly p. 409.

⁸ CD to Dr Robert Collyer, 27 Jan 1842, in House and Storey, vol. 3, pp. 22–3. Collyer was a former pupil of JE at UCH in 1833–5, who had settled in America, where he qualified in medicine and began practising as a mesmerist.

⁹ Kaplan (1975), pp. 4–5. Kaplan says at Dickens's death he had 14 volumes of works on mesmerism in his library. Two of the books by JE were inscribed: 'To Charles Dickens from his sincere friend, John Elliotson.'

¹⁰ CD, *Oliver Twist* (Ware, Herts, 1992) p. 222; *Nicholas Nickleby* (London, 1999) p. 92. Kaplan (1975) makes a full exploration of Dickens's interest in mesmerism and its influence on his fiction. Mesmerism is also discussed in Schlicke, p. 383 and in Katharina Boehm, *Charles Dickens and the Sciences of Childhood: Popular Medicine, Child Health and Victorian Culture* (Basingstoke, 2013).

¹¹ Sheldon Goldfarb, 'Ainsworth, William Harrison (1805–82)', *ODNB*, online edn, accessed 6 Nov 2015. Ainsworth to Dr James Bower Harrison (his cousin), Apr 1838, in S. M. Ellis, *William Harrison Ainsworth and his Friends* (2 vols, London, 1911), vol. 1, p. 335.

¹² William Charles Macready, *Reminiscences, and Selections from his Diaries and Letters*, ed. Sir F. Pollock (London, 1876), pp. 404, 447, 130 and 583.

¹³ UCH casebooks, UCH/MR/1/7; UCH/MR/1/9; UCH/MR/1/16, UCL archives. From July 1837 to the end of 1838, Elliotson used mesmerism on 24 patients. Of these 22 were female. In 1837 he used mesmerism on three patients – Thomas Orton, Elizabeth Okey and Caroline Shea. Lucy Clarke is not mentioned in the casebooks as she was brought in from outside. Other patients are mentioned in *The Lancet* but do not appear in the casebooks and may have been treated as out-patients. Winter estimates that one in ten of Elliotson's female patients were mesmerised in 1837–38: Winter, p. 67. The cases of Bosch, Cook, Power, Hunter and Dewberry are all detailed in UCH/MR/1/16. Power is named Peever in the casebooks but this is no doubt an error as JE calls her Power in the *Zoist*: JE, the *Zoist*, 1 (1843–44) pp. 196–7.

[14] JE, the *Zoist*, 1 (1843–44) p. 180.

[15] The quotes from JE are from the *Zoist*, 1 (1843–44), pp. 300–4. Hannah Hunter's case is also described in *The Lancet*, 26 May 1838, pp. 314–6.

[16] *Morning Post*, 2 Mar 1838.

[17] UCH casebooks, UCH/MR/1/16, UCL archives. The casebooks refer to 'Mr Herring' but this was almost certainly William Hering, who is mentioned by JE in the *Zoist* as treating another patient with mesmerism: JE, the *Zoist*, 1 (1843–44) p. 190. Hering was a member of the London Phrenological Society from 1832 and its curator from 1842.

[18] Clarke (1874), p. 168.

[19] UCH casebooks, UCH/MR/1/16, UCL archives. The patient was Mary Ann Haynes, admitted 11 May, but the experiment was frequently repeated with smaller chains.

[20] UCH casebooks, UCH/MR/1/16, UCL archives. Jane had been referred to UCH by Theophilus Thompson, who previously treated Elizabeth. Having heard of Elliotson's experiments, Thompson tried mesmerising Jane himself without success so sent her to Elliotson.

[21] Elizabeth Okey quoted in *The Lancet*, 28 Jul 1838, p. 620.

[22] I am grateful to Dr Sofia Eriksson, consultant neurologist in the Department of Clinical and Experimental Epilepsy of the National Hospital for Neurology and Neurosurgery within UCLH NHS Foundation Trust, for advice on epilepsy.

[23] My thanks to Dr Raj Sharma, head of the Hypnosis and Cognitive Therapy Unit at UCLH, for suggesting this theory. It is also possible one or both girls were subject to 'dissociative seizures', which look similar to epileptic seizures but are not caused by electrical activity in the brain. This condition may have a psychological cause and can be triggered by a traumatic event or by witnessing a sibling have an epileptic seizure. My thanks to Dr Sofia Eriksson (see note 22) for advice.

[24] Clarke (1874), p. 162–3; *The Lancet*, 15 Sep 1838, pp. 873–7. Information on Irving is from Stewart J. Brown, 'Irving, Edward (1792–1834), preacher and theologian', *ODNB*, online edn, accessed 12 Nov 2015.

[25] JE (1835–40), p. 1165.

[26] *The Times*, 29 Oct 1831, cited on UCL Bloomsbury Project website: www.ucl.ac.uk/bloomsbury-project/institutions/caledonian_church; Clarke (1874), p. 163.

[27] JE (1835–40), p. 1165.

[28] JE, the *Zoist*, 1 (1843–44) p. 176; JE (1835–40), p. 1168.

[29] JE, the *Zoist*, 1, (1843–44) pp. 90–1 and 304.

[30] *Morning Post*, 5 Mar 1838.

[31] UCH casebooks, UCH/MR/1/16, UCL archives. This occurred on 8 Apr 1838.

[32] UCH casebooks, UCH/MR/1/16, UCL archives. The patient was Lucy Shields, a 19-year-old maid, who had her tonsils removed on 20 Mar 1838.

[33] 'Animal Magnetism: second report of facts and experiments', *The Lancet*, 9 Jun 1838, p. 380.

[34] Clarke (1874), p. 163.

[35] JE (1835–40), p. 1166; the *Zoist*, 12 (1854–5), p. 132.

[36] The *Globe*, 24 Apr 1838. The report was syndicated in the *Belfast News-Letter* and other newspapers. Elliotson describes the experiments in JE (1843), p. 30.

[37] *The Lancet*, 26 May 1838, p. 320; *Morning Post*, 2 Mar 1838.

[38] JE (1835–40), p. 1167.

[39] *The Lancet*, 21 Jul 1838, p. 585; James Mouatt, the *Zoist*, 7 (1849–50), pp. 41–3.

[40] Mayo, letter to the editor, *LMG*, 28 Apr 1838, pp. 197–200. He suggested the term 'trance' on 21 Apr 1838.

[41] *The Lancet*, 9 Jun 1838, pp. 367–71; *LMG*, 31 Mar 1838, pp. 27–8.

[42] John Wilson, *Trials of Animal Magnetism on the Brute Creation* (London, 1839).

[43] *Morning Post*, 2 Mar 1838.

[44] Syndicated in the *Belfast News-Letter*, 24 Apr 1838, and elsewhere.

[45] *Satirist*, 18 Mar 1838. Previously the newspaper had ridiculed Dupotet on 5 Nov 1837. Hughes discusses the *Satirist*'s attacks on Dupotet and Elliotson in detail.

[46] S. Sandys, letter to the editor, *LMG*, 17 Feb 1838, pp. 765–7.

[47] Thomas Chandler, letter to the editor, *The Lancet*, 14 Apr 1838, pp. 81–3; Chandler to JE, the *Zoist*, 1 (1843–44), p. 166.

[48] *The Lancet*, 28 Apr 1838, pp. 168–9.

[49] *The Lancet*, 26 May 1838, pp. 314–6.

[50] Clarke (1874), p. 156.

[51] Lardner published two lengthy essays on mesmerism in the *Monthly Chronicle* for Mar–Jun and Jul–Dec 1838.

[52] JE, the *Zoist*, 1 (1843–44), p. 190. Owen had recently been appointed Hunterian Professor of Comparative Anatomy and Physiology at the Royal College of Surgeons.

[53] Faraday conducted his experiments on 10 Feb: UCH casebooks, UCH/MR/1/16, UCL archives; *Morning Post*, 2 Mar 1838; JE, the *Zoist*, 1 (1843–44), p. 306.

[54] Elizabeth Chambers Patterson, *Mary Somerville and the Cultivation of Science, 1815–1840* (The Hague, 1983); *LMG*, 26 May 1838, p. 392.

[55] *Monthly Chronicle*, Jul–Dec 1838; JE's farewell letter, the *Zoist*, 1 (1843–44), p. 92.

CHAPTER 7: THE PROPHETESS OF ST PANCRAS

[1] Anthony Todd Thomson, David Davis and Robert Liston to Richard Quain, 1 May 1838, UCH medical faculty correspondence, 102, UCL archives.

[2] Clarke (1874), pp. 305–7; Edmund A. Parkes (ed.), memoir of ATT in Anthony Todd Thomson, *A Practical Treatise on Diseases Affecting the Skin* (London, 1850); P. W. J. Bartrip, 'Thomson, Anthony Todd (1778–1849)', *ODNB*, online edn, accessed 20 Mar 2014. Information on Davis is from Norman Moore, 'Davis, David Daniel (1777–1841)', rev. Elizabeth Baigent, *ODNB*, online edn, accessed 20 Nov 2015.

[3] UCL, minutes of the management committee, 15 Mar 1838, vol. 2, 1834–39; extract of minutes of faculty of medicine, UCL, college correspondence, 4 Apr 1838, 4270 and 12 Apr 1838, 4280, UCL archives.

[4] Clarke (1874), p. 170.

[5] This rule had twice been cited in medical faculty meetings since the beginning of 1838: UCL, medical committee minutes, 12 and 19 Feb 1838, UCL archives.

[6] JE's farewell letter, the *Zoist*, 1 (1843–44), pp. 91–2.

[7] *Morning Post*, 3 Apr 1838; JE, the *Zoist*, 1 (1843–44), p. 422.

[8] Henry Crabb Robinson diaries, 29 Mar 1838, vol. 17, p. 64: Dr Williams's Library.

[9] UCH annual report 1838, UCL archives.

[10] Henry Crabb Robinson diaries, 29 Mar 1838, vol. 17, p. 64: Dr Williams's Library.

[11] JE to the medical faculty, 5 Jan 1838, *The Lancet*, 17 Feb 1838. JE claimed it was the largest medical class in the country.

[12] JE's farewell letter, the *Zoist*, 1 (1843–44), pp. 91–2.

[13] The *Zoist*, 1 (1843–44), p. 185.

[14] *LMG*, 1837–38.

[15] *Morning Post*, 5 and 7 May 1838.

[16] Henry Crabb Robinson diaries, 3 May 1838, vol. 17, p. 76: Dr Williams's Library.

[17] As described in chapter 1: *The Lancet*, 26 May 1838, pp. 282–8 and the *Morning Post*, 11 May 1838.

[18] Council minutes of the RMCS, A3 (1837–48), RSM archives.

[19] *The Lancet* and *LMG*, both 26 May 1838. Winter has confirmed there was no formal RS committee, pp. 49–52.

[20] *Morning Post*, 11 May 1838.

[21] *The Lancet*, 9 Jun 1838, pp. 367–71.

[22] The meeting took place on 28 May 1838. Minute Book of the Medical Society of London 1836–39, WL, SA/MSL/D/2/1/19. The debate is described in *The Lancet*, 23 Jun 1838, pp. 457–8. The history of the MSL is given in Penelope Hunting, *The Medical Society of London 1773–2003* (London, 2003).

[23] Solomon Gilbert Diamond and Robert D. Howe, 'Measuring Hypnosis: Relating the Subjective Experience to Systematic Physiological Changes' (2001), http://biorobotics.harvard.edu/pubs/2001/diamond_hypnometer.pdf, accessed 10 Aug 2016.

[24] *Morning Post*, 11 May and 2 Mar 1838.

[25] The *Zoist*, 2 (1844–45), p. 47. No date is given for the visit but it must have been before June 1838 when Wakefield left for Canada. David J. Moss, 'Wakefield, Edward Gibbon (1796–1862)', *ODNB*, online edn, accessed 24 Nov 2015.

[26] Both attended on 8 May 1838: *Morning Post*, 11 May 1838.

[27] JE to UCL council, 23 May 1838, college correspondence 4295; debated at the council on 26 May 1838, UCL council minutes, vol. 3 (1835–43), UCL archives. Despite this decision, on 4 August the council agreed to allow the theatre to be used for the Sicilian boy, Vito Mangiamele, to exhibit his 'powers of calculation'.

[28] Henry Crabb Robinson diaries, 26 May 1838, vol. 17, pp. 83–4: Dr Williams's Library.

[29] *The Lancet*, 16 and 23 Jun 1838, pp. 400–3 and 441–6; JE (1835–40), p. 1168.

[30] Herbert Mayo to the editor, *LMG*, 16 Jun 1838, pp. 490–8.

[31] Baron Dupotet to the editor, *LMG*, 19 May 1838, pp. 334–5.

[32] *The Lancet*, 23 Jun 1838, pp. 441–3.

[33] *The Lancet*, 9 and 16 Jun 1838, pp. 377–83 and 400–3. The weather is described in *The Lancet* report. It is sometimes difficult to tell whether Mills is referring to Elizabeth or Jane at various points though he seems to mean Elizabeth when he refers to 'O'Key'.

[34] *The Lancet*, 23 Jun 1838, pp. 441–3. The dashes in Mills's report have been filled in.

[35] Herbert Mayo to the editor, *LMG*, 16 Jun 1838, pp. 490–8.

[36] *LMG*, 30 Jun 1838, pp. 587–8.

[37] *Athenaeum*, 16 Jun 1838, pp. 417–21.

[38] *British and Foreign Medical Review*, Apr 1839, pp. 348–52. The journal was edited by John Conolly, JE's predecessor at UCL, and John Forbes, who had translated Laennec's book on the stethoscope into English in 1821.

[39] UCL, minutes of the medical committee, 2 and 6 Jun 1838, UCHoff/min/1/1, UCL archives.

[40] JE's farewell letter, the *Zoist*, 1 (1843–44), pp. 91–2.

[41] UCL, minutes of the medical committee, 9 Jun 1838, UCHoff/min/1/1, UCL archives.

[42] William Sharpey to Allen Thomson, 16 Feb 1839 in Jacyna, pp. 20–3.

[43] UCL, minutes of the medical committee, 13 Jun 1838, UCHoff/min/1/1, UCL archives; JE's farewell letter, in the *Zoist*, 1 (1843–44), pp. 91–2.

[44] UCL, minutes of the management committee, 14 Jun 1838, vol. 2, 1834–39, UCL archives.

[45] JE to medical committee, 19 Jun and 4 Jul 1838, minutes of the medical committee, 4 Jul 1838, UCHoff/min/1/1, UCL archives.

[46] *LMG*, 23 Jun 1838; *The Times*, 25 Jun 1838.

[47] *The Lancet*, Jan–Jun 1838, *passim*. More detail on Wakley's parliamentary work can be found in Brook and Hostettler.

[48] *Gentleman's Magazine*, 10 (1838), no 2, p. 106. She died on 24 May of unknown causes.

CHAPTER 8: HUMBUG! HUMBUG! HUMBUG!

[1] *The Lancet*, 18 Aug 1838, pp. 728–9.

[2] Clarke (1874), p. 160.

[3] *The Lancet*, 23 Jun 1838, pp. 443–6.

[4] *The Lancet*, 23 Jun 1838, pp. 443–6.

[5] *The Lancet*, 21 Jul 1838, pp. 585–90.

[6] *The Lancet*, 7 Jul 1838, pp. 516–9.

[7] *The Lancet*, 7 Jul 1838, pp. 517; UCH casebooks, UCH/MR/1/16, UCL archives. The woman is unnamed but it is clearly Elizabeth given the resemblance to the sketch in the casebook.

[8] *Morning Chronicle*, 20 Jun 1838.

[9] *The Lancet*, 14 Jul 1838, p. 549; *LMG*, 30 Jun 1838, p. 587. Roget asked JE to bring Elizabeth to his house in June 'to verify the simple facts exhibited by her under

mesmeric influence': Peter Mark Roget to JE, 7 Jun 1838: Townshend Manuscript Collection, Wisbech and Fenland Museum.

[10] *Penny Satirist*, 26 May 1838.

[11] JE describes these cases in a clinical lecture, *The Lancet*, 28 Jul 1838, pp. 634–7. They are also discussed in *The Lancet*, 14 Jul 1838, pp. 546–9.

[12] These three are also described in JE's clinical lecture, *The Lancet*, 28 Jul 1838, pp. 634–7.

[13] Obituary, *The Lancet*, 8 Aug 1868, pp. 203–4.

[14] JE (1835–40), p. 827. Typically he put forward various scientific theories for the frog shower.

[15] *The Lancet*, 14 Jul 1838, pp. 546–9.

[16] *Athenaeum*, 21 Jul 1838, p. 515.

[17] *Monthly Chronicle*, 2 (1838), p. 21.

[18] *The Lancet*, 21 Jul 1838, pp. 585–90.

[19] Michael Ben-Chaim, 'Gray, Stephen (1666–1736)', *ODNB*, online edn, accessed 12 Aug 2016.

[20] Mayo to the editor, *LMG*, 11 Aug 1838, pp. 771–5.

[21] *LMG*, 25 Aug 1838, pp. 842–4. This was a surgeon, William Cooke.

[22] The James Lind Library: http://www.jameslindlibrary.org/articles/who-was-james-lind-and-what-exactly-did-he-achieve/; http://www.jameslindlibrary.org/essays/2-4-the-need-to-avoid-differences-in-the-way-treatment-outcomes-are-assessed/accessed 12 Aug 2016.

[23] Wendy Moore, *The Knife Man: Blood, Body-snatching and the Birth of Modern Surgery* (London, 2005), p. 264.

[24] Dupotet, *LMG*, 23 Dec 1837, pp. 498–503; JE (1835–40), p. 687.

[25] *The Lancet*, 21 Jul 1838, pp. 585–90; Mayo to the editor, *LMG*, 11 Aug 1838, pp. 771–5.

[26] *The Lancet*, 28 Jul 1838, pp. 615–20.

[27] Mayo to the editor, *LMG*, 11 Aug 1838, pp. 771–5.

[28] JE (1835–40), pp. 1175–6.

[29] *The Lancet*, 28 Jul 1838, pp. 615–20.

[30] Clarke (1874), p. 167.

[31] *LMG*, 25 Aug 1838, pp. 842–4.

[32] *Athenaeum*, 21 Jul 1838, p. 515; *The Age*, 10 Jun 1838; *Penny Satirist*, 12 May, 26 May and 23 Jun 1838; *Figaro in London*, 9 Jun 1838.

[33] Betty A. Toole (ed.), *Ada, The Enchantress of Numbers: A Selection from the Letters of Lord Byron's Daughter and her Description of the First Computer* (Mill Valley, Calif, 1992); R. C. Terry (ed.), *The Oxford Reader's Companion to Trollope* (Oxford, 1999), p. 178.

[34] *LMG*, 14 Jul 1838, pp. 644–8.

[35] *LMG*, 25 Aug 1838, pp. 845–9.

[36] *The Lancet* reported that the committee met twice a week from the beginning of June and subjected the Okeys to experiments on 'many occasions': *The Lancet*, 25 Aug 1838, p. 780.

[37] *The Lancet*, 18 Aug 1838, pp. 727–8.
[38] *The Lancet*, 18 Aug 1838, pp. 728–30.
[39] Newman, p. 59.

CHAPTER 9: GREAT JACKEY

[1] The experiments on 16 and 17 Aug 1838 are detailed in *The Lancet*, 1 Sep 1838, pp. 805–11; Clarke, pp. 182–94; and JE (1835–40), pp. 1182–3.
[2] Andrew Byrne, *Bedford Square: An Architectural Study* (London, 1990); anon, *Architectural Association Journal*, 33 (1917), no. 365, pp. 11–5. No. 35 is now part of the headquarters of the Architectural Association School of Architecture. The drawing room forms part of the library. My thanks to librarian Eleanor Gawne.
[3] *The Lancet*, 1 Sep 1838, pp. 805–11.
[4] *The Lancet* describes Hering as 'Mr Herring' but it was almost certainly William Hering. His name was also misspelled Herring in the UCH casebooks. Clarke describes Richardson as 'Dr F. Richardson' but he is probably mistaken since the only F. Richardson at that time was a surgeon in Cheltenham. Robert Richardson graduated MD from Edinburgh in 1807: Munk's Roll, RCP, p. 134.
[5] JE (1835–40), pp. 1182–3.
[6] The group also included 'Mr B. Tipper' but it has not been possible to identify him.
[7] *The Lancet*, 1 Sep 1838, p. 811.
[8] Clarke (1874), pp. 191–4.
[9] Clarke (1874), pp. 163–4.
[10] *The Lancet*, 1 Sep 1838, pp. 811–4; *LMG*, 11 Aug 1838, pp. 771–5.
[11] *The Lancet*, 8 Sep 1838, pp. 834–6.
[12] *The Lancet*, 15 Sep 1838, pp. 873–7.
[13] *LMG*, 1 and 8 Sep 1838, pp. 908–10 and 948–51.
[14] *The Times*, 6 and 15 Sep 1838.
[15] The *Age*, 9 Sep 1838; *Penny Satirist*, 22 Sep 1838; *Satirist*, 23 Sep 1838; also published in *Cleave's Penny Gazette*, 29 Sep 1838; *The Periscope*, 1 Oct 1838, cited in Hughes, pp. 103–4.
[16] *The Lancet*, 22 Sep 1838, pp. 34–5.
[17] JE (1835–40), pp. 1182–3; the *Zoist*, 2 (1844–45), p. 176.
[18] The *Zoist*, 2 (1844–45), p. 65 and 1 (1843–44), p. 93.
[19] JE, address to his students, in *LMG*, 23 Mar 1839, p. 951.
[20] A. F. Randall, letter to the editor (23 Nov), *Hampshire Telegraph*, 3 Dec 1838.
[21] *LMG*, 6 Oct 1838, p. 54.
[22] The *Zoist*, 1 (1843–44), pp. 161 and 171–2.
[23] 'Censor', *Medical Times*, 9 Nov 1839, p. 54.
[24] *The Lancet*, 5 Jan 1839, pp. 561–2; JE, address to his students, in *LMG*, 23 Mar 1839, p. 951.
[25] JE, address to his students, in *LMG*, 23 Mar 1839, pp. 946–54; *The Lancet*, 5 Jan 1839, pp. 561–2; Clarke (1874), pp. 173–6.

[26] Minutes of hospital committee, 6 and 15 Dec 1838, in minutes of UCL Council, 22 Dec 1838, UCL archives. The original minutes of the hospital committee do not appear to have survived. The council minutes give the date of the second hospital committee as 15 Dec but Henry Crabb Robinson refers to it in his diary on 14 Dec.

[27] *The Lancet*, 5 Jan 1839, pp. 561–2.

[28] Henry Crabb Robinson diaries, 14 Dec 1838, vol. 17, p. 131, Dr Williams's Library.

[29] *The Lancet*, 5 Jan 1839, pp. 561–2.

[30] Henry Crabb Robinson diaries, 22 Dec 1838, vol. 17, pp. 134–5, Dr Williams's Library.

[31] JE to Charles Atkinson, 27 Dec 1838, college correspondence, 4454, UCL archives.

[32] *The Lancet* claimed he invited 'a very large number' of students to dinner that evening, presumably to suggest he was inciting them to protest at his resignation: *The Lancet*, 5 Jan 1839, pp. 561–2. Dickens's diary for that day says 'Dr Elliotson – Dinner – ½ past 6': House and Storey, vol. 1, p. 637.

[33] The *Zoist*, 1 (1843–44), p. 283.

[34] William Sharpey to Allen Thomson, 16 Feb 1839, cited in Jacyna, pp. 20–3.

[35] *LMG*, 22 Dec 1838, pp. 445–8.

[36] *British and Foreign Medical Review*, 5 (1839), pp. 301–52.

[37] *The Lancet*, 5 Jan 1839, pp. 561–2.

[38] *The Times*, 7 Jan 1839.

[39] *The Lancet*, 12 Jan 1839, pp. 590–7.

[40] Brougham and Goldsmid proposed that a delegation should meet Elliotson to discuss his actions but their motion was lost and the resignation was accepted by nine votes to four: minutes of UCL council, 5 Jan 1839, UCL archives. Elliotson's students continued to protest. When the council appointed a temporary replacement professor, Dr James Copland, Elliotson's devotees drowned out his introductory lecture by 'groaning and hissing'. The protest culminated in a scuffle, which resulted in a number of torn coats and black eyes: *The Times*, 15 Jan 1839; *The Lancet*, 19 Jan 1839, pp. 626–7. Copland was replaced by Charles Williams, who was formally appointed professor of medicine in July: minutes of UCL council, 20 Jul 1839, UCL archives.

CHAPTER 10: PERFECT ANAESTHESIA

[1] *The Friend of India*, 18 Apr 1839.

[2] The *Zoist*, 1 (1843–44), p. 161–2.

[3] JE, 'Intense hiccup cured by mesmerism', the *Zoist*, 2 (1844–45), pp. 42–74 and p. 318. JE refers on p. 318 to Jane Critchley as the younger sister of the woman he had treated for hiccups. She first developed a cough after hearing the pistol shot and this later developed into hiccups. Johnston is mentioned in the *London and Provincial Directory* 1851.

[4] *LMG*, 23 Mar 1839, pp. 946–53.

[5] Anon (1839), vol. 1, pp. 273–85.

[6] Minutes of UCL council, 19 Jan 1839, UCL archives; JE (1835–40), p. 1166.

[7] JE to anon, [5 April 1839?], cited in Kaplan (1975).

[8] *Blackburn Standard*, 13 Mar 1839.

[9] Anon (1839), vol. 1, pp. 273–85.

[10] Anon, *A full discovery of the strange practices of Dr Elliotson . . .* (London, c. 1842).

[11] JE (1835–40), p. 1166.

[12] Trollope, pp. 366–74.

[13] The *Zoist*, 1 (1843–44), pp. 208–9. The terms 'Okeyism' and 'Okeyites' were deployed in *The Lancet* as well as elsewhere: *The Lancet*, 6 and 27 Aug 1842.

[14] *The Lancet*, 26 Oct 1839, pp. 170–4. She was Lady Flora Hastings, former lady-in-waiting to Queen Victoria's mother, the Duchess of Kent. In fact she was not pregnant but suffering from terminal liver cancer from which she died later that year.

[15] Thomas Hood, *The Comic Annual* (London, 1842), pp. iv–v.

[16] JE (1835–40), pp. 1165–8.

[17] Trollope, p. 374.

[18] They were living in Elstree Terrace, Ossulston Street, Somers Town. The census for 1841 erroneously gives both girls' ages as 15. Elizabeth's husband was actually named William Bittlestone Bittlestone: marriage register, St James the Less, Bethnal Green, 23 Feb 1846; census 1861 and 1871; death certificate, 11 Feb 1872. Jane married Samuel Campbell but his occupation was unrecorded: marriage register, St Pancras Church, 12 Jun 1842. The date Jane died is unknown. My thanks to Jacky Worthington for her unstinting help in tracing the Okey family.

[19] Trollope, p. 374. Trollope was not sure which of the Okey sisters the daughter belonged to but as Elizabeth had only sons it must have been Jane.

[20] Captain F. Marryat to anon, 3 Aug (c. 1839), Townshend manuscript collection, Wisbech and Fenland Museum.

[21] JE to CD, May 1841 and 4 Aug 1841 in House and Storey, vol. 2, pp. 148n and 342. In Aug 1841 JE told CD he had a patient who displayed '*all* the phenomena, that you witnessed in Miss Critchley'.

[22] Trollope, pp. 367–9.

[23] The *Zoist*, 1 (1843–44), p. 177 and 2 (1844–45), pp. 194–238.

[24] The *Zoist*, 1 (1843–44), p. 161.

[25] The patients are described in the *Zoist*. Mary Ann Vergo: The *Zoist*, 1 (1843–44), pp. 197–8; Master Linnell: 1 (1843–44), pp. 199–201.

[26] The *Zoist*, 3 (1845–46), p. 322.

[27] JE to CD, Thursday evening (11 Feb 1841), HM 18486, Charles Dickens File, Huntington Library.

[28] It is not known when Symes married but by 1851 he was living with his wife, Mary, aged 25, and their three children. The eldest, Edmund, was then four, and his second son, baptised John Elliotson Symes, was three. 1851 Census, Westminster archives.

[29] Thomas Chandler to JE, 14 Aug and 3 Sep 1844, the *Zoist*, 2 (1844–45), pp. 373–6. Collyer studied under JE in 1833–35.

[30] http://www.geoffsgenealogy.co.uk/collyer/robert-hanham-collyer-chronology, accessed 15 Aug 2016.

[31] Edward Oke Spooner to JE, 23 Dec 1843, the *Zoist*, 2 (1844–45), p. 79.

[32] *Medical Times*, 18 Jan 1840.

[33] Terry M. Parssinen, 'Mesmeric Performers', *Victorian Studies*, 21 (1977–78), pp. 87–104; Gauld, pp. 203–4; Waterfield, pp. 159–60; Hall, pp. 1–2; *LMG*, 6 Aug 1841, pp. 762–5; *The Times* 20, 24 Jul and 10 Sep 1841. Winter provides the most comprehensive study of mesmeric performances in Victorian Britain.

[34] Hall; Gauld, p. 204; Winter, pp. 130–5; Gordon Goodwin, 'Hall, Spencer Timothy (1812–85)', rev. Stephanie L. Barczewski, *ODNB*, online edn, accessed 21 Jan 2016.

[35] In one case study a man with a severe stammer was cured in 10 sessions: Anthony Humphreys, 'Applications of hypnosis to anxiety control' in Heap (1988), pp. 105–14.

[36] The *Zoist*, 2 (1844–45), pp. 477–529; Winter, pp. 143–6. Alexis first visited London in 1844–45 and returned in 1849.

[37] Edmond Sheppard Symes to editor, the *Zoist*, 2, (1844–45), pp. 291–3; and pp. 477–529. *The Lancet* exposé was by John Forbes, physician to Queen Victoria's household and a lifelong opponent of mesmerism. John Forbes, 'On the pretended exhibitions in mesmerism', *The Lancet*, 3 Aug 1844.

[38] The *Zoist*, 2 (1844–45), p. 47.

[39] 'Asmodeus' to the editor, *Medical Times*, 5 Mar 1842, p. 271; the *Zoist*, 1, (1843–44), p. 280.

[40] Elizabeth Rigby, *Journals and Correspondence of Lady Eastlake* (2 vols, London, 1895), 1, p. 152.

[41] The *Zoist*, 1 (1843–44), pp. 95–100 and p. 93.

[42] Kaplan (1975); Tatar, pp. 190–1.

[43] Elizabeth Barrett to Robert Browning, 2, 3 Jul 1845, in Elvan Kintner (ed.), *The Letters of Robert Browning and Elizabeth Barrett Barrett: 1845–1846* (Cambridge, Mass, 1969), p. 114 and *passim*. Browning's poem was published in 1855: Jerome M. Schneck, 'Robert Browning and Mesmerism', *Medical Library Association Bulletin* 44 (1956), pp. 443–51. Charlotte Brontë to James Taylor, cited in Tatar, p. 190.

[44] CD to JE, 23 Oct 1839, House and Storey, vol. 1, p. 392.

[45] Schlicke, pp. 450–1.

[46] House and Storey, vol. 2, p. 343n; and JE to CD, 4 Aug 1841, vol. 2, p. 345n.

[47] Rosemary Scott, 'Townshend, Chauncy Hare (1798–1868)', *ODNB*, online edn, accessed 20 Mar 2014; Dr Peter Cave (ed.), *The Life and Times of Chauncy Hare Townshend* (Wisbech, 1998); CD to JE, n.d. (5 Aug 1840), Townshend manuscript collection, Wisbech and Fenland Museum [date according to House and Storey, vol. 2, pp. 109-10]. Townshend to CD, 24 Jul 1841, House and Storey, vol. 2, pp. 342 and 342n. CD to John Forster, 1, 2, 3 Apr 1842, House and Storey, vol. 3, p. 180. CD's interest in mesmerism is fully explored in Kaplan (1975).

[48] Kaplan (1975), pp. 75–95; Tomalin, pp. 160–3; CD to Emile de la Rue, 26 Dec 1844, House and Storey, vol. 4, p. 243.

[49] CD to Douglas Jerrold, 24 Oct 1846, House and Storey, vol. 4, p. 645.

[50] Countess of Blessington and Count D'Orsay attended demonstrations by Lafontaine and Alexis; they were friendly with JE: Wolff, p. 240; Count D'Orsay to JE, 16 Aug 1841, Misc Ms 3173, Pforzheimer Collection, NYPL; CD to Countess of Blessington, 23 Nov 1841 and D'Orsay to CD, 11 Dec 1841, House and Storey, vol. 2, pp. 425–6. JE details Lady Mary Bentinck's work in the *Zoist*, 3 (1845–46), pp. 344 and 363. Initially he describes her as 'a lady of rank, the daughter of a duke' who treated people in Nottinghamshire but later says she introduced a patient to him. Since Bentinck was married to Sir William Topham, the barrister who mesmerised James Wombell (see note 57), her identity is clear. JE says the Duke of Marlborough saw one of his patients and he mentions being called to Blenheim on 16 Aug 1841: the *Zoist*, 1 (1843–44), pp. 450 and 2 (1844–45), p. 198. Prince Albert: Gauld, p. 206. The 'British court' is mentioned in William Lang, *Animal Magnetism or Mesmerism* (New York, 1844), p. 108.

[51] *The Times*, 24 Jul 1841.

[52] James Braid, *Neurypnology, or the rationale of nervous sleep, considered in relation to animal magnetism* (London, 1843). Alan Gauld, 'Braid, James (1795–1860)', *ODNB*, online edn, accessed 20 Mar 2014; Gauld, pp. 279–82; Crabtree, p. 125. The quotes are all from Braid except for *Medical Times*, 12 Mar 1842, p. 283. According to Waterfield the term 'hypnotisme' was first used 35 years earlier by Étienne Félix d'Henin de Cuvillers but Braid was the first to introduce the term in English and popularised it: Waterfield, p. xxx.

[53] *Medical Times*, 29 Jan 1842, pp. 212–3.

[54] The *Zoist*, 3 (1845–46), p. 345.

[55] JE (1835–1840), p. 1166; the *Zoist*, 2 (1844–45), p. 88.

[56] Obituary, William Collins Engledue, *BMJ*, 29 Jan 1859. Details of the operation are given by Engledue in the *Zoist*, 2 (1844–45), pp. 271–2 and by Elliotson in JE (1843), pp. 74–5. Engledue's address to the Phrenological Association which led to the protest was published in *Phrenological Journal*, 15 (1842), pp. 289–381. The association, a rival to JE's society, had been founded in 1838.

[57] W. Topham and W. Squire Ward, *Account of a Case of Successful Amputation of the Thigh, During the Mesmeric State, without the Knowledge of the Patient* (London, 1842); JE (1843), pp. 5–11. Topham was married to Lady Mary Bentinck; JE said she had first suggested mesmerism for the case. William Wood assisted at the operation.

[58] JE (1843), pp. 12–62; JE, 'False accusation in the Royal Medical and Chirurgical Society against a poor man because he suffered no pain while his Leg was amputated in the mesmeric coma', the *Zoist*, 9 (1851–52), pp. 88–106; Minutes of the RMCS 1840–49, MCS/B7, 22 Nov and 13 Dec 1842, RSM archives. Since neither Topham nor Ward were members, their paper was presented by a friend, Edward Stanley, although they attended the meeting.

⁵⁹ This was Dr James Copland, Elliotson's temporary replacement at UCL: JE (1843), p. 59.

⁶⁰ *The Lancet*, 22 Nov 1842, pp. 357–61; *Provincial Medical and Surgical Journal* (later *BMJ*), 29 Apr 1843, pp. 92–3; *MCR*, 1 Jul 1843, pp. 147–50.

⁶¹ JE, 'False accusation . . . ' the *Zoist*, 9 (1851–52), pp. 88–106. The claim was made by Marshall Hall at the RMCS in Dec 1850 and published in the *Medical Times*, 20 and 28 Dec 1850, and *The Lancet*, 28 Dec 1850. An affidavit was subsequently taken from Wombell stating that he had not felt pain during the operation and signed with a cross on 22 Mar 1851, published in JE, 'False accusation . . . ' the *Zoist*, 9 (1851–52), pp. 97–8.

⁶² The *Zoist*, 2 (1844–45), pp. 101–3; pp. 100–1; pp. 96–8; p. 107.

⁶³ The *Zoist*, 2 (1844–45), pp. 121–2; pp. 115–9; pp. 390–403; pp. 410–29; and 3 (1845–46), pp. 385–6.

⁶⁴ *Exeter and Plymouth Gazette*, 31 May 1845, cited in Purland Album, vol. 4, NLM.

⁶⁵ The *Zoist*, 2 (1844–45), pp. 103–4 and 119–20; 3 (1845–46), pp. 380–4. The Jamaican case is from 2 (1844–45), pp. 98–100.

⁶⁶ Esdaile (1846 and 1856). The quote from the professor of anatomy is from (1856), p. 20. Biographical information is from D. G. Crawford, *Roll of the Indian Medical Service 1615–1930* (London, 1930), p. 103; Stephen and Lee, vol. 18, pp. 1–3; Waltraud Ernst, 'Esdaile, James (1808–59)', *ODNB*, online edn, accessed 3 Apr 2013. Esdaile married a third time in 1851, to a widow named Sophia Ullman, and brought her back to Scotland: St John's Church, Calcutta, parish register.

⁶⁷ James Esdaile, *Record of Cases treated in the Mesmeric Hospital, from Nov 1846 to May 1847* (Calcutta, 1847).

⁶⁸ James Esdaile to JE, 4 Oct 1849, in Purland Album, vol. 4, NLM.

⁶⁹ Martineau; T. M. Greenhow, *Medical Report of the case of Miss H—M—.* (London, 1845); JM to Capt J. James, 11 Dec 1845, the *Zoist*, 3 (1845–46), p. 536; Wolff, pp. 87–92. Biographical information from Webb; and R. K. Webb, 'Martineau, Harriet (1802–76)', *ODNB*, online edn, accessed 20 Mar 2014.

⁷⁰ CD to William Darwin Fox, 20 Dec 1844, Darwin Correspondence Database, www.darwinproject.ac.uk/entry-801 accessed 2 Feb 2016.

⁷¹ Gauld, p. 211.

⁷² *PMSJ*, 11 Feb 1843, pp. 398–402; J. B. Estlin, president's address, 15 Jul 1843, *PMSJ*, pp. 303–8; Hall, p. 61.

⁷³ Jane Carlyle to Mary Russell, 29 [30] Dec 1844, in Carlyle, vol. 18, pp. 306–8.

⁷⁴ Charles Radclyffe Hall, 'On the rise, progress, and mysteries of mesmerism', *The Lancet*, 1 Feb to 3 May 1845.

⁷⁵ Martineau, pp. vi–vii; Webb, p. 231.

⁷⁶ JE, *The Harveian Oration, delivered before the Royal College of Physicians, London, June 27ᵗʰ, 1846* (London, 1846). He did not deliver it in English as some writers have suggested nor did he give it at UCL as asserted by Hughes. W. J. Bishop and F. N. L. Poynter, 'The Harveian Orations, 1656–1947', *BMJ*, 18 Oct 1947, pp. 622–3. *The Lancet*, 13 Jun and 4 Jul 1846, pp. 662–3 and 16–8.

[77] JE, the *Zoist*, 1 (1843–44), p. 93.

CHAPTER II: PANDORA'S BOX

[1] Details of the operation are from William Squire, 'On the introduction of ether inhalation as an aesthetic in London', *The Lancet*, 22 Dec 1888, pp. 1220–1; Cock (1911b); Merrington, pp. 31–5. The duration of the operation was given by three different pupils as 25, 26 and 28 seconds. Ether was used in an operation in Paris on 15 Dec 1846, administered by a Boston medical student, but was only partially successful: Warren, p. 22.

[2] Sir J. Russell Reynolds, *Essays and Addresses* (London, 1896), p. 274.

[3] Information on the history of anaesthesia is from Stanley; Stratmann; Snow; Keys.

[4] Crawford W. Long, 'An account of the first use of sulphuric ether by inhalation as an anaesthetic in surgical operations' (1849), reprinted in Frank Cole (ed.), *Milestones in Anesthesia: readings in the development of surgical anesthesia, 1665–1940* (Lincoln, Neb, 1965), pp. 109–15. This was probably the first ever operation under ether, although William E. Clarke, a chemistry student at Rochester University, New York, is said to have administered ether to a woman who had a tooth extracted in Jan 1842: Henry M. Lyman, *Artificial Anaesthesia and Anaesthetics* (London, 1882), p. 6; Lyman gives no source. Biographical information on Long is from Bynum and Bynum, vol. 3, p. 812.

[5] 'Surgical operations performed during insensibility', *The Lancet*, 2 Jan 1847, pp. 5–8. This report includes the paper read by surgeon Henry Jacob Bigelow to the Boston Society of Medical Improvement on 9 Nov 1846 which had been sent to Boott by Bigelow's father, Jacob Bigelow.

[6] Cock (1911b). The volunteer, Dr Montague Duncan, wrote to Cock to describe his role.

[7] *LMG*, 18 Dec 1846, pp. 1085–6.

[8] Cited in the *Zoist*, 6 (1848–49), p. 211. The original of the letter is said to be lost but was published in the *North British Review* (1847).

[9] Thomas W. Baillie, 'The first European trial of anaesthetic ether: the Dumfries claim', *British Journal of Anaesthesia*, 37 (1965) pp. 952–7. According to Baillie, the ship's surgeon on the same ship that brought Bigelow's letter to Boott informed Scott of the discovery. An account of the operation was reported in the *Dumfries and Galloway Courier*, 18 Jan 1847, but gave no date. Scott made his claim in a letter to *The Lancet* dated 15 Oct 1872.

[10] *The Lancet*, 2 Jan 1847, pp. 5–8 and 16–7. *The Lancet* gave a brief report of the Boston operation on 26 Dec 1846, p. 704. *LMG*, 1 Jan 1847, pp. 38–9.

[11] *The Lancet*, 9, 16, 23, 30 Jan and 6 Feb 1847; *LMG*, 8, 22 Jan and 5 Feb 1847. The operations described were all performed in January.

[12] *The Lancet*, 16 Jan 1847, p. 80; Snow, p. 32; *The Lancet*, 23 Jan 1847, p. 99; *The Lancet*, 16 Jan 1847, pp. 79–80. The case of the miner is from James Robinson, *A Treatise on the Inhalation of the Vapour of Ether* (London, 1847), p. 47.

[13] Squire, ibid; *The Times*, 15 Jan 1847.

[14] *The Times*, 12 Jan 1847: the first was an arm amputation, the second the removal of a breast tumour.

[15] *LMG*, 12 Mar 1847, pp. 460–3; *The Lancet*, 10 Apr 1847, pp. 392–3.

[16] Snow; Sandra Hempel, *The Medical Detective: John Snow and the Mystery of Cholera* (London, 2006).

[17] *The Times*, 19 Mar 1847; *LMG*, 26 Mar and 2 Apr 1847, pp. 563–7 and 585–90. The operation took place on 9 Mar and she died two days later.

[18] *The Lancet*, 16 Oct 1847, pp. 410–1.

[19] Information on Simpson and chloroform is from James Young Simpson, *Account of a New Anaesthetic Agent, as a Substitute for Sulphuric Ether in Surgery and Midwifery* (Edinburgh, 1848); Simpson, *Answer to the Religious Objections Advanced Against the Employment of Anaesthetic Agents in Midwifery and Surgery* (Edinburgh, 1848); J. Duns, *Memoir of Sir James Y. Simpson* (Edinburgh, 1873); Stratmann; Snow.

[20] Eve Blantyre Simpson, *Sir James Young Simpson* (Edinburgh, 1896), pp. 50–1. Simpson gives no date for the letter although Duns dates it to 1837. However, JE refers to Simpson visiting him in July 1842 when he took him to see Rosina: the *Zoist*, 2 (1844–45), p. 225. Simpson is quoted on 25 June 1842 saying he had witnessed some demonstrations at JE's house that morning: *The Lancet*, 2 Jul 1842.

[21] Liston to James Miller, 17 Nov 1847, cited in Duns, p. 216.

[22] *The Lancet*, 'Fatal application of chloroform', 5 Feb 1848, pp. 161–2; J. Y. Simpson, 'The alleged case of death from the action of chloroform', *The Lancet*, 12 Feb 1848, pp. 175–6.

[23] *London Daily News*, 5 Jul 1848, cited in Keith Sykes, 'References to Anaesthesia in 19th-century British Regional Newspapers', *Proceedings of the History of Anaesthesia Society*, 41 (2009), pp. 28–35.

[24] Tomalin, p. 216; Snow, p. 70; Stanley, p. 305.

[25] Cited in the *Zoist*, 5 (1847–48), p. 375.

[26] John L. Hunt, 'Untamed editor: F Knight Hunt MRCS (1814–54)', *Journal of Medical Biography*, 5 (1997), pp. 210–20.

[27] Leaflet on opening of Exeter mesmeric infirmary, c. 1850, in Esdaile (1852).

[28] The *Zoist*, 5 (1847–48), pp. 78–82.

[29] The *Zoist*, 8 (1850–51), pp. 208–9.

[30] The *Zoist*, 5 (1847–48), pp. 197–201.

[31] Keys, p. 29.

[32] Esdaile (1852); Esdaile, *Record of Cases Treated in the Mesmeric Hospital, from Nov 1846 to May 1847* (Calcutta, 1847).

[33] Esdaile, 'Account of "A review of my reviewers"', 26 Jan 1848, the *Zoist*, 6 (1848–49), pp. 158–71.

[34] The *Zoist*, 7 (1849–50), p. 35; Esdaile, 'On the operation for the removal of scrotal tumours, etc., the effects of mesmerism and chloroform compared', the *Zoist*, 9 (1851–52), pp. 114–24.

[35] The *Zoist*, 6 (1848–49), p. 114. In addition to charting Esdaile's catalogue of

success, the *Zoist* publicised details of mesmeric surgery in Britain. Altogether it would report a total of 16 amputations, 28 operations to remove tumours and 150 other surgical operations along with countless dental extractions and midwifery cases. Bernard Hollander, 'Hypnosis and Anaesthesia', *Proceedings of the RSM*, 25 (1932), no. 4, pp. 21–34.

[36] Esdaile (1852), pp. 5–9.

[37] JE, 'On the art of suddenly restoring the moral feelings and intellect to activity in large masses of mankind', the *Zoist*, 5 (1847–48), pp. 44–50; JE, 'On medical anti-mesmerists', the *Zoist*, 7 (1849–50), pp. 370–89.

CHAPTER 12: THE SWEETEST SLEEP

[1] The LMI was 'founded' in June 1846 when subscribers met at Lord Ducie's house, but did not open until Jan 1850. Bedford Street is now Bayley Street. The first five annual reports are published in the *Zoist* while the sixth was separately published. Details of patients in 1855 are from *Report of the Sixth Annual Meeting of the London Mesmeric Infirmary, 8 June 1855* (London, 1856).

[2] Report of the Sixth Annual Meeting.

[3] Report of the Sixth Annual Meeting. Mrs Granger's condition could have been caused by Meigs' Syndrome. It is possible her illness resolved because the ovary untwisted itself. My thanks to Dr Nicholas Cambridge for advice.

[4] Thomas Capern, *Mesmeric Facts* (London, 1870).

[5] Ibid. Capern later returned to the West Country to practise independently and claimed to have cured more than 600 people by 1864.

[6] Wendy Moore, 'Faith Healing', *Observer*, 15 Dec 2002; *BBC Horizon*, 'The Power of the Placebo', shown 29 Jun 2015; T. Kaptchuk et al, 'Placebo effects in medicine', *New England Journal of Medicine*, 373 (2015), no. 1, pp. 8–9; Irving Kirsch, 'Hypnosis and placebos', *Anales de Psicologia*, 15 (1999), no. 1, pp. 99–110.

[7] The *Zoist*, 9 (1851–52) p. 129; Report of the Sixth Annual Meeting.

[8] JE, the *Zoist*, 13 (1855–56), pp. 113–21; Purland, *Painless Removal of the Female Breast in the Mesmeric Trance* (London, 1854). Purland, who worked as a mesmerist at the LMI, was an eccentric character who compiled scrapbooks of memorabilia. One of these albums is devoted to mesmerism: Purland Album, vol. 4, NLM. He kept a photograph of Mrs Flowerday and a letter from her thanking him for his kindness.

[9] *The Times*, 2 May 1854.

[10] *The Lancet*, 8 Aug 1846, p. 164.

[11] Report of the Sixth Annual Meeting; JE to Harriet Martineau, n.d. (c 1861), HM 285, Cadbury Research Library, Special Collections, University of Birmingham. The donations from Dickens and Baillière are recorded in the sixth report.

[12] Ruth Brandon, *The Spiritualists: the passion for the occult in the nineteenth and twentieth centuries* (London, 1983).

[13] Wolff, pp. 244–5; Trollope, p. 376. Both were attending events organised by Daniel Home at his house in Ealing.

[14] James Braid to Michael Faraday, 22 Aug 1853, Frank A. J. L. James (ed.), *The Correspondence of Michael Faraday* (6 vols, London, 1991–2012), vol. 4, pp. 560–1.

[15] JE, the *Zoist*, 12 (1854–55), p. 175. The *Zoist* ran numerous articles discrediting spiritualism. Braid described JE's explanation as 'Elliotson's Mesmeric residuum force theory'.

[16] CD to Thomas Serle, 2 Jan 1844, and CD to Forster, 30 Nov 1846, in House and Storey, vol. 4, p. 8 and 669.

[17] William Charles Macready, *The Journal of William Charles Macready, 1832–51*, ed. J. C. Trewin (London, 1967), p. 276.

[18] Gordon N. Ray (ed.), *The Letters and Private Papers of William Makepeace Thackeray* (4 vols, Cambridge, Mass., 1946), vol. 2, pp. 595, 610, 704; J. M. Schneck, 'John Elliotson, William Makepeace Thackeray, and Doctor Goodenough', *International Journal of Clinical and Experimental Hypnosis*, 11 (1963), pp.122–30. Thackeray to JE, n.d. (Nov 1850), Townshend manuscript collection, Wisbech and Fenland Museum. The quotes are from Thackeray, *The History of Pendennis*, ed. Donald Hawes (Harmondsworth, 1972), pp. 539–42.

[19] Application on behalf of Maria Goodluck: BL Loan 96 RLF 1/1310. Elliotson supported numerous other applications to the RLF preserved in this archive.

[20] CD to Macready, 21 and 24 Aug 1841, in House and Storey, vol. 2, pp. 363 and 368; M. Clare Loughlin-Chow, 'Overs, John A. (1808–44)', *ODNB*, online edn, accessed 20 Mar 2014.

[21] Bulwer-Lytton, *A Strange Story* (London and Berkeley, 1973), p. 380. JE wrote to thank Bulwer-Lytton for his tribute: JE to B-L, 8 Feb 1862, Hertfordshire archives, DE/K/C4/2.

[22] JE (1835–40) p. 646; Wilkie Collins, *The Moonstone* (London, 1967) pp. 410–3.

[23] Elizabeth Inchbald, *Animal Magnetism* (Dublin, 1777); Ben P. Robertson, *Elizabeth Inchbald's Reputation: A Publishing and Reception History* (London, 2015), p. 81.

[24] Winter, pp. 122–4; Tomalin, pp. 277–82. The first performance on 6 Jan was staged with *Animal Magnetism*: Robert Louis Brannan (ed.), *Under the Management of Mr Charles Dickens: His Production of 'The Frozen Deep'* (Ithaca, 1966).

[25] M. C. Rintoul, *Dictionary of Real People and Places in Fiction* (London, 1993), p. 393.

[26] *Morning Post*, 3 Aug 1868.

[27] *Association Medical Journal* (now *BMJ*), 5 Jul 1856, pp. 574–6.

[28] The *Zoist*, 13 (1855–56), p. 441.

[29] *The Lancet*, 14 Nov 1863, p. 581.

[30] Hostettler, pp. 144–6; Brook, p. 175.

[31] The *Zoist*, 3 (1845–46), pp. 317–8; 2 (1844–45), p. 66.

[32] Alan Gauld, 'Home, Daniel Dunglas (1833–1886)', *ODNB*, online edn, accessed 15 Dec 2014; D. D. Home, *The Complete D. D. Home* (2 vols, Worksop, 2007), vol. 2, pp. 109–112 and vol. 1, 330–2.

[33] Munk's Roll, RCP, pp. 258–62.

[34] Three photographs of JE – two full length seated in a studio and one head and shoulders – survive in a collection of letters preserved in the Science Museum

Library: MS 2108/26b. One of them is dated 1861 but they were probably all taken at the same time. JE to Dr William Munk, 27 Jun 1864: RCP archives, ALS/E21. Munk was the Harveian Librarian at the RCP who compiled biographical records of the fellows, now known as Munk's Roll.

[35] *The Times*, 14 Apr 1868; *The Lancet*, 18 Apr 1868, p. 518; *Morning Post*, 15 Apr 1868. *The Times* premature obituary triggered a raft of death notices in the regional newspapers.

[36] Will of Eliza Elliotson, proved 13 Mar 1885. It is not known whether Elliotson's spiritualist friends attempted to contact him after death but he lives on – in some ways at least. An American neurosurgeon, Norm Shealy, believes he is the reincarnation of Elliotson: http://tinyurl.com/jq2gc6c, accessed March 2017. And the video game Assassin's Creed Syndicate, set in Victorian London, features Elliotson as a malevolent doctor.

[37] Wolff, p. 238.

[38] *The Times*, 14 Apr 1868; *Morning Post*, 3 Aug 1868; *The Lancet*, 8 Aug 1868.

[39] The *Zoist*, 2 (1844–45), p. 196.

[40] Gauld, pp. 287, 297–301, 306–50.

[41] *BMJ*, 29 Jul 1893, p. 277.

[42] Hunting, pp. 422–4.

[43] Pintar and Lynn, pp. 112–34; G. F. Wagstaff, 'Current theoretical and experimental issues in hypnosis: overview' in Heap (1988), pp. 25–39; Brian J. Fellows, 'The use of hypnotic suggestibility scales' in Heap (1988), pp. 40–50.

[44] UCLH established a hypnosis service for patients with various conditions based at the former Royal London Homeopathic Hospital, now the Royal London Hospital for Integrated Medicine. Prior to this a hypnotherapy service for patients with IBS was set up in Manchester. A report by the British Psychological Society, 'The Nature of Hypnosis', published in 2001, outlines the benefits of hypnosis for various conditions: http://ukhypnos.wpengine.netdna-cdn.com/wp-content/uploads/2015/01/The-Nature-of-Hypnosis_0.pdf, accessed December 2014.

[45] Pintar and Lynn, pp. 166–8. The Cochrane Centre, which conducts systematic reviews of health research, cites eight studies of hypnotherapy, including for smoking, labour pain and IBS, and concludes that none show strong evidence of effectiveness: http://www.cochrane.org/search/site/hypnotherapy, accessed 8 Mar 2016. This result says as much about study design as hypnosis effectiveness. In 2008 the National Institute for Health and Care Excellence (NICE) recommended hypnosis in its guidelines for patients with IBS.

[46] Albrecht H. K. Wobst, 'Hypnosis and Surgery: Past, Present and Future' in *Anesthesia & Analgesia*, 104 (2007), no. 3, pp. 1199–1208.

[47] Ibid.

[48] Marie-Elisabeth Faymonville, Professor of Anaesthesiology, University of Liege, 'The use of hypnosis in preparing patients for surgery', RSM hypnosis and psychosomatic medicine section conference, 11 May 2015; M. E. Faymonville, 'Psychological approaches during conscious sedation', *Pain*, 73 (1997), no 3, pp. 361–7.

SELECT BIBLIOGRAPHY

MANUSCRIPT SOURCES

Cadbury Research Library, Special Collections, University of Birmingham
Carl H. Pforzheimer Collection of Shelley and his Circle, New York Public Library, Astor, Lenox and Tilden Foundations
Combe correspondence, NLS
Dr Williams's Library, London
Edinburgh University Library Special Collections
MS Huntington, Huntington Library, San Marino, California
Medical Society of London archives
National Archives (TNA), London
Purland Album, Theodosius Purland Collection of Materials on Mesmerism, National Library of Medicine, US
Royal College of Physicians of London archives
RSM archives
St Thomas' Hospital archives at KCL archives
St Thomas' Hospital archives at LMA archives
Science Museum Library
Townshend Manuscript Collection, Wisbech and Fenland Museum
UCL College Archives, UCL Library Services, Special Collections
Wellcome Library

WORKS BY JOHN ELLIOTSON IN CHRONOLOGICAL ORDER

The Institutions of Physiology (London, 1815, 1817, 1820, 1824)
The Introductory Lecture of a Course upon State-Medicine (London, 1821)
Lumleyan Lectures, 1829 (London, 1830)
Human Physiology (London, 1835–40)
Numerous Cases of Surgical Operations Without Pain in the Mesmeric State (London, 1843)

OTHER PUBLISHED SOURCES

Anon, *A Full Discovery of the Strange Practices of Dr Elliotson on the Bodies of his Female Patients!* (London, 1842)

Anon, *Physic and Physicians* (2 vols, London, 1839)

Anglesey, George Charles Henry Victor Paget, Marquess of, *One-Leg: The Life and Letters of Henry William Paget, First Marquess of Anglesey, K. G. 1768–1854* (London, 1961)

Brook, Charles, *Battling Surgeon: A Life of Thomas Wakley* (Glasgow, 1945)

Bynum, W. F. and Bynum, Helen (eds), *Dictionary of Medical Biography* (5 vols, Westport, Conn, 2006)

Bynum, W. F. and Porter, Roy, *Medical Fringe and Medical Orthodoxy 1750–1850* (London, 1987)

– *Companion Encyclopaedia of the History of Medicine* (Oxford, 1993)

Carlyle, Thomas and Jane Welsh, *The Collected Letters of Thomas and Jane Welsh Carlyle*, Sanders, Charles Richard (gen. ed.), (Durham, NC, London, 1970–95)

Clarke, James Fernandez, *Autobiographical Recollections of the Medical Profession* (London, 1874)

Clarke, Linda, *Building Capitalism: Historical Change and the Labour Process in the Production of the Built Environment* (London, 1992)

Cock, William, 'Anecdota Listoniensia', *University College Hospital Magazine*, 2 (1911a), no. 1, pp. 55–60

– 'The first operation under ether in Europe', *University College Hospital Magazine*, 1, (1911b), no. 4, pp. 127–44

Colquhoun, J. C., *Report of the Experiments on Animal Magnetism made by a Committee of the Medical Section of the French Royal Academy of Sciences* (Edinburgh, 1833)

Cooper, Bransby Blake, *The Life of Sir Astley Cooper, bart.* (2 vols, London, 1843)

Cooter, Roger, *The Cultural Meaning of Popular Science: Phrenology and the organization of consent in nineteenth-century Britain* (Cambridge, 1984)

– *Phrenology in the British Isles: An Annotated Historical Biobibliography and Index* (Metuchen, NJ, 1989)

Dickens, Charles, *Oliver Twist* (Ware, 2000)

Dupotet, Baron de Sennevoy, *An Introduction to the Study of Animal Magnetism* (London, 1838)

– *Le Magnétisme opposé à la Médecine* (Paris, 1840)

Esdaile, James, *Mesmerism in India, and its Practical Application in Surgery and Medicine* (London, 1846; 1989)

– *The Introduction of Mesmerism (with the Sanction of the Government) into the Public Hospitals of India* (Perth, 1852, 1856)

Ford, John M. T., *A Medical Student at St Thomas's Hospital, 1801–1802: the Weekes family letters* (London, 1987)

Forster, John, *The Life of Charles Dickens* (London, 1892)

Gauld, Alan, *A History of Hypnotism* (Cambridge, 1992)

Hale-White, Sir William, *Keats as Doctor and Patient* (Oxford, 1938)

Hall, Spencer T., *Mesmeric Experiences* (London, 1845)

Heap, Michael (ed.), *Hypnosis: current clinical, experimental and forensic practices* (London, 1988)

– (ed.), *Hypnotherapy: a handbook* (Maidenhead, 2nd ed, 2012)

Hostettler, John, *Thomas Wakley: An Improbable Radical* (Chichester, 1993)

House, Madeline and Storey, Graham et al (gen. eds), *The Letters of Charles Dickens* (12 vols, Oxford, 1965–2002)

Hughes, William, *That Devil's Trick: Hypnotism and the Victorian Popular Imagination* (Manchester, 2015)

Hunting, Penelope, *The History of the Royal Society of Medicine* (London, 2002)

Jacyna, L. S. (ed.), *A Tale of Three Cities: The Correspondence of William Sharpey and Allen Thomson* (London, 1989)

Kaplan, Fred, *Dickens and Mesmerism: The Hidden Springs of Fiction* (Princeton, 1975)

– (ed.), *John Elliotson on Mesmerism* (New York, 1982)

Keys, Thomas E., *The History of Surgical Anesthesia* (New York, 1963)

Lawrence, Susan C., *Charitable Knowledge: Hospital Pupils and Practitioners in Eighteenth-Century London* (Cambridge, 1996)

Lehman, Amy, *Victorian Women and the Theatre of Trance: Mediums, Spiritualists and Mesmerists in Performance* (Jefferson, NC, 2009)

Mackay, Charles, *Memoirs of Popular Delusions* (London, 1841; 1852)

Martineau, Harriet, *Letters on Mesmerism* (London, 1845)

Merrington, W. R., *University College Hospital and its Medical School: A History* (London, 1976)

Miller, J., 'A Gower Street Scandal', *Journal of the Royal College of Physicians of London*, 17 (1983), pp. 181–91

Moscati, F. M., *Mr Moscati and John Elliotson, or, the Revengeful Attack of* The Times *Explained and Refuted* (London, 1834)

Newman, Charles, *The Evolution of Medical Education in the Nineteenth Century* (Oxford, 1957)

Nicolson, Malcolm, 'The art of diagnosis: medicine and the five senses' in Bynum and Porter, (1993), vol. 2, pp. 801–25.

Pintar, Judith, and Lynn, Steven Jay, *Hypnosis: A Brief History* (Chichester, 2005)

Ridgway, Elizabeth S., 'John Elliotson (1791–1868): a bitter enemy of legitimate medicine?' parts I and II, *Journal of Medical Biography*, 1 and 2 (1993 and 1994), pp. 191–8 and 1–7.

Schlicke, Paul (ed.), *Oxford Reader's Companion to Charles Dickens* (Oxford, 2011)

Snow, Stephanie, *Blessed Days of Anaesthesia: How Anaesthetics Changed the World* (Oxford, 2008)

South, John Flint, *Memorials of John Flint South*, ed. C. L. Feltoe (London, 1884)

Sprigge, Samuel, *The Life and Times of Thomas Wakley* (London, 1897)

Stanley, Peter, *For Fear of Pain: British surgery, 1790–1850* (Amsterdam, 2003)

Stephen, Sir Leslie and Lee, Sir Sidney (eds.), *Dictionary of National Biography* (London, 1885–1900)

Stratmann, Linda, *Chloroform: The Quest for Oblivion* (Stroud, 2003)

Tatar, Maria, *Spellbound: Studies on Mesmerism and Literature* (Princeton, 1978)

Tomalin, Claire, *Charles Dickens: A Life* (London, 2011)

Trollope, Thomas Adolphus, *What I Remember* (London, 1887)

Warren, John Collins, *The Influence of Anaesthesia on the Surgery of the Nineteenth Century* (Boston, 1906)

Waterfield, Robin, *Hidden Depths: The Story of Hypnosis* (London, 2002)

Webb, R. K., *Harriet Martineau: A Radical Victorian* (London, 1960)

Winter, Alison, *Mesmerized: Powers of Mind in Victorian Britain* (Chicago, London, 1998)

Wolff, Robert Lee, *Strange Stories and Other Explorations in Victorian Fiction* (Boston, 1971)

INDEX

Mesmerism and me:
how hypnosis changed my life

People often imagine that writing a book must be a life-changing experience. Writing *The Mesmerist* really did change my life – immeasurably for the better – for it brought me a cure for headaches.

All my adult life I have been plagued by headaches. They began when I was in my teens and by the time I reached my fifties I was suffering two or three headaches a week. Sometimes the excruciating, stabbing pains seemed to be triggered by stress or tiredness or alcohol, but at other times those factors had no effect at all.

Various doctors over the years diagnosed 'tension headaches' and prescribed a succession of medication or therapies, but none of these brought lasting relief and over-the-counter painkillers were useless. My working life was blighted, my weekends often obliterated, my holidays frequently dominated by the searing pains. And then in May 2016 my headaches suddenly stopped and – apart from three or four brief episodes – they have not returned. The solution was not a new miracle drug or a change of lifestyle – it was hypnosis.

Ordinarily I would never have considered undergoing hypnosis. As a medical journalist I am generally sceptical of so-called complementary therapies and always insistent on evidence of effectiveness before trying any remedy, whether orthodox or alternative. But writing *The Mesmerist* led me into uncharted territory. I was lured into writing about mesmerism – effectively hypnosis – by the extraordinary story of the Okey girls who enthralled Victorian London with their strange performances. At first I was fairly sure the two sisters were just brilliant actors who managed to hoodwink medical experts and literary society alike. I wanted to know how they achieved this audacious deceit. Delving deeper, however, I became less sure that the girls were tricksters and more convinced there was something stranger going on;

there might be something in hypnosis after all.

The more I researched the story, the more I realised I needed to try hypnosis for myself. As a writer I'm always keen to walk in my subject's footsteps, though this is not always easy. Researching my first book, *The Knife Man*, about the eighteenth-century surgeon John Hunter, I forced myself to visit a modern-day dissection class. Just as crossing the threshold of a dissecting room was a challenge, so I felt a deep-rooted fear of undergoing hypnosis.

Like most people, my expectations of hypnosis had been fuelled by stage shows and television programmes in which men in slick suits convinced unwitting volunteers to rob banks or eat onions. I viewed hypnotism as something either to laugh about or to recoil from. Yet researching the science of hypnosis convinced me to discount the popular myths.

Although much about hypnosis remains unexplained, brain scans reveal that people under hypnosis show a unique pattern of brain activity. Whether this is a special state, or 'trance', is still hotly debated. Studies suggest that ninety per cent of us are susceptible to hypnosis but experts agree that nobody can be hypnotised against their will or compelled to do something they don't want to do. At the same time, there is some good evidence that hypnosis can help break habits such as smoking and over-eating, treat certain conditions, such as anxiety and irritable bowel syndrome, and relieve pain. Hypnosis is even being used as an alternative – or adjunct – to chemical anaesthesia for surgery and dental procedures just as in the days of John Elliotson.

Finally I took the plunge. In May 2016 I visited Dr Rumi Peynovska, a qualified medical doctor and psychotherapist as well as a hypnotherapist, who had helped with some of my research. Even then I had no intention of trying hypnosis for my headaches. It was only when Rumi said I needed to focus on a goal that I mentioned them at all.

The session was disarmingly straightforward and down-to-earth. There was no couch, no swinging watch, no command to look into Rumi's eyes. Instead I sat in an armchair while she took me through a series of relaxation techniques. In a loud, melodic voice, she told me to imagine I was holding a heavy book in my outstretched hands. Naturally my arms fell to my lap. Then I had to visualise walking down steps to a relaxing place – unimaginatively I chose a favourite beach – before opening a door into a room where I would see a dial that controlled my headaches. Whenever I felt any pain, I should turn down this dial. Finally, she commanded me to walk back up the steps and open my eyes. At no point did I think I was in a 'trance' or had lost control; I felt fully aware throughout. As I left I certainly felt relaxed but had no serious expectations.

Yet since that one session I have had almost no headaches. Now whenever I feel a headache threatening I take myself through the same steps – essentially self-hypnosis – for five or ten minutes. Within half-an-hour or so the symptoms have usually gone. On the few occasions a full-blown headache has developed I've lain down in a dark room and methodically gone through the same process. An hour or so later my headache has lifted.

Obviously it is impossible to be absolutely certain hypnosis was the cure. Other factors may have been responsible. Yet the fact that I now feel able to prevent or control my headaches suggests hypnosis was the key. For me – as a writer of stories – it makes perfect sense. In the past I saw myself as someone who had headaches and therefore I expected headaches to occur. Now I have broken that cycle. I tell myself a different story: I'm no longer someone who has headaches. And I'm forever grateful, both to Rumi and to the experience of writing *The Mesmerist*, that my life has been changed for the better.

Wendy Moore
September 2017

If you want to try hypnosis it is advisable to find a hypnotherapist with medical training through a reputable organisation such as the UK Council for Psychotherapy, British Society of Clinical and Academic Hypnosis or National Hypnotherapy Society.

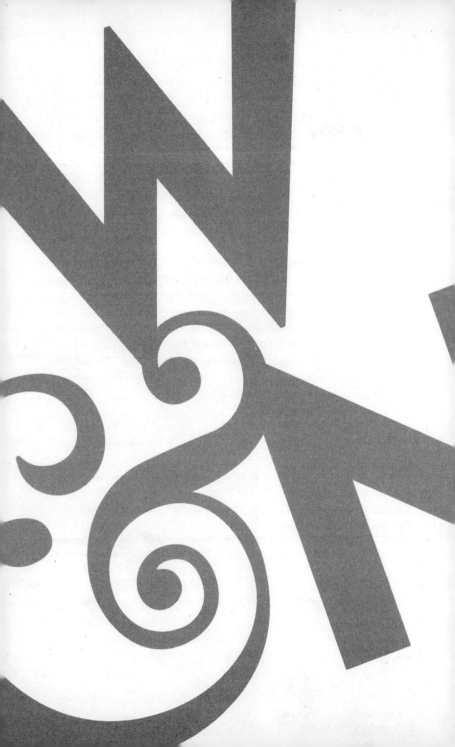